Cases
in Bioethics

SELECTIONS FROM
THE HASTINGS CENTER REPORT
Second Edition

Prepared by

Bette-Jane Crigger

Editor, Hastings Center Report

St. Martin's Press

New York

Senior editor: Don Reisman
Manager, publishing services: Emily Berleth
Project management: Peter Feely, Publication Services, Inc.
Cover design: Levavi & Levavi

Library of Congress Catalog Card Number: 92-50009

Manufactured in the United States of America.

7 6 5 4 3

f e d c b a

For information, write:
St. Martin's Press, Inc.
175 Fifth Avenue
New York, NY 10010

ISBN: 0-312-06746-1

Note to the Reader

The purpose of this book is not to report actual incidents, but to pose ethical dilemmas. A few of the cases are nevertheless drawn from the public record. These are "A Demand to Die"; "The Woman Who Died in a Box"; "Sterilizing the Retarded Child"; "In Organ Transplants, Americans First?"; and "A Prisoner in Need of a Bone Marrow Transplant." Even in some of these cases, the names are omitted or altered. The remaining cases are not intended to be and should not be read as reports of actual incidents. Some of these cases were inspired by actual incidents, but the names and many of the facts have been changed to provide both anonymity and greater clarity in presenting the ethical issues. The others were designed as paradigmatic examples of common ethical dilemmas or composites of a number of cases posing similar problems, and thus were not derived from any particular incidents. None of these cases should be read as reports of actual events.

Acknowledgments

Acknowledgments and copyrights are continued at the back of the book on page 297, which constitutes an extension of the copyright page. All citations refer to the *Hastings Center Report*. It is a violation of the law to reproduce these selections by any means whatsoever without the written permission of the copyright holder.

1. Vol. 14, No. 6, December 1984, pp. 30-31
2. Vol. 17, No. 2, April 1987, pp. 25-26
3. Vol. 22, No. 2, March-April 1992, pp. 56-57
4. Vol. 20, No. 6, November-December 1990, pp. 33-35
5. Vol. 21, No. 5, September-October 1991, pp. 29-31
6. Vol. 12, No. 1, February 1982, pp. 27-28
7. Vol. 10, No. 3, June 1980, pp. 22-24
8. Vol. 11, No. 1, February 1981, pp. 10-11

Contributors

Virginia Abernethy is Professor of Psychiatry (Anthropology), Vanderbilt University Medical School.

Terrence F. Ackerman is Professor and Chair, Department of Human Values and Ethics, College of Medicine, University of Tennessee.

Lori B. Andrews is a Research Fellow at the American Bar Foundation.

Paul S. Appelbaum is A.F. Zeleznik Professor of Psychiatry, University of Massachusetts Medical Center.

Henry Aranow Jr. (deceased) was Lambert Professor Emeritus of Medicine, College of Physicians and Surgeons, Columbia University.

Mila Ann Aroskar is Associate Professor, School of Public Health, University of Minnesota.

Roger A. Balk is the Chairman of the subcommittee on ethics, Animal Care Committee at McGill University, Montreal, Quebec.

Marc D. Basson is Postdoctoral Research Fellow, Department of Surgery, Yale University.

Margaret Battin is Professor of Philosophy, University of Utah.

Robert C. Benfari is lecturer in Psychology, Harvard School of Public Health, and Visiting Professor at Tufts University.

Robert A. Berenson is a physician in private practice in Washington, DC.

Kåre Berg is Chairman of the Institute of Medical Genetics, University of Oslo.

Ellen W. Bernal is Hospital Ethicist, St. Vincent Medical Center, Toledo, Ohio.

J. David Bleich is Talmud Professor of Jewish Law and Ethics, Cordoza School of Law, Yeshiva University.

Richard B. Brandt is Professor Emeritus of Philosophy, University of Michigan.

Anthony Breuer is a contributor to this volume.

Dan W. Brock is Professor of Philosophy and Professor of Human Values in Medicine, Brown University.

Baruch Brody is Leon Jaworski Professor of Biomedical Ethics, Baylor College of Medicine.

Daniel Callahan is Director of the Hastings Center.

Michael L. Callen is a founding member of People with AIDS Coalition and Community Research Initiative, New York.

Howard Caplan is a physician (geriatrics) in private practice in Los Angeles.

Ronald A. Carson is Kempner Professor and Director, Institute for the Medical Humanities, University of Texas Medical Branch at Galveston.

Christine Cassel is Chief, Section of General Internal Medicine, University of Chicago Medical Center.

Eric J. Cassell is Clinical Professor of Public Health, Cornell University Medical College.

Luther A. Cloud is former Director, Alcoholism Rehabilitation Center, St. Mary's General Hospital Corporation.

Robert L. Cohen is former Vice President for Medical Operations, New York Health and Hospital Corporation.

Morris F. Collen is a consultant in the Division of Research, Kaiser Permanente, Oakland.

Andrew Czeizel is a medical geneticist at the National Institute of Hygiene in Budapest, Hungary.

Norman Daniels is Professor and Chairman, Department of Philosophy, Tufts University.

Mannette Dennis is Patent Attorney with Ostrolenk Faber in New York City.

Nancy Dickey is a physician in private practice in Richmond, Texas.

Strachan Donnelley is Director of Education and Associate for Environmental Ethics, The Hastings Center.

Nancy Neveloff Dubler is Director, Division of Legal and Ethical Issues in the Health Care Department of Epidemiology and Social Medicine, Montefiore Medical Center/The Albert Einstein College of Medicine.

Gerald Dworkin is Professor of Philosophy, University of Illinois at Chicago.

Harold Edgar is Professor of Law, Columbia University School of Law.

H. Tristram Engelhardt, Jr. is Professor in the Center for Ethics, Medicine, and Public Issues, Baylor College of Medicine.

Ebun O. Ekunwe is Senior Research Fellow, Institute of Child Health and Primary Care, College of Medicine of the University of Lagos, Nigeria.

Cheryl Eth is Assistant to the Director, Emanuel Streisand School, Venice, California.

Spencer Eth is Associate Chief of Psychiatry, VA Medical Center, West Los Angeles, California.

David Fassler is Clinical Director, Otter Creek Associates, Burlington, Vermont, and Instructor in Psychiatry, Cambridge Hospital, Harvard Medical School.

Herbert Fingarette is Professor of Philosophy, University of California, Santa Barbara.

Joseph J. Fins is Associate for Medicine, The Hastings Center, and Fellow in Medicine, New York Hospital-Cornell Medical Center.

John C. Fletcher is Director, Center for Biomedical Ethics, and Professor of Biomedical Ethics and of Religious Studies, University of Virginia.

Brian Folker is Research Associate in the Division of Library and Information Management, American Medical Association.

Lachlan Forrow is Coordinator of teaching programs, Division of Medical Ethics, Harvard Medical School, and Beth Israel Hospital.

Cory Franklin is Director of Medical Intensive Care, Cook County Hospital, and Assistant Professor of Medicine and Medical Ethics, University of Health Sciences, Chicago Medical School.

Benjamin Freedman is Professor of Medicine and Philosophy at the McGill Center for Medicine, Ethics and Law, and Clinical Ethicist, Jewish General Hospital of Montreal.

Charles Fried is Professor of Law, Harvard University, and former Solicitor General, Department of Justice, Washington, D.C.

Willard Gaylin is a psychiatrist and President of The Hastings Center.

Marie-Claude Goulet is Law Clerk for Justice Peter Cory, Supreme Court of Canada.

James M. Gustafson is Henry R. Luce Professor of Humanities and Comparative Studies, Emory University.

Sally Guttmacher is Professor, Department of Health Education, New York University.

Arthur W. Hafner is Director of the Division of Library and Information Management, American Medical Association.

Michael R. Harrison is Director, Fetal Treatment Program, Department of Surgery, University of California at San Francisco.

Mary Sue Henifin is a lawyer with the firm Debevoise & Plimpton, New York City, Editor of *Women and Health*, and a member of the Reproductive Rights Law and Policy Project, Rutgers University.

Lawrence Hessman was formerly Clinical Instructor in Medicine and Community Medicine, Tufts University School of Medicine.

Angela R. Holder is Clinical Professor of Pediatrics (Law), Yale University School of Medicine, and Counsel for Medicolegal Affairs, Yale-New Haven Hospital and Yale University School of Medicine.

Patricia S. Hoover is the Undergraduate Advisor, Undergraduate Nursing Program, University of Toledo.

Kim Hopper is Assistant Professor, City University of New York Medical School.

David A. Hyman an attorney with Mayer, Brown & Platt in Chicago, Illinois.

Kenneth V. Iserson is Associate Professor, University of Arizona Health Sciences Center, Section of Emergency Medicine.

David L. Jackson is Clinical Professor of Preventive Medicine, Ohio State University.

Michael Jellinek is Chief of Child Psychiatry Service and Director of Outpatient Psychiatry, Massachusetts General Hospital.

Deborah G. Johnson is Associate Professor of Philosophy, Department of Science and Technology Studies, Rensselaer Polytechnic Institute.

Olga Jonasson is Professor and Chair, Department of Surgery, Ohio State University Hospital.

George A. Kanoti is Director of the Office of Bioethics, Cleveland Clinic Foundation.

Sahar Kayata is Assistant Professor of Pediatrics in the Medical College of Wisconsin.

Herbert J. Keating III is Associate Chair and Residency Director, Department of Medicine, Medical Center of Delaware.

Michael J. Kelly is Dean of the University of Maryland School of Law.

M. Margaret Kemeny is Chief of Surgical Oncology, St. Vincent's Hospital and Medical Center, and Associate Professor of Surgery, New York Medical College.

Ross Kessel is former Acting Dean of Graduate and Interprofessional Studies and Research, University of Maryland at Baltimore.

Kathy Kinlaw is Associate Director, Emory University Center for Ethics in Public Policy and the Professions.

Nicholas N. Kittrie is Edwin A. Moders Scholar and Professor of Law, The American University.

Howard Klar is former Director of Inpatient Psychiatrics, VA Medical Center, Bronx, N.Y.

John I. Kleinig is Professor of Philosophy, Department of Law and Police Science, John Jay College of Criminal Justice, City University of New York.

Hans-Georg Koch is Research Associate and Director of the Department of Law and Medicine, Max Planck Institute for Foreign and International Criminal Law in Freiburg, Germany.

Douglas P. Lackey is Professor of Philosophy, Baruch College and the Graduate Center, City University of New York.

The Honorable Richard D. Lamm is Professor, Center for Public Policy and Contemporary Issues, University of Denver and former governor of Colorado.

Sheldon H. Landesman is Associate Professor in the Department of Infectious Diseases, SUNY Downstate Medical Center, Brooklyn, NY.

John La Puma is Director, Center for Clinical Ethics, Lutheran General Hospital.

Daniel H. Lederer is Clinical Assistant Professor of Medicine, Brown University.

Carol Levine is Executive Director of The Orphan Project, New York.

Robert J. Levine is Professor of Medicine and Lecturer in Pharmacology, Yale University School of Medicine.

A-J Rock Levinson is former Executive Director, Concern for Dying, New York.

Robert E. Litman is Co-Director of the Suicide Prevention Center in Los Angeles.

Abbyann Lynch is Director, Bioethics Department, Hospital for Sick Children, Toronto, Canada.

Joanne Lynn is Senior Associate, Center for Evaluative Clinical Sciences, and Professor of Medicine and Community and Family Medicine, Dartmouth Medical School.

Darryl Macer is foreign Professor in the Institute of Biological Sciences, University of Tsukuba, Japan, and a bioethics consultant to the Department of Scientific and Industrial Research and the Ministry for the Environment, New Zealand.

Thomas B. Mackenzie is Associate Professor of Psychiatry and Medicine, Department of Psychiatry, University of Minnesota.

Daniel C. Maguire is Professor of Moral Theology, Marquette University.

Mary Mahowald is Senior Scholar, Center for Clinical Medical Ethics, The University of Chicago.

Don Marquis is Associate Professor in the Department of Philosophy, University of Kansas.

J. Joel May is Senior Consultant, The Pennington Group, Titusville, New Jersey.

Kevin M. McIntyre is Associate Clinical Professor of Medicine, Harvard Medical School.

Gilbert Meilaender is Professor of Religion, Oberlin College.

Robert Michels is Professor and Chairman, Department of Psychiatry, Cornell University Medical College, and Psychiatrist-in-Chief, The New York Hospital.

David H. Miller is Associate Professor of Medicine at Cornell University Medical College.

Robert I. Misbin is Associate Professor of Medicine, The University of Florida.

Theodore C. Nagel is Associate Professor of Obstetrics and Gynecology, University of Minnesota.

Richard H. Nicholson is a physician and Editor of the *Bulletin of Medical Ethics*, London, England.

Kathleen Nolan is Visiting Associate for Medicine, The Hastings Center.

Jeffrey Paul is Associate Director and Professor of Philosophy, Social Philosophy and Policy Center, Bowling Green State University.

Richard M. Pauli is Associate Professor of Pediatrics and Medical Genetics, University of Wisconsin at Madison.

Joy Hinson Penticuff is Associate Professor of Nursing, The University of Texas at Austin School of Nursing.

Robin Levin Penslar is a Research Associate at the Poynter Center, Indiana University.

Francis C. Pizzulli is an attorney in Santa Monica, California.

Jeffrey M. Prottas is Deputy Director, Bigel Institute for Health Policy, Heller Graduate School, Brandeis University.

Ren-Zong Qiu is Associate Professor, Department of Philosophy of Science and Director of the Program in Bioethics, Institute of Philosophy of the Chinese Academy of Social Sciences, Beijing.

Frederic G. Reamer is Professor in the School of Social Work at Rhode Island College.

Nancy K. Rhoden (deceased) was Professor of Law at the University of North Carolina.

Knut Ringen is Technical Advisor Coordinator, Labor Health and Safety Fund, Washington, D.C.

Judith Wilson Ross is Associate Director of UCLA Medical Center's Program in Medical Ethics, and Associate at the Center for Bioethics, St. Joseph Hospital System, Orange County, California.

Barbara Katz Rothman is Professor of Sociology, Baruch College, and the Graduate Center, City University of New York.

Cappy Miles Rothman is a urologist in private practice in Los Angeles, California.

Fenella Rouse is Executive Director, The Mayday Fund, New York.

William Ruddick is Professor of Philosophy, New York University.

James E. Sabin is Associate Director, Teaching Center, Harvard Community Health Plan, Cambridge, Massachusetts.

Francisco M. Salzano is Professor of Genetics, Federal University of Rio Grande do Sul, Porto Alegre, Brazil.

Dennis F. Saver is a physician in private practice in Newburg, West Virginia.

Sylvan J. Schaffer is Assistant Professor of Psychiatry, Albert Einstein Medical School, and Coordinator of Law and Psychiatry Services, Long Island Jewish Medical Center.

Kenneth F. Schaffner is Co-Director, Center for Medical Ethics, University of Pittsburgh.

R. B. Schiffer is Associate Professor of Psychiatry and Neurology, University of Rochester.

Lawrence J. Schneiderman is Professor of Community & Family Medicine, University of California at San Diego, School of Medicine.

Ferdinand Schoeman (deceased) was Professor of Philosophy, University of South Carolina.

Daniel H. Schwartz is Special Assistant to the President, Montefiore Medical Center.

Mark Sheldon is Associate Professor of Philosophy and Adjunct Associate Professor of Medicine at Indiana University.

Mark Siegler is Professor of Medicine and Director, Center for Clinical Medical Ethics, The University of Chicago.

Steven Sieverts is former Vice President of Blue Cross and Blue Shield of Greater New York.

Lewis M. Silverman is an emergency physician in New York City.

Ethel S. Siris is Associate Professor of Clinical Medicine, Department of Medicine, Columbia University College of Physicians and Surgeons.

David A. Smith is Director of Legal Services, Choice in Dying, Inc., New York.

Peter P. Sordillo is Associate Professor of Medicine, Mount Sinai School of Medicine.

Grant E. Steffen is a member of the Ethics Committee, Swedish Medical Center, Englewood, Colorado.

Bonnie Steinbock is Associate Professor of Philosophy and Public Policy, State University of New York at Albany.

Lance K. Stell is a medical ethicist at Charlotte Memorial Hospital and Medical Center, Charlotte, N.C., and Chairman of the Philosophy Department, Davidson College.

Ron Stephens is Professor of Medicine, Division Director, University of Kansas Medical Center.

Robert E. Stevenson is Director, American Type Culture Collection, Rockville, Maryland.

Carson Strong is Associate Professor of Human Values and Ethics, College of Medicine, University of Tennessee.

Carol A. Tauer is Professor of Philosophy, The College of St. Catherine, St. Paul, Minnesota.

Joe E. Thornton is former Professor of Psychiatry, Stanford University Medical Center.

Hans O. Tiefel is Professor of Religion, The College of William and Mary.

Tatjana Ulshoefer is Scientific Collaborator, Department of Law and Medicine, Max Planck Institute for Foreign and International Criminal Law, Freiburg, Germany.

Jan van Eys is Mosbacher Chair in Pediatrics and Head, Division of Pediatrics, University of Texas, M.D. Anderson Cancer Center.

Robert M. Veatch is Professor of Medical Ethics, Kennedy Institute of Ethics, Georgetown University.

Sophia Vinogradov is Research Fellow, Biological Psychiatry, Department of Psychiatry, Stanford University Medical School.

Leroy Walters is Director, Center for Bioethics at the Kennedy Institute of Ethics, Georgetown University.

Mary Anne Warren is a Lecturer in Philosophy, San Francisco State University.

Jeffrey Wasserman was former Pew Health Policy Fellow, The RAND Graduate School. Robert Weikart is Substance Abuse Therapist, Chelsea Hospital, Chelsea, Michigan.

Robert Weikart is Substance Abuse Therapist, Chelsea Hospital, Chelsea, Michigan.

Dorothy C. Wertz is Research Professor in Public Health, Boston University.

Robert B. White is Marie B. Gale Professor of Psychiatry, Department of Psychiatry and Behavioral Sciences, The University of Texas Medical Branch at Galveston.

William P. Whitely is Director of Information Analysis, American Medical Association.

Morton E. Winston is Associate Professor of Philosophy, Trenton State College and Adjunct Professor of Ethics, Johns Hopkins University School of Continuing Education.

Sally M. Winston is Director, Anxiety Disorders Program, Shepard and Enoch Pratt Hospital, Towson, Maryland.

Stuart J. Youngner is Associate Professor of Medicine, Psychiatry, and Biomedical Ethics, School of Medicine, Case Western Reserve University.

Preface

In many ways, cases are the lifeblood of bioethics, moments when ethical theory must join with the practical realities of the clinic to resolve real-life dilemmas. Since it was first published in 1971, the *Hastings Center Report* has regularly featured case studies in bioethics and related fields, which have been widely used as educational tools by clinicians, teachers, ethics committees, and others.

The case studies published in the *Report* are designed not to offer "right" answers to moral dilemmas in medicine and the life sciences, or to expose outrages in medical practice or research, but to illustrate how thoughtful individuals approach such problems, bringing to bear the perspectives of different academic and professional backgrounds and varying ethical traditions. Thus the editorial staff of the *Report* has chosen difficult cases about which people of good conscience may disagree, and asked commentators to explore how they would resolve the issues raised and why they reason as they do.

This second edition of *Cases in Bioethics* reflects the evolving—and newly emerging—concerns of bioethics. New cases have been incorporated that raise issues in new and troubling contexts, such as whether and when physicians may override a patient's wishes as expressed in an advance directive in an emergency situation ("Whether 'No' Means 'No'"), or the tension between protecting both the patient and the interests of the family and its members when a physician suspects the patient has been abused ("The Usual Suspects"). So too, cases address new issues of professional conduct, including the impaired professional ("When the Doctor Is on Drugs") and potential conflicts of interest as physicians become entrepreneurs ("When Opportunity Knocks"). Others speak to concerns emerging from the new molecular biology—how to balance patient confidentiality and family members' right to know when a devastating genetic disease like Huntington's is diagnosed ("The Price of Silence"), or the limits to human intervention in creating "chimera" animal species ("New Creations?"). Still others take up policy issues that become ever more pressing: The claims a noncompliant, drug-abusing patient has to scarce medical resources when her drug abuse contributes to her medical needs ("The Noncompliant Substance Abuser"); the assurance that patients receive the range of care they need when third-party payers hesitate to pick up the tab ("When Is Home Care Medically Necessary?").

Some of the cases presented here have been drawn from material in the public record, as listed in the "Note to the Reader" on the copyright page. Others are fictional insofar as names and details are concerned. Yet all reflect the experiences of those who must make the "hard choices"—physicians, nurses, patients, and families; courts, legislators, and administrators. However fictional they may be in their particulars, these cases are intended to raise the kinds of ethical dilemmas that we confront in the real world of medical practice and research.

This volume is the fourth such collection of cases originally published in the *Hastings Center Report*. It is an updated edition of *Cases in Bioethics: Selections from the Hastings Center Report* prepared by Carol Levine, former editor of the *Report*, and incorporates cases published since that edition appeared in 1989.

(The two earliest collections, *Cases in Bioethics from the Hastings Center Report*, were published by The Hastings Center in 1982 and 1984.)

I have not attempted to improve upon the organizational structure of the earlier edition. Thus, as are their predecessors, the case studies in this volume are organized into topical categories that emphasize the primary focus of the case, such as "Privacy and Confidentiality" or "Decisions about Death." To be sure, many cases speak to more than one issue and could be classified in other ways. As a guide for readers, the secondary topical table of contents on pages xxi–xxii reflects other possible groupings of these cases.

Cases and commentaries are reprinted largely as they originally appeared in the *Report*. Contributors' identifications have, however, been updated and gathered together in an alphabetical listing on pages iii–ix, while other supplementary material that appeared with the cases has been omitted. Where cases are not identified with the author's byline, they were prepared by the editorial staff or individuals who prefer to remain anonymous. Each part concludes with a *Selected Bibliography* to guide the reader to relevant literature. A *Glossary* (pp. 293–296) defines basic terms in bioethics; it is not intended to be definitive, but to introduce readers to important terms that occur regularly in the cases.

Many individuals have contributed to the evolution of the case studies over the history of The Hastings Center and the *Report*, notably Daniel Callahan, Director of the Center; Robert M. Veatch, originator of the case study format and former Center Associate; Peter Steinfels, Margaret O'Brien Steinfels, and Courtney S. Campbell, all former editors of the *Report*; and Arthur L. Caplan, formerly Associate for the Humanities. Others have contributed editorial and administrative skills, among them Hilde L. Nelson, Associate Editor, and Amy Menasché and Mary Grace Pagaduan, Editorial Assistants.

I owe a special debt, however, to Carol Levine, former editor of the *Report* and now Executive Director of The Orphan Project. Carol played a major role in shaping the development of case studies during her tenure with the *Report* and as editor of the previous edition of this volume. In preparing this new edition, I have done little more than incorporate cases published after her departure from The Hastings Center.

And, of course, we must thank not least the contributors whose cases and commentaries appear here, thoughtful individuals who were willing to share their reflections with readers of the *Hastings Center Report* and this new volume.

B-J.C.

The following reviewers for St. Martin's Press provided helpful comments: Robert V. Andelson, Auburn University; Luther J. Binkley, Franklin & Marshall College; William Bywater, Allegheny College; Patricia Fauser, Illinois Benedictine College; Albert Flores, California State University–Fullerton; Gerry C. Heard, Louisiana College; Margaret Reed Holmgren, Iowa State University; Lawrence Koehler, Central Michigan University; Jackie Litt, Allegheny College; Ronnie Littlejohn, Belmont College; Douglas C. Long, University of North Carolina; David Ozar, Loyola University of Chicago; Robert F. Rizzo, Canisius College; Mark Sheldon, Indiana University; Carl Skrade, Capital University; Alan Soble, University of New Orleans; and Larry R. Taylor, New Mexico Highlands University.

Topical Contents in Brief

Topical Table of Contents

Part Two: Reproductive Rights and Technologies

Part Three: Death and Dying

Part Four: Research with Living Subjects

Part Five: Mental Incompetence

Part Six: Allocation and Health Care Policy

Alternate Topical Table of Contents

Health Care Professionals' Responsibilities and Patients' Rights

INTRODUCTION

What does it mean to be a physician—or nurse, counselor, or other caregiver—in an age of technologically sophisticated medicine? What values inform professionals' relationships with their patients, and what obligations do they owe to the vulnerable individuals under their care? The relationship between doctor and patient has traditionally been a privileged one, in which physicians share intimate knowledge of and exercise considerable power over their patients' lives, in virtue both of their expertise as healers and of the special moral authority conferred upon them by society.

Professional codes of ethics have governed physicians' conduct from the Hippocratic tradition of ancient Greece to the present day. Yet where "medical ethics" once referred largely to what physicians should (or should not) do to promote patients' best interests as medically defined, it is now directed more toward questions of how patients and caregivers ought properly to work together to determine what is in the patient's interests and to share decision making. Changes in the health care system—including the prominence of high technology, tertiary care, and third-party payment—and the rise of the patients' rights movement over the last twenty to thirty years have combined to create dilemmas not envisioned by the Hippocratic Oath. The cases that follow explore dimensions of the relationships between patients and caregivers that are especially problematic in contemporary medical practice.

Cases in the first section—"Professional Conduct"—address questions of the special moral character of professional roles. They discuss in various forms dilemmas for caregivers in understanding their professional duties—to patients, colleagues, and others. Questions include not only how the scope of the

1

professional-patient relationship is defined, but also how factors outside that relationship, such as physicians' investment in diagnostic centers, influence it.

The second section—"Informed Consent"—explores questions about how decisions regarding medical treatment are best made, and who is best situated to make them. For example, do patients need to know how experienced their physician is before they can give truly informed consent? Can physicians withhold treatment they believe is futile without discussing that decision with patients? Case studies also examine how decisions are made for patients, such as children, who cannot decide for themselves.

Cases in the concluding section—"Privacy and Confidentiality"—consider especially the privileged character of the relationship between patient and caregiver and professionals' duty to safeguard confidential information. Among the questions raised in this section are how to balance the potential harm done to the patient by divulging privileged information against the possible harm of not telling others who may be profoundly affected by that information.

When the Doctor and the Minister Disagree

Mary Clarkson is fifty-five years old; for the past eight months her husband, Bill, has been in California settling the estate of a relative. He comes home once every two months for a weekend visit and then returns to California. Mrs. Clarkson has been feeling depressed and lethargic; she voluntarily admits herself to the psychiatric unit of a community hospital seventy-five miles from home.

Mrs. Clarkson is very religious and has been attending church with her sister and brother-in-law. Upon admission to the hospital Mrs. Clarkson calls her minister, Rev. Tark, and asks him to visit her.

During the visit Mrs. Clarkson tells him about her marital problems: she and her husband constantly argue about his absences and how to deal with their thirty-year-old son who has had recurrent emotional and financial problems. Mrs. Clarkson feels guilty about not having given her son more money and support, and she wants to help him solve his problems. Her husband, however, wants nothing more to do with him. Rev. Tark offers her absolution after her "confession," and prays with her for strength to get well and to return home.

The next day Rev. Tark receives a call from Mrs. Clarkson's psychiatrist, Dr. Vern. Dr. Vern wants to know if Rev. Tark has visited Mrs. Clarkson and what was said. Rev. Tark explains that he saw Mrs. Clarkson at her request and that he heard her confession and offered her absolution.

Dr. Vern states that Mrs. Clarkson would be better off if she saw only him for counseling during her three-week stay as an inpatient. He feels that her depression is the result of a failed marriage and that she can only recover when she acknowledges that fact and begins proceedings for separation. Rev. Tark disagrees that the marriage should be ended. His goal is to help resolve the difficulties, which he thinks began when Mr. Clarkson retired from his factory job, at the age of fifty-five, about a year and a half earlier.

A few days later Rev. Tark's superior receives a letter from Dr. Vern, in which he states that Rev. Tark "must get clearance from the attending psychiatrist for any contact he is to have with the patient during hospitalization." After Mrs. Clarkson is sent home she will be free to choose whom she wants to see for counseling, the letter continues, but in the hospital the presence of her minister will only undermine her medical treatment.

Should Rev. Tark return to see Mrs. Clarkson in spite of Dr. Vern's ban? Does Mrs. Clarkson have the right to choose her counselor? Do patients "belong" to any professionals?

COMMENTARY
Robert Weikart

The case suggests several ethical issues: informed consent, autonomy vs. paternalism, beneficence, and respect for differing belief systems. The patient is directly involved in the first and last issues, while the psychiatrist and clergyman are involved in the middle two.

In considering informed consent, it would be helpful to know what Mrs. Clarkson was told upon admission to the hospital. Was she told that her visitors would be limited? Was she told that the psychiatrist would determine whom she could see? The case does state that Mrs. Clarkson called Rev. Tark "upon admission to the hospital" and requested a visit. Either she was informed of a visitor rule and had disregarded it or was not informed and subsequently invited specific people to visit her. Since she was depressed and lethargic upon admission, it could be a positive sign if she has called upon those who can offer her support with or without the approval of her psychiatrist.

Assuming that Mrs. Clarkson is competent and was not told that her visitors would be restricted, she was treated paternalistically. Paternalism usually protects someone from hurting himself or herself or others or protects the individual who is incompetent to make decisions. Paternalism presupposes that the physician will act only in the patient's best interests. It also gives the patient the right to negotiate the bounds of such paternalism. But in this case the patient's best interests were not served when her minister was asked not to return, with no negotiation about the extent of paternalism.

Those who would favor paternalism in this case might argue that Mrs. Clarkson does not know what is good for her and needs the guidance of a professional. However, if we accept this argument, was she competent to admit herself initially to the hospital and to ask her minister to visit? If she is conditionally or intermittently competent, who makes that diagnosis?

The psychiatrist also faced a conflict of interest. Can a psychiatrist who works for a hospital psychiatric unit be beneficent toward patients while also being an agent of the institution? If the institution prohibits visitors for new patients but the psychiatrist deems visitors helpful for patients, which side will he uphold?

At the crux of this discussion are Mrs. Clarkson's religious beliefs. Since she has been attending church with her relatives, it appears that religion is important to her. She also seems to believe in the sacrament since she participated in confession and absolution with Rev. Tark.

Her faith raises several questions. How does Mrs. Clarkson view divorce? If she views it as a sin, and is encouraged by Dr. Vern to leave her husband, she may have feelings of guilt and a sense that she has lost grace with God.

There is some overlap between what clergy and psychiatrists do, and this seems to be part of the problem. In this instance, the minister is dealing with the sacramental aspect of her life, which affects how she lives her life. The psychiatrist is concerned with her marital situation, but needs to consider her religious values as well.

After the inpatient treatment is finished Mrs. Clarkson will need ongoing support. She will probably see Rev. Tark as she did before. There is some question, however, about whether she will continue to see Dr. Vern since he is affiliated with a hospital far from her home. Rev. Tark can provide continuity of care as well as support for her religious beliefs.

If Dr. Vern thinks it unwise for Mrs. Clarkson to see Rev. Tark, he should meet with Rev. Tark and explain his reasons. Dr. Vern also should enlist Rev. Tark's help in resolving any guilt generated by Mrs. Clarkson's decision, if she makes it, to divorce her husband.

I believe that Mrs. Clarkson has the right, especially if she was not previously informed otherwise, to see the professionals she chooses. Her beliefs are important to her and need to be sustained as a resource both for the present and the future.

COMMENTARY
Howard Klar

Psychiatric disorders, more than any other group of medical problems, are shaped and influenced by the social and cultural milieu in which they occur. When changes in a person's emotional life lead that person to seek treatment, the psychiatrist's obligation is to consider sociocultural factors, as well as many others that may be contributing to the patient's problem. After carefully assessing the problem from these different frames of reference, the physician can integrate biological, social, and psychodynamic factors in order to arrive at a plausible explanation. Then, with the patient's consent, effective treatment can begin.

Dr. Vern did not fulfill this responsibility to his patient and Rev. Tark could not, due to a different orientation, fulfill this responsibility either. As a result, a travesty of clinical care occurred.

Mrs. Clarkson is a woman with a shaky marriage, a troubled son, a guilt-ridden conscience, and perhaps, a biologic propensity toward depression. Given the turmoil in her personal life, it would not be surprising if Mrs. Clarkson were also troubled by thoughts and feelings that are at odds with her strong religious beliefs. Despite her regular attendance at church services, she is unable to find solace from her depression solely through religion. She then voluntarily seeks medical care in a hospital. Implicit in this decision is Mrs. Clarkson's belief that Rev. Tark's counseling alone could not help her overcome her depression.

When patients enter the hospital they have the right to expect that the medicine practiced there will be grounded in science and that the practitioners in the hospital will be credentialed professionals. They further have the right to assume, in most cases, that they will participate in all decisions regarding their care, including decisions about who can and cannot provide care in the hospital. Patients do not retain the right to choose anyone to treat them in a hospital, particularly if they seek a treatment not acceptable by the hospital's standards.

We never know if Rev. Tark views himself as a practitioner, only that Dr. Vern finds him intrusive. Interestingly, both men seem to have a point of view regarding Mrs. Clarkson's marriage. One wants to save the marriage, the other seeks to end it. What does the patient want? Neither Rev. Tark nor Dr. Vern seems to care. Mrs. Clarkson is not mentally incompetent, therefore she does not need to be told what to do. She may require time to struggle toward a decision about her marriage, but it is *her* decision to make. The two men are engaged in a struggle to impose their points of view on Mrs. Clarkson, not in a discussion of how to help the patient.

Banning the minister from seeing Mrs. Clarkson is Dr. Vern's trump card in this test of wills. There is no question regarding a hospital's right to restrict visitors if the visit is harmful to the patient's condition. Whether Dr. Vern was correct in interpreting Rev. Tark's visit as harmful is another matter. Certainly, "confession and absolution" are not medical treatments for depression. However, religious beliefs obviously play an important role in understanding Mrs. Clarkson's problems, and the potentially positive role Rev. Tark could play in her treatment should not be underestimated.

Rev. Tark was fulfilling his professional role and attempting to help his congregant. We should not expect him to be aware of the complex issues involved in the treatment of depression, that is, to behave like a physician. We may even be inclined toward a more forgiving stance toward his trying to "save the marriage," without placing Mrs. Clarkson's wishes first.

Dr. Vern was wrong to deny the minister his right to visit Mrs. Clarkson. While the minister may have been misguided, he was clearly not dangerous or harmful to the patient. As a psychiatrist, Dr. Vern's professional obligation to his patient is to be aware of the multiple factors impinging on her clinical condition. To suddenly deny her access to her minister, without even consulting her, is clearly an abridgment of her rights.

Physicians in the hospital setting are granted enormous authority over the care and management of their patients. It is reasonable to expect that this authority will be used fairly and in the interests of the patient, not to prevent the patient from hearing points of view that differ from the physician's.

Hospitals rightly impose limitations on the freedom of patients to choose both treatments and "treaters." While this restriction protects patients from snake-oils and charlatans, it also requires that the physician in charge exercise judgment regarding the role of "nonscientific" factors, like religion, in a patient's treatment. If Rev. Tark and Dr. Vern cannot work out their differences, then Rev. Tark should call Mrs. Clarkson and explain the dilemma. Mrs. Clarkson would then be free to discuss it with Dr. Vern and seek another medical opinion, or even to leave the hospital.

Every profession carries with it a set of values and obligations. The conflict in this case occurred when the professional values of Rev. Tark collided with those of Dr. Vern. While both men lost sight of the patient's right to find her own way, even within the constraints of being in a hospital, Dr. Vern lost sight of the values of his profession—namely, to make use of the patient's values and psychosocial supports in her care, rather than to further alienate her from them.

2

The Nurse's Appeal to Conscience

Alice Howard is a registered nurse at Hillside Nursing Home where she cares for Jane Barnes, a sixty-three-year-old woman who has terminal colon cancer. Mrs. Barnes is in considerable pain, which has been increasingly difficult to control. The attending physician, Dr. Jones, has ordered moderate doses of morphine. The family understands that at these doses morphine may depress respiratory effort, thus hastening death.

In the past months Mrs. Barnes and her family have moved toward acceptance of death. Some member of her family is with her constantly to comfort her. She is receiving morphine as often as every three hours and her sleeping respiratory rate is now very slow.

Most of the nurses see no problem with giving morphine to Mrs. Barnes. However, Nurse Howard disagrees. She believes that the morphine will cause Mrs. Barnes to die earlier than she would have otherwise; thus she cannot, in good conscience, give the injection. The other nurses resent interrupting their busy schedules to "cover" for Nurse Howard. Dr. Jones regards her refusal as a potentially serious form of disobedience.

One night, Nurse Howard is the only R.N. on duty. Mrs. Barnes has been very restless, and unable to sleep, even though she received her medication. In obvious discomfort, Mrs. Barnes presses the call button and asks for more medication. Her daughter pleads with Nurse Howard to help her mother. Nurse Howard hesitates. She is the only person on the night shift who is legally qualified to give this injection; if she refuses, she will have to bother Dr. Jones with a late-night call and suffer the consequences.

Do nurses have the right to refuse medical orders or to ignore the wishes of the patient and family on grounds of conscience?

COMMENTARY
Ellen W. Bernal and Patricia S. Hoover

Alice Howard has made an appeal to conscience the basis for her ongoing refusal to administer the morphine. Such an appeal should be founded on a prior judgment of the rightness or wrongness of an action. The action, if taken, will violate one's integrity; thus the deciding factor is personal rather than external sanction. For the nurse, an appeal to conscience also requires consideration of professional obligations. Nurse Howard believes that giving morphine injections is wrong because it may hasten Mrs. Barnes's death.

Nurse Howard should examine the factual basis for this belief and current nursing practice recommendations with respect to pain control. In order to give competent care, the nurse must understand the pharmacology of the medications she administers. Respiratory distress is an important potential side effect to consider when administering morphine. It is difficult to say with absolute certainty how much morphine might lead to severe respiratory distress or the death of a patient.

Nurse Howard can decrease this risk by carefully assessing Mrs. Barnes's condition *each time* the analgesic is to be given. She needs to consider the following: When did Mrs. Barnes get the last dose of morphine? How has she responded to previous doses? What is her mental status? What are her vital signs, especially respiratory rate and depth? What subjective and objective symptoms of pain does she exhibit? The answers will guide Nurse Howard in deciding whether giving the morphine is safe. However, no blanket assurance can be given that the morphine she administers will not hasten Mrs. Barnes's death.

Nurse Howard should also consider the American Nurses' Association Code for Nurses (1985). The Code states that nurses have a moral obligation to "take all reasonable means to protect and preserve human life when there is a hope of recovery or reasonable hope of benefit from life-prolonging treatment." But nurses also "may provide interventions to relieve symptoms in the dying client even when the interventions entail substantial risks of hastening death." When analgesics such as morphine are administered for alleviating pain, this should be done on a regularly scheduled basis and before the pain occurs or increases significantly. We see no indication that Nurse Howard attempted to assess or anticipate her patient's need for morphine or to explore other means of pain relief such as positioning, relaxation exercises, or imagery.

It is the nurse's duty to remain faithful to the implicit promises she has made to her patient. One implicit promise is Nurse Howard's obligation to respect Mrs. Barnes's autonomy. At the beginning of this illness and at her admission to the nursing home, Mrs. Barnes could have expressed her values and plans. Nurse Howard should have based nursing treatment on the informed decisions of her patient. Allowing Mrs. Barnes to be as fully involved as possible in planning for pain relief can have an added benefit; increasing Mrs. Barnes's control over the situation may reduce her perceived pain.

If after such discussions Nurse Howard finds that she cannot give the morphine, she should explain, nonjudgmentally, her own moral position regarding the use of morphine. She should then assure Mrs. Barnes that another nurse will give the medication. Nurse Howard is also obligated to make her refusal known to the nursing home, "in advance and in time for other appropriate arrangements to be made for the client's nursing care" (ANA Code, 1985).

A second implicit promise is the obligation to "be with" the patient both physically and psychologically. But Nurse Howard's conscientious objection to administering morphine seems to stand in the way of a trusting, healing relationship; perhaps she should remove herself from Mrs. Barnes's care. She should also persist in her attempt to resolve the situation with Dr. Jones and the nursing home administration. If she is unable to reach an understanding, then she may have to consider employment elsewhere.

While Nurse Howard hesitates, Mrs. Barnes suffers. We believe her basic nursing duty should override her appeal to conscience in the immediate situation. It is inexcusable that she has allowed herself to be placed in this avoidable position. She should formulate a plan of action before other such emergencies occur.

COMMENTARY
Mila Ann Aroskar

Nurses (and the public) agree that nurses have a primary obligation to relieve the pain and suffering of dying patients. Such a position is supported by the American Nurses' Association Code for Nurses (1985). Meeting this obligation is one way of demonstrating respect for persons and advocacy in support of a dying patient's comfort and best interests.

Alice Howard cannot appeal to external authority such as the nursing code to support her position and she has not done so. Her appeal is to her own conscience and her concepts of right and wrong. This also assumes that she is basing her refusal on accurate and complete information about Mrs. Barnes's clinical situation, knowledge about drugs such as morphine, and so forth.

Nurses who refuse to participate in certain patient care procedures or treatments and who base their refusals on an appeal to conscience are still responsible for the consequences to patients of their decisions. They are responsible for assuring that patients' lives and safety are not jeopardized by such decisions. Simply abandoning identified patients is never morally justifiable.

At the same time, patient advocacy has some limits. Nurses do not have an absolute moral obligation to do unquestioningly whatever is requested by patients, families, or other health professionals or to take actions that violate deeply held moral beliefs. (Legally, nurses and other health professionals cannot be required to participate in abortions or sterilizations.) If such an absolute obligation existed, it would negate the idea of nurses as moral agents who are responsible for making decisions and taking into account the possible consequences of those decisions.

Nurses, like patients, are persons worthy of respect. As such, they should never be treated solely as means to the ends of others even if the "others" are patients or clients to whom nurses are primarily accountable. Nurses may be subjected to various forms of coercion ranging from threats to peer pressure if they refuse to carry out the physician's "orders," particularly when other nurses do not question them. Such actions or an environment that condones such actions may jeopardize an individual nurse's personal and professional integrity in any practice setting and require change.

Alice Howard has several obligations as a moral agent, including explicit consideration of both positive and negative consequences of her decision. No one can guarantee that there will be no negative consequences for refusing to carry out patient care that other nurses in a similar situation do perform. She must also be aware that nurses have moral obligations for advance planning to assure that Mrs. Barnes's welfare is not jeopardized by her refusal to give the morphine as ordered.

Mrs. Barnes's situation clearly requires effective pain relief. If Alice Howard has used every available nursing means to reduce Mrs. Barnes's pain and suffering without effect, then the injection of morphine is a last resort, which has been ordered by Mrs. Barnes's physician with the support of her family. We do not know if the patient has made any specific choices about pain control or if she is able to participate in such planning. Since Alice Howard is the only one who can legally give the morphine, she must either give it herself, find someone else who can give it legally (unlikely at 2:00 A.M.), or notify Dr. Jones and accept the consequences of doing so—possibly at serious risk of losing her job.

While patient care institutions would be unable to continue providing services if everyone refused to carry out standard interventions designed to reduce pain and suffering of dying patients, there should be mechanisms by which staff can be heard if they disagree with patient care decisions based on an appeal to conscience. Institutions should develop an explicit policy for managing such situations. Nurses do not have an obligation to carry out "orders" that jeopardize patients' safety and welfare. In fact, they clearly have a professional and moral obligation to question such written or verbal orders to stop such actions.

Nursing practice or ethics committees can discuss this and similar issues before they end up in the courts. Nurses should be allowed to refuse to carry out particular procedures or treatments based on an appeal to personal conscience and ideas of right and wrong if the decision is founded on accurate and complete information, acceptance of consequences, and advance planning. The patient's safety and welfare remain the primary consideration.

3

The Usual Suspects

Mr. and Ms. N. had ruefully come to think of the hour just before dinner as the naughtiness hour. That was the time of day when Alexander, aged five and emotionally troubled, was most apt to pick fights with his sister Fanny, almost three. They were a little tired, a little hungry, and generally at loose ends, clamoring for attention while their mother and father did their best to get dinner on the table.

Tonight the children were such a nuisance underfoot that Ms. N. sent them out of the kitchen to quarrel elsewhere while she mashed the potatoes and Mr. N. made the gravy. Two minutes later there was a crash from upstairs, followed by a thud. Mr. and Ms. N. took the stairs two at a time to Alexander's room. Fanny's right arm hung at an unnatural angle and she was bleeding freely from a cut above her right eye. The skin along the cheekbone had already begun to swell. Two drawers stood open like stairsteps in Alexander's chest of drawers, and the toys he kept on top had been swept to the floor. "Did you do this?" Mr. N. demanded.

Alexander nodded, terrified. "It wasn't my fault. She made me. She climbed up on my drawers and started messing with my stuff, so I went up after her and pushed her off. She's not even s'posed to be in here!"

On the way to the emergency room, under cover of Fanny's steady sobbing, Ms. N. laid her hand on her husband's sleeve. "Do you remember what happened to the Thompsons last year when Katie broke her collarbone? When the doctors didn't believe them? There were social workers all over their house and they had to go to their lawyer to keep her out of foster care. It could happen to us, too. What are we going to tell the doctor about how Fanny got hurt? What if they took Alexander away from us?"

"I don't know. He really has gotten more violent. It's been building up over the last couple of months and then he socked that kid at school last week. We've got no choice but to get him into therapy." "If they let us. What if they report us?"

After much discussion, Mr. and Ms. N. agreed to say that Fanny had gone alone into her brother's room and had hurt herself while trying to get a toy down from his chest of drawers. They had heard too many horror stories of burned-out case workers and bureaucratic bungling to risk upsetting their already troubled son even further through state intervention. They resolved to watch over Fanny more carefully and to find a good psychotherapist for Alexander immediately.

Unfortunately, Mr. and Ms. N. are not accomplished liars. As Dr. E. examines Fanny they tell their story too completely, as if they had rehearsed it. When Ms. N. repeats for the third time that Alexander wasn't in his room at the time, Dr. E. begins to suspect their account of what happened, and she also has some idea why they might be lying.

Are Mr. and Ms. N. justified in their attempts to protect their family with a lie? Further, should Dr. E. report her suspicions?

COMMENTARY
Kenneth V. Iserson

Unlike the charitable picture of the family painted in the case history, the physician has only the obviously false history, the parents' aberrant behavior, and the seriously injured two-year-old on which to base her actions. This is child abuse until proven otherwise. Morally and legally the incident must be reported and steps taken to protect the defenseless child until the situation can be investigated.

What is omitted from the case description, and not considered by parents who lie about a child's injury, is that the experienced physician will usually *ask the child* how the accident happened. Children do talk, and it is hard to get them to go along with a lie. If this type of discrepancy is discovered, the child would usually be immediately removed from the home, at least temporarily. If no other choice exists or the child is suspected of having other injuries, he or she is admitted to the hospital for protection and further evaluation.

Even if the physician knows that five-year-old Alexander is emotionally volatile and prone to violence, would she still be obligated to report the situation as child abuse? The case history suggests that the physician "has some idea why they might be lying." Two factors govern her behavior. The first is to identify her patient; the second is to assess, as best she can, her patient's risk of further injury. Although physicians experienced in caring for ill and injured children do attempt to involve the entire family when possible, none forget that their patient is the child, a defenseless victim of abuse. The patient, then, is two-year-old Fanny, and her welfare must dictate the physician's behavior. Is she at risk? Even with a suspicion that a sibling rather than an adult injured the child, the parents' aberrant behavior (easily exposed by experienced clinicians) suggests that they will not follow through to protect the injured child, and may even be abetting the abuse. It would be Utopia if the clinician could be all things to all people, but she can't. Her duty lies with protecting her patient and she must report her suspicions.

What if the parents had told the truth about the accident, as they understood it? How should the physician proceed? Child abuse is not defined by the age of the perpetrator. Sibling spats are common and injuries do occur; many are seen daily in emergency departments and physician offices. Some require sutures, others casts, and many, merely reassurance. The difference is that the behavior is seen both by the parents and the physicians as normal for age and circumstances. Unfortunately, a mentally disturbed five-year-old can do a great deal of damage to a two-year-old sibling, and the parents' discussion in this case suggests that they believe their son is mentally disturbed. It is the parents' responsibility to protect both of their children, yet these parents did not seem to be considering how to protect their daughter. Yes, they would possibly seek counseling for Alexander, but what does the now-casted Fanny do in the meantime? The emergency physician would proceed based upon her discussions with Mr. and Ms. N., Fanny, and perhaps Alexander. She may counsel Mr. and Ms. N. about protective measures needed to assure Fanny's safety, or direct them to a child counselor for Alexander. She may decide not to call child protective services, or may indicate that this is merely "a notification" rather than a need for immediate action.

That is the final point. Notification of protective services is normally a graded response, determined by the physician seeing the child and the prior history of reports with the services. Rather than being all or nothing, notification may initiate various activities. Some notifications lead to immediate police involvement and arrest of suspected abusers (usually in cases of death or severe injury), others to immediate on-site investigation by the social worker or police, others to an investigation the next day with follow-ups, and still others to only a record being made in case future events occur. While the federal government found that only about 53 percent of reported cases of child abuse or neglect were "validated," the key for a physician faced with questionable circumstances is to err in her patient's favor and protect the child.

COMMENTARY
Ferdinand Schoeman

The parents of the children are worried about their emotionally disturbed and violently prone boy being taken from them and placed in an ineffective social service agency. Are the parents justified under the circumstances in lying to prevent an investigation and minimize the prospect that their child will be taken away from them and put in a dysfunctional service setting?

The two-year-old Fanny was left unprotected by the parents, though not necessarily in a way that we could confidently say that the parents were neglectful. Her older brother's aggression seems to be emerging as a problem, but reasonable parents would not necessarily have been able to anticipate this degree of aggression from their son. His aggressive behavior would not on its own seem aberrant, but given his handicap, we can say his parents owe him special care.

Mr. and Ms. N. fear that an inept social service agency will further damage their emotionally disturbed son's prospects for constructive treatment. They believe they can provide this service for Alexander and now appreciate the need of doing so to protect everyone: their son, their daughter, their own survival as a family capable of caring for their children, and their cohesiveness as a family. We don't know how accurate the parents are in assessing the social service alternatives, though what they fear seems reasonable in many settings. We don't know how assiduous they will be in actually following through with their plans for private therapy for Alexander. We don't know what a private therapist might recommend to help Alexander with his emotional handicap. The therapist could recommend an alternate site placement. But even if that is so, the parents could be more confident about that judgment being in their son's interest than were the same judgment made by social services. By beginning with private consultation, they feel they can protect their son.

How might social services fail? Social services might err in not intervening when intervention is called for; they might err in intervening in a way more drastic than is appropriate. They might err in intervening in a way that exacerbates rather than ameliorates Alexander's emotional problems.

Let's now make some assumptions. The parents are right in mistrusting social services; they are right in believing they will provide private therapy and will follow through with whatever the therapist recommends. They are right in thinking that they can protect Fanny from Alexander's aggressiveness while home. Then it seems to me it is legitimate for them to lie about how

Fanny got hurt. (Here I am factoring out that they are bad liars, something that makes deliberation about the legitimacy of lying moot. If they won't be believed anyway, there is not much point to lying.)

Now as we change the assumptions, the outcome may change. Say they are wrong about social services, or about their own willingness to provide private therapy, or about their capacity to protect Fanny while in the house with Alexander, or about the difference that private therapy could make, or their willingness to follow the therapist's advice, whatever it is. In the case of any of these events, Mr. and Ms. N.'s lying would not actually protect their son or their daughter.

Would their lying in this case protect some other legitimate interest like family integrity? Is there such a thing as family integrity that is distinct from concern for the well being of the individual members? I believe that there may be such a good, but do not think the immediate case reflects this, or provides us with grounds that legitimize parental discretion in this case. I would think, for instance, that were some body part necessary to save one of the children and the other child were the only available donor, the parents could allow the transplant even though it jeopardizes the interests of the donor child. In this instance, being part of a family makes a difference in what sort of discretion to tolerate. But in the case before us, it is very unclear how the family in any sense is being helped by the lying. It is the son rather than the family that is legitimately protected by the lie. Mr. and Ms. N. are trying to care for Fanny, but they must protect Alexander too. In the case before us, they are right to lie.

4

When Opportunity Knocks

Dr. A. is a general practitioner in a small city. He was recently approached by a promoter who offered him the opportunity to invest in a free-standing radiology center. The center, to be staffed by a qualified radiologist, will provide x-rays and diagnostic imaging for all of Dr. A.'s patients.

Dr. A. is asked to put up $10,000 per share. He is told that he will earn 25 percent or more annually on his investment. The promoter tells him that the rest of the doctors in town are investing and shows him financial data from another facility that earned 80 percent annually after two years of operation. Dr. A.'s return will be calculated based on his investment. However, the profitability of the center will depend on the total number of patients that are referred — a fact that the promoter makes crystal clear to Dr. A.

Dr. A. already owns stock in several publicly traded companies that sell drugs he prescribes to his patients. He has always told himself that the companies are so large (and his practice so small) that his judgment could never be affected by stock ownership. Furthermore, medicine is a field in which he has special knowledge—why shouldn't he use that knowledge to pick up good stock?

Dr. A. is less certain about investing in an imaging center, even though he has often been envious of the income of radiologists. The promoter reassures him that everything is legal and the American Medical Association (AMA) is on record that these arrangements are not unethical. "Everyone is doing it—opportunity knocks only once" are the last words Dr. A. hears from the promoter.

What should Dr. A. do? Are there any ethical or legal limits on physician investments of this sort?

COMMENTARY
Robert A. Berenson

For all the delivery system variations in an increasingly complex, pluralistic health structure, the activity characterizing American medicine today is entrepreneurship, and a focus on the bottom line. It is debatable whether the public is well served by having physician energies spent pursuing entrepreneurial activities. However, the premises for this debate should not presuppose a simplistic dichotomy between serving the public good versus professional avarice; the Federal Republic of Germany provides health insurance for its citizens, directly controls physician spending and, nevertheless, permits vigorous entrepreneurial competition among non-hospital-based physicians. The relevant point here is, as the promoter correctly suggests to Dr. A., that in the United States health care system today virtually everybody is involved in entrepreneurialism. The deal proposed by the promoter, while more visible than other entrepreneurial activities and therefore a target of scrutiny, is refreshingly wholesome compared to other kinds of current economic practices in health care.

What are some of the structural and systemic parameters within which Dr. A. must make his decision? A typical, small-city general practitioner such as Dr. A. will earn about $90,000 for working a 58-hour week, or about $32 per hour. A radiologist in the center that currently provides radiology services in his small city will earn nearly two and a half times more per hour. So it is little wonder that Dr. A. occasionally finds himself envious. In addition, the disparity in earnings between the two will show a continual increase.

In all likelihood, many of Dr. A.'s primary-care colleagues perform x-rays in their own offices. No ethical problems arise in this situation, they inform him. After all, internal self-referral is an accepted professional activity; one cannot be accused of kickbacks to oneself. Notwithstanding their lack of training, they interpret their own x-rays because their license to practice medicines gives them that privilege. Indeed, providing in-office x-rays has become a major profit center for many primary care physicians.

Dr. A.'s income may also have declined in recent years partly because he has entered contracts with managed care organizations that use marketplace leverage to have him discount his services. In contrast, the radiology center may have the franchise for radiology services in the city's hospital and therefore control a major barrier to market entry of potential competitors. The center would effectively have a monopoly on radiology services for the area, and their prices will reflect a monopoly market, not a competitive one.

In short, general physicians who perform x-rays in their own offices and radiology facilities with market dominance are able to engage in entrepreneurial activities and generate income in ways that appear ethically acceptable but may not serve the public interest.

With these systemic constraints and realities in mind, is the proposed deal jaywalking or crossing with the light? Nothing in the arrangement resembles a kickback, because Dr. A.'s prospective profits are neither directly nor indirectly dependent on the volume of his own referrals. Importantly, his share of profits appears to be proportional to his own equity in the company. Nevertheless, would his financial interest in the radiology center provide Dr. A. an unsavory inducement to generate referrals?

Assuming the quality of the center is acceptable, ethical concern would be focused not on the existing volume of Dr. A.'s x-ray referrals, but primarily with the marginal referral, the one that he otherwise would not have made. In fact, Dr. A.'s benefit from a marginal referral is negligible, at most coming to a few cents, because his $10,000 investment certainly cannot represent even 1 percent of the equity in such an enterprise. This entrepreneurial arrangement is thus not dissimilar to his owning shares in the publicly traded pharmaceutical companies where his own prescribing pattern produces a negligible impact on his own investment. By comparison, Dr. A.'s colleagues who perform their own x-ray procedures by self-referral achieve marginal profits close to 100 percent of reimbursement.

Dr. A., being an ethical physician and a smart businessman, would still demand a series of additional safeguards about the referral arrangement. First, no physician investor can own more than, say, 5 percent of the outstanding shares. Second, physicians as a group should make up a minority interest of shareholders, and have minority representation on the Board of Directors, but should be encouraged to advise directly on the clinical aspects of the center's operations. Third, physician investors must prominently disclose their investment to all patients whom they might refer to the center, in the knowledge that patients may request referral elsewhere. Finally, the center must conduct quality assurance and utilization review programs open to outside scrutiny.

Even with these protections in place, Dr. A. would refer his patients to the center only if it provided quality services; the loss of his investment would be insignificant compared to patient perceptions that he was compromising their care to foster an investment. With the requisite safeguards, Dr. A. should have no *ethical* qualms about investing in the center. The test of whether society would benefit from Dr. A.'s investment is whether the new facility has a pro-competitive impact on the health-care delivery in his city. Given the utter lack of competition for radiology services in most areas, it is just possible that Dr. A. and his patients would benefit together.

COMMENTARY
David A. Hyman

Any system for compensating physicians necessarily creates a conflict of interest and some inappropriate incentives. Critics have long recognized this problem, although its importance has grown as cost containment has become a significant issue. The difficulty was acidly stated by George Bernard Shaw in his introduction to the (aptly titled) *Doctor's Dilemma:*

> That any sane nation, having observed that you could provide for the supply of bread by giving bakers a pecuniary interest in baking for you should go on to give a surgeon a pecuniary interest in cutting off your leg, is enough to make one despair of political humanity. But that is precisely what we have done. And the more appalling the mutilation, the more the mutilator is paid. He who corrects the ingrowing toe-nail receives a few shillings: he who cuts your inside out receives hundreds of guineas, except when he does it to a poor person for practice.

Against this backdrop, what is one to make of the promoter and his arrangement? Is this just a variant of fee-for-service practice, raising no new issues? Or is it something altogether less acceptable?

Professional organizations have attempted to provide some guidance as to the ethical acceptability of these "deals." The AMA has sanctioned such arrangements, noting that "physician ownership interest in a venture with the potential for abuse is not in itself unethical." However, the AMA does require full disclosure of the economic interest to all referred patients, a fact conspicuously omitted from the promoter's prospectus. The AMA also has the most entrepreneurially inclined ethical code of any physician organization. The American College of Physicians is less enthusiastic about such arrangements, concluding that "the physician must avoid any personal commerical conflict of interest that might compromise his loyalty and treatment of the patient." Similarly, the American College of Radiology (ACR) recently stated that "referring physicians should not have a direct or indirect financial interest in diagnostic or therapeutic facilities to which they refer patients." The ACR's position is markedly less compelling if one recalls that arrangements like Dr. A.'s have dramatically cut into radiologists' income and referral base.

The most fundamental criticisms of these arrangements point to their effect on Dr. A.'s professionalism, and on the difficulty Dr. A. will experience trying to disassociate the patient's medical needs from his own economic interests. Two related but distinct arguments inform this point of view. The most obvious argument against these ventures is financial—critics fear that the cost of health care will skyrocket as more and more tests are ordered. Economic incentives exist because they influence behavior, and the effect on Dr. A. is likely to be substantial. What empirical evidence there is tends to confirm the obvious conclusion—rewarding a particular clinical decision (such as ordering an x-ray) tends to result in that decision being made more frequently. The dramatic growth in the Medicare budget indicates that physicians do not routinely violate the predictions of economists.

Although Dr. A.'s return does not vary directly with his referral behavior, such ventures typically have mechanisms such as peer pressure to encourage high utilization. Encouragement may not even be necessary in many instances—"a piece of the action" has always helped ensure maximal effort. Having just learned an expensive lesson the hard way about the effects of a system of open-ended reimbursement, it seems foolhardy to repeat the same mistake. A study performed by the Inspector General of HHS concluded that excessive testing by physicians with ownership interest in facilities to which they referred patients cost the Medicare program $28 million in 1987. More of these facilities will only worsen the pressure on the budget, and money that could have been spent on necessary health care will be diverted to noncostworthy testing. Efforts at cost containment will be unsuccessful unless they can counter the effect of these ownership interests—presumably by providing still more incentive payments, which will worsen the budgetary constraints even more.

One can also argue that these arrangements will corrupt the decision-making process and undermine professionalism. The full implications of this claim must be understood in the context of a typical doctor-patient relationship. A physician in some ways in nothing more than the agent of his patients, providing services that the principal desires or requires. Like all employees, the physician deserves compensation for his efforts, and, like all dealings between agent and principal, compensation creates a variety of incentives, for both good and evil. Yet, the situation has an implicit conflict of interest because a physician is more than just an agent. Because a physician recommends services and then provides them (or at least stands to profit by the recommendation), he is at once agent and principal, counselor and consumer. Even without this duality, treating physician and patient as arms' length contracting parties is simply misplaced, because patients rarely have the knowledge or inclination to monitor their physician's performance or scrutinize his recommendations. Fiduciary obligations bind the physician because trust is fundamental to the doctor-patient relationship.

Because of the duality of the physician's role, any form of compensation creates an unavoidable conflict of interest. Yet that observation is not a license to create any compensation system. Conflict of interest admits of degrees—of better and worse. The question reduces to a more pragmatic one: what sort of conflict will we tolerate? We allow fee-for-service practice and captitated care even though they create unhealthy incentives for over- and underutilization. However, patients are quite familiar with the ways in which their physician's judgment may be affected in these circumstances, and they consider it when they assess his recommendations. Entrepreneurial activities are rarely disclosed. Even if they were, few patients understand that the physician receives an increased economic return for every patient he refers.

What does all this mean in practical terms? Suppose Dr. A. is following a patient with yearly CT scans. Might the patient now require biannual or quarterly scans? After all, Dr. A. is simply being more cautious. If the only available appointment is at 2:00 A.M. three weeks later, while another facility is perpetually vacant, well, Dr. A. simply has a great deal more confidence in the skill and professionalism of his own imaging center. Certain types of facilities will be "overbuilt," as every physician with a referral pool seeks to enter these arrangements. Skimming of paying patients to these facilities is also likely. What one means by "abuse" is likely to require a new definition, to account for the subtle (and not so subtle) effects of these ownership interests. Perhaps Shaw, once again, understood the difficulty best—

> What other men dare pretend to be impartial when they have a strong pecuniary interest on one side? Nobody supposes that doctors are less virtuous than judges, but a judge whose salary and reputation depended on whether the verdict was for plaintiff or defendant, prosecutor or prisoner, would be as little trusted as a general in the pay of the enemy. To offer me a doctor as my judge and then to weight the decision with a bribe of a large sum of money and a virtual guarantee that if he makes a mistake it can never be proved against him, is to go wildly beyond the ascertained strain which human nature will bear.

Shaw is perhaps too pointed—it is foolish to suggest that physicians should receive no payments for their treatment of patients. Yet he is also perfectly accurate—it is foolhardy to allow these sorts of conflict of interest and expect the quality and cost of health care to remain stable, or to expect the public to esteem those with such conflicting allegiances. Dr. A.'s misgivings are well founded. If this is opportunity, he should be glad it only knocks once, and might have hoped it never knocked at all.

5

When the Doctor Is on Drugs

You are both personal physician and friend to another physician, Dr. G. He has seemed withdrawn, irritable, and distracted recently. You have heard rumors through the hospital grapevine that not long ago he made a serious error in calculating a medication dosage, but that the error was caught by the pharmacist before the drug was dispensed.

Dr. G. has resisted your gentle explorations and expressions of concern during casual encounters, so you are surprised when he blurts out while seeing you for a routine office visit that he is using cocaine daily. You encourage him to enter a detoxification and addiction treatment program but he declines, saying that he can "handle it" by himself. Unfortunately, his personality changes persist, and even though he assures you that he is now drug-free you strongly suspect that Dr. G.'s drug abuse continues. No further obvious medical errors occur, but stories are circulating in the hospital about his abusive responses to late-night telephone calls. When you directly confront him with your suspicions, he cuts off all further contact between you.

You wish to intervene, but are uncertain how to proceed. You believe you should at least raise your concerns to the quality assurance committee of the hospital medical staff or to the impaired physicians committee of the state medical society, if not to the state licensing board. Are you justified in doing so on the basis of your current information? Won't Dr. G. just deny everything and accuse you of possessing an economic motive? Should his admission of cocaine use to you during a professional contact be kept confidential? What are the moral and legal implications of breaking confidentiality?

If you do not reveal everything that you know, you have no convincing evidence to present. You realize you have no proof that Dr. G. has harmed any patient, but wonder if your social duty extends to protecting his patients from the possibility of future damage. What if you're wrong, and he is no longer using drugs? If being irritable is a crime, the hospital medical staff is going to be decimated! If you intervene, there is a real chance that Dr. G. will end up the victim of rumors in the community and perhaps have his name listed in the National Practitioner Data Bank. How can you sort through your duties to him as his friend, his physician, and his colleague, while remembering that you have duties to society as well?

COMMENTARY
Herbert J. Keating III

In this wonderful country where the media is hungry for medical man-bites-dog stories and televised lawyers encourage every patient to consider himself a malpractice plaintiff, physicians are understandably reluctant to find fault with their colleagues. One never knows who else might be listening.

Doctors are particularly afraid to bring the faults of their colleagues to public attention. They are afraid that they will be sued, afraid that their own shortcomings will be revealed or that someone will accuse them of a self-serving economic interest. They are also afraid that they might unjustly deprive a person of his livelihood. When, as here, the faulty colleague is also a friend and a patient, someone who has put his trust and confidence in you, and when his faulty conduct arises out of a potentially reversible but addictive disease, one associated with manipulative and sociopathic behavior, an enormously complicated situation arises for the ethical physician. What should be done?

In Dr. G.'s case the time for action would seem to be now. His behavior has changed noticeably. He has made a potentially serious mistake in prescribing, and his effectiveness as a clinician is being undermined by his abusive manner and the resulting rumor mill. Undoubtedly, patients will be injured by this physician should he continue to use cocaine.

The principle of *primum non nocere* (or nonmaleficence) incorporates the requirement that physicians prevent conditions likely to be harmful to patients.

There is also the compelling duty to maintain the quality of the profession. A colleague who does drugs is not respectable, and a physician who may be perceived as covering up for him brings the profession into disrepute.

All of this said, it nonetheless seems that the duties arising from the doctor-patient relationship take precedence in this case. This relationship was established prior to Dr. G.'s cocaine problem. Doesn't Dr. G. also deserve compassionate care, especially for a disease that may have arisen by the stresses of his profession? Besides, there is the possibility that an effective plan may be able to resolve the problem of the cocaine use that renders Dr. G. potentially harmful to patients.

If the physician caring for Dr. G. has a therapeutic relationship with him, one that results in Dr. G. becoming free of cocaine, then the physician can maintain confidentiality, and should not report him.

If there is no such therapeutic relationship, or if the therapeutic relationship breaks down, then I believe that the physician is obligated to report Dr. G. to appropriate authorities. In some states, my own included, this is not only ethically correct but it also required by law. This action will result in Dr. G. being reported to the National Practitioner Data Bank. In California, and perhaps other states, a specific "diversion" program exists, allowing treatment of the impaired physician in a program outside of legal or licensing processes. This would be an ideal step if Dr. G. were willing to commit himself.

In this case it is not clear whether Dr. G. is anyone's patient anymore. We are told that he has "cut off all further contact." In this situation, severance of the doctor-patient relationship should be more formalized. The physician should contact Dr. G. immediately and insist on a clarification of their relationship, preferably in person, although telephone contact may be the only feasible way. The question for Dr. G. should be framed simply: "Are you still my patient?" Ideally, Dr. G.'s answer should be witnessed by someone impartial. If the answer is "yes," then the physician should insist that Dr. G. be enrolled in a program which would enable him to be drug-free, corroborated by urine testing to assure compliance.

If the answer is "no," then the physician must insist on immediate referral to another competent physician to supervise Dr. G.'s drug-free rehabilitation. The physician should also insist that the copies of a record certifying Dr. G.'s compliance, preferably including urine testing results, be forwarded to him to insure that Dr. G. is undergoing successful therapy.

The physician should not tolerate any half-way measures. Dr. G. must understand unequivocally that anything short of immediate steps to becoming drug-free will result in his being reported.

COMMENTARY
Terrence F. Ackerman

The physician faces two difficult questions regarding a colleague whom he suspects is chemically dependent. He must decide whether to disclose his suspicions and must determine which third party should be informed.

Disclosure of the fact that Dr. G. regularly uses cocaine is morally constrained by the obligation to treat confidentially information revealed in the therapeutic relationship. However, this obligation may be overridden when necessary to prevent serious harm to others. Moreover, physicians have a role-specific duty to apprise appropriate authorities of colleagues who practice medicine in an incompetent manner, including those impaired by chemical dependency. Thus prevention of serious harm to others is a relevant factor in determining permissible violations of confidentiality.

The physician does not have direct evidence that Dr. G. is endangering the welfare of his patients. Nevertheless, recent changes in his behavior, conjoined with the admission of regular cocaine use, raise legitimate suspicions that he may be chemically dependent. Conclusive evidence is not necessary to justify disclosure. Fuller assessment of Dr. G.'s medical condition and ability to practice medicine safely is a role responsibility assigned to specific third parties, such as physician impairment programs. Thus reasonable suspicion of chemical dependency is sufficient for considering disclosure.

Before deciding on disclosure the physician should be reasonably certain there is no alternative way to assure that Dr. G. is properly evaluated. Unfortunately, Dr. G. has spurned his expression of concern. Moreover, fierce denial is typical of persons who are chemically dependent. It is exceedingly unlikely that the physician could break through such denial and secure Dr. G.'s voluntary commitment to undergo diagnostic assessment. Outside assistance is needed.

Other moral conditions that must be satisfied in breaking confidentiality also provide guidance in deciding who should be informed. The party to whom the disclosure is made should be able to minimize the impact of the violation of confidentiality on Dr. G.'s rights and welfare. In addition, this third party should have the capacity to protect Dr. G.'s welfare by providing appropriate medical assistance if he is chemically dependent. The third party must also be able to ensure that the risks to his patients are effectively minimized. Finally, the physician should choose a plan for disclosure that allows him to ameliorate the effects of violating confidentiality in his subsequent interactions with Dr. G.

These conditions are best satisfied by disclosing the information to the state impaired physicians program. First, the procedures it follows in investigating and managing cases will carefully circumscribe any further disclosure of information about Dr. G. This involves discretion in making further limited contacts for securing information and expert judgment in determining when the data is sufficient to justify intervention. If Dr. G. is chemically dependent, the impaired physicians program will withhold this information from disciplinary bodies provided that his treatment progresses satisfactorily.

Second, the impaired physicians program possesses the resources to protect and promote Dr. G.'s welfare. If the diagnostic assessment is positive, he can be referred to an appropriate addiction treatment program. This will help assure that Dr. G. achieves long-term remission of his disease and is able to resume medical practice after a suitable period of treatment. In addition, if Dr. G. is already threatened with disciplinary action, the impaired physicians program can provide advocacy to protect his position of employment or staff privileges conditional upon successful completion of treatment.

Third, the impaired physicians program can ensure that the risks to Dr. G.'s patients are effectively minimized. If Dr. G. needs therapy, he will be required to sign a contract that details treatment expectations for a period of approximately two years. His recovery could be monitored by random drug screens and regular review of his progress by a case monitor. An important component of the contract would be the stipulation that if Dr. G. fails to maintain remission, the impaired physicians program may refer the matter to the state licensing board for disciplinary action. These conditions guarantee that any relapse into active disease is recognized and promptly addressed.

Finally, disclosure to the impaired physicians program may allow the physician to ameliorate the effects on Dr. G. of his decision to break confidentiality. This referral places the matter in a therapeutic rather than a disciplinary context, thereby defusing any imputation by Dr. G. of malicious intent. Moreover, if the initial investigation suggests that further action is warranted, the physician might join the group conducting the intervention to express his concern for Dr. G.'s welfare. This may reassure Dr. G. that he remains a loyal friend.

The investigation or diagnostic assessment may fail to establish that Dr. G. is chemically dependent. In this case, the impaired physicians program can recommend appropriate counseling for Dr. G. regarding his use of cocaine and its potential consequences. It can also follow the case to assure that Dr. G. does not become chemically dependent.

Concern for the welfare of physicians and the patients they serve fully justifies a well-funded and professionally staffed program for impaired physicians, fully supported by the state medical society and licensing board.

6

The "Student Doctor" and a Wary Patient

Marc D. Basson

Like many medical schools, State Medical College permits its third-year students to rotate through Anesthesiology for a month. During the first week, students follow Anesthesiology residents as they visit patients. Then students are assigned their own patients. After obtaining informed consent, they administer anesthesia under supervision.

James Denton is one such third-year student, rotating through the Smithville VA, an affiliated hospital. His first solo patient is Robert Criswell, a sixty-four-year-old man with metastatic prostate cancer who is scheduled to undergo bilateral orchiectomy (castration) in the morning. Criswell has a history of heavy smoking and poor pulmonary function, so James reasons that a spinal anesthetic would be safer than general anesthesia.

The attending anesthesiologist tentatively agrees to this plan. "You've done lumbar punctures before, haven't you?" the anesthesiologist asks. James says that he has done one spinal tap previously, but had great difficulty with it. He adds that he has seen three others performed. "Well, you've got to learn some time," responds the anesthesiologist. "Don't worry, I'll be with you."

James returns to the ward and finds Mr. Criswell. The residents have advised him to introduce himself as "Doctor" Denton so as not to frighten the patient unnecessarily. Some of James's fellow students use deliberately ambiguous phrases such as "one of the anesthesiology team that will be taking care of you." James selects a popular alternative, introducing himself as "a student doctor from Anesthesiology."

James tells Mr. Criswell that he would like to use spinal anesthesia and explains the procedure for lumbar puncture. "You should know," he says as he fills in the consent sheet, "that like any other medical procedure a lumbar puncture has risks, including bleeding, infection, paralysis, pain, and perhaps even death. Also, a few people develop severe headaches after such a procedure and we will ask you to lie flat for twenty-four hours afterwards to lessen the chances of this happening."

"Tell me, Doctor," Criswell asks, "have you ever had any of these problems with your patients?" James feels uneasy at being called a doctor and at Criswell's assumption that he has done many lumbar punctures before, but he decides that this is not the time to bring up his inexperience. "No, never, although I have seen one moderately severe spinal headache lasting for three days in a friend's patient," he responds.

"That's OK, I can take a headache," Criswell says as he signs the consent form. "I didn't want to insult you or anything. It's just that I've heard all kinds of stories about those medical students from the university coming over here to practice on the vets and leaving them paralyzed for life."

How should James Denton introduce himself? Is he morally or legally obligated to discuss his inexperience in obtaining an informed consent? Would it make a difference if the patient had never raised the issue of experience?

COMMENTARY
Gerald Dworkin

Considering the frequency with which situations similar to the one described in this case arise in everyday medical practice, it is surprising that the legitimacy of what occurs has not occasioned greater ethical scrutiny. Perhaps this is a specific instance of the generalization that the amount of attention paid to ethical issues is inversely proportional to their frequency in practice. Abortions performed because the life of the mother is threatened by pregnancy account for a miniscule proportion of the total, but occupy a fairly high proportion of the philosophical literature. This case, involving the training of students by allowing them to practice technical procedures on patients under supervision, occurs routinely. Yet the only public discussion I have seen concerned the bizarre case of a salesman from a medical instrumentation company who was allowed to operate on patients—without their knowledge—in order to demonstrate the nature and value of his company's products.

We are not faced here with a moral dilemma. This is not a situation in which there are good reasons of a fairly weighty nature for and against a certain course of action. A patient is being misled as to the qualifications, experience, and competence of his "healer." He thinks that James is a doctor (when he is not). He thinks that James has performed this procedure many times before (when he has not). He thinks that James has fairly wide experience with the possible side effects of the procedures (when he has not). While the violation of informed consent is not as gross as that which occurs very commonly when a surgeon does not tell his patient that the operation will actually be performed by a resident or intern (under the surgeon's supervision), the interference with the patient's ability to make an informed choice is clear. In the absence of exceptions to the principle of informed consent, we must condemn this practice.

By exceptions to the principle of informed consent, I mean factors such as impossibility (the patient is unconscious or an infant), waiver (the patient has waived the right to be informed), external justification (getting the consent of the patient would violate more important rights of others), internal justification (the ends served by the rule would be better served by making an exception).

In this case I do not see that such factors are present, and I conclude therefore that James ought to inform his patient of his status, experience, and qualifications. The patient then could either decide to go ahead or ask for a more experienced physician. The fact that the patient has explicitly raised the issue of experience is only relevant insofar as it offers empirical evidence that this patient is particularly worried about this matter. But it is reasonable to assume that all patients have a concern about their doctor's experience and competence, and would want to know that this is the first time he or she is performing a fairly risky procedure.

This answer to the particular issue does not, however, address the more general concern underlying the practice; namely, that we would all be worse off if surgeons and anesthesiologists could not be trained and training requires "hands on" experience. The solution is not deception, but finding ways to make it attractive for patients to agree to being the subjects of such training. It is reasonable for teaching hospitals to claim that the quality of care they provide is better than that of nonteaching hospitals, and that the "price" for this is that patients agree to being part of the training process. As long as this is done forthrightly, and patients have some degree of choice as to the hospitals they enter, I see no objection. Or perhaps there could be a price differential, depending on whether a doctor performed the operation or merely supervised it. This is common practice for analysts-in-training, who charge their patients a greatly reduced fee.

It is worth noting that the problem of "hands on" training is not confined to the medical profession. Airline pilots, automobile mechanics, sushi chefs, student drivers, hairdressers, psychotherapists—all have to impose risks on others in order to learn their skills. But those who bear the risks ought to be aware that they are doing so and be compensated in some fashion for their cooperation.

COMMENTARY
Eric J. Cassell

The case raises two distinct questions. The first is how the medical student, James Denton, should respond to the patient who questions his qualifications. The second is the more general question of whether medical educators are justified in allowing trainees to have primary responsibility for the care of the sick when more qualified physicians are available.

James Denton is obligated to tell the patient, Robert Criswell, the truth. But that is not the end of the matter, it is merely the beginning. Ethical issues such as truth-telling are too often dealt with as though they stood alone and timeless, like public monuments. These problems achieve their importance because of their place in human relations—of persons to themselves and to others. In medical practice, telling the truth serves something larger than itself. It is, for example, an important aspect of trust, and trust is fundamental in the doctor-patient relationship. But trust is a complex, poorly understood matter and so it is easier to discuss truth-telling in the same oversimplified way that we often discuss other ethical issues like autonomy.

Consider this case again. Robert Criswell has metastatic cancer of the prostate and he is about to have his testicles removed. From this history we do not know much about him, but if he is like most of us, he may be frightened by his situation. He is in a VA hospital where the care is sometimes impersonal and where his need for reassurance and for the information that might reduce his uncertainties may not be met.

Into that setting walks James Denton, third-year student-cum-anesthesiologist, also frightened and unsure. The way this case history is recounted suggests that they are adversaries. On the contrary, they are natural allies (like many, perhaps most, doctors and sick patients) because they need each other. Should Denton be honest? Of course he must tell the truth. But then he must actively set out to win Criswell's trust because both he and the patient need it. He must make it clear that he is a novice, but just because of that he will be more attentive and more concerned about Criswell's well-being than another, more experienced anesthesiologist might be. For this and other reasons (including the fact that information can itself be therapeutic when properly employed) he will carefully explain what is to be done, why it is being done, and what it means to Criswell, answering each of the patient's questions (and getting the correct information when he does not know). He will point out that the attending physician will be watching over them to make sure nothing goes wrong, and that he, James Denton, will visit Criswell while he is in the hospital.

For the rest of his life, if he takes care of patients, James Denton will be talking people into doing things that, while for their benefit, may be fraught with risk and fear. And on many of those occasions he will be pursued by doubts and well aware that others might do things better. That is the nature of medical care. Of course, when trust has been created and nurtured, it must not be betrayed because that is worse than lying.

This case does not describe an isolated instance, although "see one, do one, teach one" is an exaggeration of the problem. It is the strength of American medical education that physicians learn while taking care of patients under the guidance of more experienced teachers. However, the teachers, especially attending physicians, could often give better, more efficient, and less costly care to a particular patient than their trainees. Indeed, the student or house officer may be learning on someone who has been the patient of the teacher for many years. In that case the attending physician further helps the doctor in training by including him or her within the bonds of trust that have developed over those years. How, then, can we justify this method of education? Without this system of supervised learning by doing, teachers themselves would not be well trained and the qualifications of the whole profession would suffer.

What I have touched on so briefly describes a complex system of relationships and bonds that are part of the moral nature of the institution of medicine. Many would be quick to point out the ethical error if James Denton lied to Robert Criswell about his professional status. Those same critics, both inside and outside of the profession, might consider it old-fashioned, "hierarchical," or too conservative to worry about such important moral flaws as the failure to give deference to attending physicians and patients, the failure to protect the bonds of trust between patient and doctor, and the failure to protect both the past and the future of the profession of medicine. But a lie by James Denton threatens only Denton and Criswell, while those other "old-fashioned" flaws endanger the integrity of the profession without which no one would take this case seriously.

7

Proxy Consent for a Medical Gamble

Dennis F. Saver

Norma Walker left her job when six months pregnant. Nine days after the baby was born she experienced severe headache, fever, and a mild reaction to light. The next day, Sunday, she met with her obstetrician in the hospital emergency room. He found no abnormalities and felt strongly that further evaluation by an internist was imperative.

Since Mrs. Walker did not know an internist, she and her husband were worried about finding a physician who would come to the emergency room on a Sunday morning. Dr. Stanley, a physician whom they both knew personally, happened to be in the emergency room at the time, and Mr. Walker asked him to assume care of his wife. Her obstetrician agreed.

Dr. Stanley learned that the Walkers' two-year-old child had recently had viral meningitis, as had several other children and adults living near their home. When reached by phone, their pediatrician confirmed that two children had been proven by lumbar puncture to have aseptic meningitis and had been treated conservatively at home. During the interview the Walkers expressed anger about the impersonal and unpleasant way Mrs. Walker had been treated by hospital personnel in the labor and delivery suite a week earlier. Mr. Walker was especially bitter and was certain she would have had better care at home.

The results of laboratory tests showed that Mrs. Walker probably had a just-beginning viral meningitis (for which no specific treatment is necessary), but may have had a bacterial meningitis (a life-threatening illness requiring treatment with intravenous antibiotics).

The test findings were carefully explained to the Walkers. Dr. Stanley stated that because of the circumstances, the chances of Mrs. Walker having viral meningitis were very high. But the result of the spinal fluid test raised the possibility of bacterial meningitis. The physician argued that, if he or his wife were the patient, he would play it safe and go into the hospital for two days of intravenous antibiotics until the spinal fluid culture was complete.

Mrs. Walker felt too ill to think clearly—she would, she said, do whatever her husband decided. Mr. Walker was determined to be involved in the decision. He was clearly concerned for his wife, but wasn't sure whether "playing it safe" was the best course of action. He appreciated the personal favor of the physician who had agreed to undertake her care on short notice and had given a detailed explanation of the medical evaluation. However, her recent hospitalization had left a bad impression. Also the couple had no insurance. Was the small chance really much of a gamble? Mr. Walker needed time to think and went for a walk.

Upon returning, he announced his decision—to take the gamble. He would take his wife home, fully aware of the risks and of Dr. Stanley's discomfort with his decision. Who ought to have made the decision about treatment in this case? Was Mr. Walker's decision justifiable?

COMMENTARY
Ronald A. Carson

Hospital care is often brusque and inconsiderate, at times even unkind. Patients understandably recoil from such treatment and seek to avoid it. Patients also, increasingly, want to take part in determining the shape of their care. The sophisticated patient expects a full explanation of what ails him or her and wants to contribute to decisions made regarding the course of treatment. The unsophisticated, too, often want to know—not the detail, perhaps, and all the possible options, but certainly the odds and the risks. They, too, often wish to say, and have taken into account, how much discomfort and what degree of suffering they are prepared to undergo for this or that outcome.

While sensitive physicians are trying to be responsive to these sorts of expectations, an important and useful distinction ought not to be sloughed over, namely, the distinction between treatment decisions and decisions about the course of treatment. Treatment decisions are medical decisions in the strict sense, decisions predicated on the special knowledge of the medically trained. Assembling relevant evidence, examining it, and interpreting it is the proper business of physicians and should be left to them. Acting on an interpretation of that evidence to treat a patient in distress is also the physician's responsibility. Difficulties arise in cases such as Mrs. Walker's not in diagnosis or treatment, but on the way from one to the other. It is at this point that the physician must consider the treatment options available and weigh their probable outcomes. It is at this juncture that competent adult patients rightfully become partners with their physicians in the decision-making process.

Course-of-treatment decisions are not medical decisions but life decisions. At issue are the physical, psychological, and social effects this or that treatment is likely to have on this particular patient and those nearest him or her. Gauging those effects does not require medical expertise but rather knowledge of the patient's circumstances "from the inside." Choices about the course a treatment should take (and, indeed, the choice between treatment and no treatment) are most appropriately made by those who stand to bear the consequences of the decision.

The decision required in this case is a medical one. This does not mean that the patient and her husband should be excluded from the discussion. But, knowing the consequences of bacterial meningitis, Dr. Stanley was right in recommending hospitalization for prophylactic treatment until lab results conclusively ruled out a bacterial infection. He had to consider the possible effects of Mrs. Walker not receiving adequate care at home (antibiotics, administered intravenously) and of her being at home with what might turn out to be a contagious disease. True, the evidence for viral meningitis was all but overwhelming, but it was also circumstantial. The presence of those white cells caused Dr. Stanley to hesitate and recommend precautionary treatment.

It is clear that Mr. Walker considered the decision one he had to make (a course-of-treatment decision) and that the physician saw it as a treatment decision. What is not clear is the degree of forcefulness the physician used in recommending hospitalization. If the proper interpretation of symptoms and test results is what is at issue, the recommendation to hospitalize and initiate prophylactic therapy should be insisted upon by the physician. The Walkers may, in the face of that insistence, take it upon themselves to go home, but the physician will not have encouraged that decision by offering them a choice which is not theirs to make.

COMMENTARY
Henry Aranow Jr.

I have conducted my medical practice on the assumption that competent adults have the right and the responsibility to make final decisions about their own medical care. They may, if they so desire, delegate this responsibility to another competent adult of their choosing.

The inflammation of the covering of the brain designated by the term "meningitis" is almost always accompanied by some inflammation of the adjacent brain substance. This latter, if of sufficient extent and degree, may cause disturbances in thinking. Some patients with meningitis are manifestly mentally incompetent to make a reasoned decision about their treatment options. The case description states, "Mrs. Walker felt too ill to think clearly—she would, she said, do whatever her husband decided." The portion of the history of the patient's illness given in the abstract is very scanty, nor are any of the details of the physical examination performed by Dr. Stanley included. The statement that her obstetrician found no abnormalities seems to refer to abnormalities of her reproductive system, since he felt that further evaluation by an internist was *imperative* [my emphasis]. Such information might have been of value in attempting to evaluate Mrs. Walker's mental competence.

When the decision of a person given the responsibility of making a therapeutic decision on behalf of another differs sharply from that recommended by the physician charged with the patient's care, I believe it is the duty of the physician to present to the patient himself or herself the considerations that led to the recommendations rejected by the patient's delegate. Under such circumstances, the mental competence of the patient is of utmost importance.

The case description leads me to believe that Dr. Stanley felt that Mrs. Walker was competent to delegate the decision-making responsibility to her husband. This competence means to me that, when Mr. Walker's decision differed so strikingly from his own, he should have re-presented his arguments to Mrs. Walker, explaining the bases of his professional recommendations, informing her of the risks inherent in the course chosen by her husband, persuading her to withdraw the delegation of decision-making authority from him, and deciding for herself to accept Dr. Stanley's advice.

In my view, the medical arguments for in-hospital treatment are over-whelming until the test results definitely exclude bacterial meningitis. Bacterial meningitis can be a fulminating illness in which a delay in therapy for even a few hours may lead to death or permanent disability. To permit the mother of two children, who has a central responsibility in their care and upbringing, to run such a risk because of her anger and that of her husband "about the impersonal and unpleasant way she had been treated by hospital personnel in the labor and delivery suite a week earlier" strikes me as, in the highest degree, unwise and irresponsible.

We are asked, "Was the small chance really much of a gamble?" My answer is that for such stakes, "It is an appalling one!"

The wisdom of any medical intervention may be evaluated by computing the cost/benefit ratio to the patient and, less importantly, to her family and to society. With the possibility of the death or serious disability of a young mother in one pan of the balance, against two days of undesired and possibly unnecessary hospitalization in the other, the indicator bangs against the end of the scale in the direction of hospitalization and treatment.

It is clear that I do not believe Mr. Walker's decision was justifiable. The fact that Dr. Stanley was only "accidentally" involved in Mrs. Walker's care raises the possibility in my mind that he might have pushed his recommendations much harder with both the Walkers had he been their "regular" or "personal" physician.

COMMENTARY
Nancy K. Rhoden

Competent adults can, in general, refuse medical treatment even when their refusal is unwise, ignorant, or life-threatening. Such situations are agonizing, but more agonizing, and much more complicated, are situations where third parties refuse treatment for others. In the case at hand, Mr. Walker is making a decision with potentially disastrous consequences for his wife's life and health.

Initially, at least, he has the right to make this decision, since his wife has delegated decision-making power to him. There should be a strong presumption in favor of a proxy's decision when he has recently, and competently, been authorized to decide by the patient herself. But this presumption should not be absolute. Any third-party decision maker has an obligation to promote the patient's best interests and to make a decision which the patient could reasonably have made herself. Decisions by parents or court-appointed guardians which violate this duty can be challenged. Decisions by authorized proxies should be subject to similar scrutiny, to guard against unreasonable decisions or decisions based upon ulterior motives.

In this case, despite the couple's lack of insurance, the facts as presented suggest that Mr. Walker acted from concern for his wife. Obviously, if his motives were suspect, Dr. Stanley should take further action. But the real problem here is not Mr. Walker's motive, but the reasonableness of his decision.

Given the facts at hand, is his decision justifiable? Such decisions can be evaluated in several rather disparate ways. They can be considered in purely medical terms—what is the probable diagnosis, what are the relevant risks of alternative courses of treatment, and so on? By these criteria, Mr. Walker's decision is probably unjustifiable. Competent physicians would likely agree as to the need for hospitalization here, at least for observation, because bacterial meningitis can very quickly become life-threatening.

Mr. Walker's decision, however, should not be evaluated solely on medical grounds. Individuals do not make personal treatment decisions in exactly the same way doctors do: rather, their decisions are necessarily, and properly, influenced by their personal values, needs and preferences. Though proxy decision makers are, correctly, given less leeway to be idiosyncratic, their decisions should not automatically be deemed unjustifiable whenever they differ from medical judgment. Rather, we should ask if the proxy's decision is based on factors which the patient would find relevant and important, and if his weighing of risks is one a reasonable person could make.

Thus it is not inappropriate for Mr. Walker to consider his wife's subjective response to hospitalization, since it is a factor which would probably have influenced her decision, even though it is irrelevant to a purely medical judgment. Nor is it inappropriate for Mr. Walker, in weighing the risks, to take into account that his wife's illness was probably viral. The more unlikely that she has bacterial meningitis, the more reasonable his gamble becomes. Additionally, since one reason for recommending hospitalization is to provide careful observation and ready access to treatment, he can consider how closely he will be able to monitor his wife's condition, and how quickly he could get her to a hospital should changes occur.

Mr. Walker, of course, has an obligation to weigh these factors against the risks of taking her home. To do this, he must be accurately apprised of the risks. From the presentation of facts in this case, it is hard to tell exactly how grave Dr. Stanley believed the risks to be. Although the Walkers were told that bacterial meningitis is a life-threatening illness, we do not know whether they were told that it can progress very rapidly to the critical stage, so that a delay in treatment may be fatal or may cause permanent neurological damage. If Mrs. Walker had been told this, it is less likely that she would have been genuinely uncertain as to what to do: there is no indication that her values are so unusual that she would prefer death in a friendly environment to cure in an impersonal one. If Dr. Stanley feels that he inadvertently characterized the risks of going home as less serious than they are, or that Mr. Walker interpreted them wrongly, he should at least try to re-present the facts to both of them before accepting Mr. Walker's decision. And if Mr. Walker remains steadfast, perhaps Dr. Stanley should also try to get Mrs. Walker to take the responsibility herself.

If, however, Dr. Stanley believes that, in his best medical judgment, his characterization of hospitalization as simply "playing it safe" (rather than medically imperative) does not minimize the risks, then he might be constrained to find Mr. Walker's decision, though far from ideal, justifiable. If this is the case (perhaps because Dr. Stanley feels virtually certain that Mrs. Walker's case is viral, or because the couple live very near the hospital), then he should respect Mr. Walker's decision. He should, however, carefully alert both of them to what changes to look for, and impress upon them the importance of an immediate return to the hospital should such changes occur.

8

Faith Healing for Childhood Leukemia

Within twenty-four hours a ten-month-old boy was transferred from a small local hospital to a university hospital and then to its affiliated cancer center with a presumptive diagnosis of leukemia. Because the diagnosis had not been confirmed by bone marrow examination, information on the type of leukemia — needed for an outline of a specific therapy and a more accurate prognosis — was not available.

When the baby was admitted on a Saturday afternoon, only his mother was present. The child was not acutely ill, and the severe anemia that had concerned the referring physician had been corrected by transfusion before the transfer. The baby seemed much better, according to his mother. However, there were significant signs of tumor. The medical approach currently considered optimal is hydration, medication to counteract excess uric acid, and careful characterization of the leukemia. After that, specific therapy can be offered. The characterization could not begin until after the weekend but some therapy could begin immediately.

This information was explained first to the mother, and a few hours later to the father. After two hours of deliberation, they told the attending physician that they refused therapy. They would, they said, place their faith in God. They had recently seen sight restored to the baby's great-grandmother when she was taken to a healing service after a debilitating stroke.

They felt that all the cancer center measures would very likely fail and they would then take the child to a faith-healing service. It made more sense to them to refuse the therapy and take the child to the faith-healing service right away. They had prayed for a sign from God to help them make this decision, and took the nurse's failure to start an intravenous infusion on the first attempt as just such a sign.

The physician asked the father why God would allow cancer centers to exist if prayer were a more appropriate mode of exercising parental responsibility. The father replied, "Cancer centers are part of God's plan, so that children of parents who do not believe still have a chance." The parents were then asked whether they could muster a perfect enough faith to mediate the healing. The answer was that such a faith was not necessary — they had a perfect God.

The child was discharged without therapy with a return appointment at the center's clinic, but the family did not keep the appointment.

Did the attending physician take the right course of action by acceding to the parents' desires so easily? Should other staff have been requested to negotiate with the family? Should legal remedies have been sought to ensure treatment for the child? What are the limits of religious freedom and parental authority when a child's medical care is at stake?

COMMENTARY
Baruch Brody

I must confess that I have little sympathy for the parents' decision. Coming from a Jewish theological background, I find their position objectionable on theological grounds. The objection was best put by Rabbis Akiva and Ishmael when they said: "Just as if one does not weed, fertilize, and plow, the trees will not produce, and if fruit is produced but is not watered or fertilized it will not live but die, so with regard to the body. Drugs and medicines are the fertilizer and the physician is the tiller of the soil." It is strange to find people actively intervening through natural means to produce desired results in all areas but matters of life and death, and insisting that in those areas alone man should merely pray and leave himself in the hands of God.

My views about the family decision, and the views of the readers of this case study, are not, however, what is immediately crucial here. That issue is a different one, namely, who has the right to make the decision for the ten-month-old boy. Only if we decide that we as a society, or some agents of ours (the physician, the hospital, the courts), should be making the decision will it be relevant to ask what *we* think should be done for the child.

One other preliminary point. There are those who believe that adults should not be allowed to refuse medical treatment *even for themselves* in such cases. They believe that society, through its agents, should insist upon making the judgment even for an adult patient. The many people who hold this view will certainly not want to allow the parents the authority to decide to refuse treatment for the child. So this case is a difficult one *only* for those, like myself, who think that adult patients can choose for themselves to rely upon faith healing rather than medical treatment. The question then becomes whether they can also make this decision for their child who is incapable of deciding for himself.

What is the extent of parental authority over the child and to what extent should society intervene to override certain parental decisions? I know of no adequate theoretical answer to this question. We can, however, reject as inadequate two often-held but nevertheless crude models. One maintains that making decisions for the child is a right of the parents, and when society or its agents intervene, they violate these parental rights. The other maintains that making a decision for the child is an obligation placed by society upon the parents, and society may intervene whenever it judges it to be in the best interest of the child.

I would like to advocate a third model for the parental role. In this model, parents do have a right to make decisions for their child. At the same time, the child has a right against the parents that the parents not use their capacity and right to make decisions in ways that are harmful to the child. Society's role here is part of its general role to adjudicate between members with conflicting rights. If we adopt this model, what shall we say about this case? All parties involved believe that the continued life of the child is the value to be promoted; the dispute is about the efficacy of different ways of pursuing this value. (This differentiates the present case from Jehovah's Witnesses cases.) Therefore, it seems to me perfectly appropriate for society to say (a) if there is ever a case where the child's right to protection takes precedence, it is where the child's life is at stake; (b) in this conflict, where the dispute is about efficacy, and not values, we can easily decide that medical treatment is likely to be the more efficacious; and (c) we therefore expect our agencies (doctors and hospitals acting with the approval of the courts) to protect the child by insisting upon treatment.

But what about the religious freedom of the parents? Surely, if anything is settled in this area, it is that freedom of action (as opposed to belief) where the rights of others are seriously challenged is not justified merely on the grounds that the action is backed by a religious belief.

COMMENTARY
Jan van Eys

Parents' responsibility for the care of infant children is total. Their absolute authority can be overruled, however, if the state decides that parental decisions are not in the best interest of the child. Such state action is a lengthy process, which stirs wide debate unless the action is based on generally unacceptable behavior by the parents, such as overt physical abuse. In the case of life-threatening illness in a child, the choice of medical care by the parents is based on their perception of the illness. It is frequently argued that an inadequate understanding of the disease may prevent parents from making a valid and reasoned decision. Nevertheless, the state does not intervene a priori in making such decisions.

In this case, involving leukemia in an infant, the parents' perception of the probability of poor outcome was not unreasonable. Chemotherapy is never an easy road to follow and is often more difficult in infants. The outcome does vary with the type of leukemia and a prognosis could not be given. But even in the type of leukemia with the most optimistic prognosis, an optimistic outcome would be statistically less certain in an infant than in a four- or five-year-old.

The judgment that a parent is making a decision in the best interest of the child is usually based on the medical personnel's perception of whether parents are seeking a mode of care that has curing as a goal. The harshest judgments are given to those parents who forgo the application of proven or near-proven effective therapy. In this case the parents chose to substitute one mode of treatment with curative intent—chemotherapy—for another—faith healing—thereby creating the dilemma.

There is in the United States a strict separation of church and state. In matters spiritual the parents' decision-making power is even more absolute than in matters physical. Not to feed a child would be considered child abuse; not to give a child spiritual instruction is the business of the parents and not of the state. In addition, although the state makes judgments about what constitutes adequate nutrition, there are very few state judgments about what constitutes adequate spiritual sustenance.

Does separation of church and state imply a separation of church and medicine? Is medicine in fact allied with the state or with the spiritual realm? There is no doubt that the treatment offered the child was wholly biological. However, this does not mean that medical therapy lacks a strong component of faith, even at its most overtly physical, such as in cases of surgery. Clearly medical and spiritual matters are not nearly as separate in the eyes of patients as they are in the eyes of many physicians.

The juxtaposition of faith healing and medicine puts the burden of response squarely on the physician. Does the physician accept the proposition that these are comparable alternatives? As an analogy, Laetrile and classical chemotherapy for cancer are comparable alternatives in the sense that both are attempts to cure the disease. Given such a choice, the decision can be based on recorded past experience. Presumably, an objective decision can then be made about the preferability of conventional chemotherapy over Laetrile.

Obviously the juxtaposition of faith healing and classical medicine does not readily allow an objective evaluation. On the other hand, to reject faith healing a priori as an element of care by the parents would force the physician to confront his or her own belief system. To reject faith healing as an alternative that is outside the system of organized medicine, and thereby to argue that faith healing is not a selection of care but a rejection of medicine, demands an a priori rejection of the concept of faith.

Usually parents use faith healing as a form of support, a "hedging of one's bets." As such it can be ignored, endorsed, or condoned by physicians. In this case the confrontation was stripped of any smokescreen, and the question was presented in its barest form. The parents rejected the concept of classical medicine and faith healing as complementary modes of care: classical medicine, they said, is God's plan for those of little faith.

The fact that an infant is involved in this argument is not as important as the argument itself. Its application to infants recalls the long-standing theological debate over infant baptism. There are arguments that a child should not be baptized until he or she can purposefully make that choice. However, if there is no time to let the child select the alternatives, such debates become irrelevant. The implications inherent in faith healing are clear: the parents feel a responsibility to ensure that their child follow their convictions. No doubt different physicians would have reacted and responded to this challenge differently. The response is clearly dependent on the physician's own deep-seated spiritual beliefs. Any absolute solution would reflect the attitude of the person who proclaims such wisdom, not a fundamental truth about human existence and parental responsibility.

9

Who Speaks for the Patient with the Locked-in Syndrome?

Before his stroke, Mr. B. was an alert and active resident in an intermediate care nursing home. The staff described him as fiercely independent and deeply religious. They routinely try to assess residents' wishes concerning Living Wills and resuscitation measures, but Mr. B. consistently refused to discuss these matters.

His stroke was caused by a clot in the large artery at the base of the brain and was accompanied by paralysis of nearly all voluntary muscles. He could neither speak nor move except for opening and closing his eyes. He was, however, alert and able to understand conversation. He was, in neurological terms, "locked in," aware of himself and his surroundings but unable to communicate effectively with his relatives or the health care team.

Using a simple code of open eyes for "yes" and closed eyes for "no," the staff was able to get answers to simple questions. However, when a question with even minimal emotional content was asked—Do you recognize your niece?—Mr. B. would begin to cry and was unable to give a clear response. Further, his capacity to respond to simple questions waxed and waned.

The diagnosis of brain stem stroke was confirmed by two neurologists who agreed that the prognosis for even minimal recovery of function was near zero. In this situation, long-term survival depends largely upon the vigor with which complications such as pneumonia are treated.

By the fourth hospital day Mr. B.'s condition had stabilized and he was able to breath without ventilator assistance. But he remained "locked in" and unable to speak or move.

How vigorously should the staff press Mr. B. with questions on resuscitation or restoration of the ventilator for treatment of pneumonia? Given the difficulty in communicating, can Mr. B. be considered competent to consent to or to refuse treatment? How might his guardian justify consent to or refusal of vigorous, life-sustaining therapy? Might the attending physician write a Do Not Resuscitate (DNR) order without approval of the patient's guardians?

COMMENTARY
Grant E. Steffen

Is Mr. B. competent to give or withhold consent to treatment? This is the central question, for if it is answered "no," then the answer to the first question—how vigorously the staff should question him—is "not at all." It would be pointless to push Mr. B. for answers only to discard them as the views of an incompetent person.

But probably one must ask such questions in order to *determine* if Mr. B. is competent. Competence to consent to or refuse treatment involves (1) the capacity to understand and reason about choices; (2) the capacity to communicate one's choice; and (3) the possession of a stable set of values and goals upon which to base one's choice. While most questions of competence focus upon the first element, for Mr. B. the second element is the problem.

We are told that Mr. B. can communicate with a simple yes/no code by blinking his eyes but that this strategy fails when questions with emotional content are asked. This, along with his waxing and waning capacity to respond, probably makes Mr. B. incompetent to give or withhold consent. Nevertheless, I feel that an attempt should be made to test his desire and capacity to enter into a dialogue about treatment choices.

One need not ask him directly about DNR orders, but may gently ask if he would like to discuss treatment options. This question should be asked on at least two different occasions. If the answers are both positive and consistent, then Mr. B. is probably competent and discussions about specifics should proceed. Further questioning may well uncover confusion and inconsistency. If these persist, then I would stop the dialogue.

Even then, such a discussion may be of questionable value. A stroke, whether or not it causes loss of speech, may commonly affect the intellect and make any response questionable. So we may not know that even a consistent response is what Mr. B. really means.

Concerning the third element of competence we are told that Mr. B. is deeply religious. While this gives no clue about the content or the stability of his religious beliefs, we may nevertheless assume that Mr. B. does possess that stable set of goals and values. However, to the extent that they involve questions of Living Wills, he has refused to talk about them. Does this past refusal give us an adequate reason not to ask about treatment choices? I do not think so, since we are not told who asked what questions or how the questions were asked in the nursing home. Now Mr. B.'s situation has changed and he should have one more chance at this dialogue.

The last two questions in the case description suggest that in fact Mr. B. was ruled incompetent. Who, then, may speak for Mr. B.? A competent family member such as Mr. B.'s niece, though having no legal status, may give consent to treatment. If the niece is aware of Mr. B.'s wishes, she could give consent on that basis. But there is no record of a Living Will and Mr. B. has refused to talk about such matters. So there seems to be no basis for a substituted judgment.

To determine if the niece is capable of or likely to make decisions in Mr. B.'s best interest, I would want to know if her relationship to her uncle was close and caring, cordial but distant, or one of indifference or hostility. Will she benefit by his death? While the nursing home staff may be able to clarify this relationship, the answers to the questions may remain unclear; if so, the physician should ask the court to name a guardian.

The guardian has the same problem as the niece—to decide what is in Mr. B.'s best interest. If the neurologists are correct in their prognosis of no chance of significant recovery, then I believe that most people in Mr. B.'s predicament would decline vigorous life-sustaining therapy. For the quadriplegic life is restrictive, frustrating, and grim; but there is at least communication and a sharing of memories, feelings, and hopes with one's friends. But for the person who is "locked in," communication is severely restricted and life would offer little more than discomfort, frustration, and despair.

I feel that the quality of Mr. B.'s life is minimal, the burden of his illness intolerable, and that life-sustaining therapy should not be given. This analysis claims neither a logical nor an empirical basis. It is simply my intuition that the difference between the benefits of treatment—prolonged life—and the burden of that life is too great.

The last question is not whether a DNR order is appropriate but rather if it may be written without the guardian's approval. If the attending physician does not think that cardiac or respiratory arrest is imminent, then there is no reason to exclude the guardian from sharing in that decision. If a guardian has not been appointed and if arrest is thought to be imminent, then the physician may write the order with the niece's approval. If the niece refuses to be involved in the discussion or is not available, then the physician may write the order on his own.

Though writing a DNR order should be, whenever possible, a shared decision between the physician and the competent patient, or between the physician and the incompetent patient's family, if this sharing is impossible the physician is not thereby relieved of the duty that exists in all clinical settings—namely, to act in the patient's best interest.

In that classic tale of revenge, *The Count of Monte Cristo*, Alexandre Dumas gives us two examples of locked-in people. Though the hero, Edmund Dantes, was locked in the Chateau D'If for fourteen years, his prison was outside himself. He could still walk and talk and plot his escape. M. Noirtier de Villefort was also locked in, but his prison, like Mr. B.'s, was his body. M. Noirtier could communicate with eye signals and quite effectively influence and sometimes even control his family.

Given the primitive state of medical care in nineteenth century France, I assume that the character of M. Noirtier was not copied from life, but rather constructed from Dumas's superb imagination. I know of no locked-in patient with a long-term survival and a level of function similar to those displayed by Monsieur Noirtier. Mr. B.'s only escape from being locked in (the Monte Cristo syndrome) is death.

COMMENTARY
Cory Franklin

The central issue in this case is whether life-sustaining care should be delivered to this patient. This decision depends primarily on two factors: the ability to ascertain the patient's wishes and the outcome if such care is delivered or withheld. The facts strongly suggest that vigorous, life-sustaining therapy should be applied.

In most situations, the definitive indication not to administer aggressive support (endotracheal intubation, cardiopulmonary resuscitation, intensive care) involves either a prior declaration by the patient to that effect (not present here) or a discussion with the patient where he refuses these measures. To be valid, this type of communication must meet certain standards: the patient must understand the nature of his disease and the proposed therapies. He must further understand the potential consequences of refusing these therapies. Finally, the caregivers must be reasonably confident that the patient is expressing his true wishes, that is, his understanding and refusal are not compromised by pain, fear, anger, depression, or denial.

Mr. B. can only answer yes or no by blinking. His answers to simple questions are unclear. According to the standards, the caregivers cannot render a reliable clinical judgment on Mr. B.'s competence to refuse therapy given the limitations on communication. The problem is simply too complex for yes or no answers.

Mr. B., like other locked-in patients, is conscious, alert, and can understand what is being said to him. To deny him the option of life-sustaining therapy because he cannot communicate is to apply an unfair standard. Similar patients unable to speak or write, such as quadraplegic, ventilator-dependent patients would not (and should not) be denied aggressive therapy on this basis. Where doubt exists concerning a patient's wish to be resuscitated, the principle in most cases is "to err on the side of life." Without his prior request, Mr. B. should not have aggressive support withheld simply because his consent cannot be clarified.

When the patient's wishes cannot be ascertained, we must revert to other criteria to determine whether aggressive support is warranted. In this case, the most important issue is the patient's prognosis. Mr. B.'s problem illustrates the axiom that "good facts promote good ethics." The information presented states that, soon after the stroke, two neurologists agreed that Mr. B.'s prognosis for even minimal recovery was poor. This point deserves further scrutiny.

Locked-in state is a relatively new syndrome, first described in the medical literature less than twenty years ago (see F. Plum and J. Posner, *The Diagnosis of Stupor and Coma*, 1966). (Ironically, the condition may have been first mentioned by Alexandre Dumas, describing M. Noirtier de Villefort in *The Count of Monte Cristo* over 100 years ago.) Though the condition was originally considered uniformly fatal, several studies reported in the *Annals of Neurology* and *Transactions of the American Neurological Association* in the last five years have documented patients who have recovered. Many of those who recovered suffered from the same type of cerebrovascular disease as Mr. B. Some patients recovered almost complete function (walking, talking, bowel and bladder control) and were discharged from the hospital.

In several cases, patients' paralysis and loss of speech persisted for three months before recovery began. The largest series of patients with locked-in syndrome described in the literature comprise less than ten patients. This is far too few to permit identification of clinical signs associated with future recovery. As is true with other neurologic disorders, early prediction of the extent of recovery for individual patients is difficult, if not impossible.

Numerous authors and at least one current neurology text (*The Clinical Neurosciences* edited by R. N. Rosenberg, 1983) recommend vigorous medical support early in the course of locked-in syndrome, since potential for significant recovery exists. Measures to prevent pneumonia and other pulmonary complications are considered standard medical care. When these patients require life-sustaining care there is no medical justification for withholding it. For Mr. B., one potential future scenario illustrates this: at some point he may require a tracheotomy to control his lung secretions and avoid asphyxiation. If this were not performed, he might suffocate on his own secretions while conscious, alert, and unable to notify anyone.

Mr. B. may not recover from the locked-in syndrome. Ultimately he may be completely dependent on others and require lifetime institutional care. This situation might last weeks, months, or even years. He may not be completely helpless. Some patients with the syndrome have learned to communicate through Morse Code and computers. (Language interaction with Mr. B. and patients like him presents a challenge to our future computer technology.) The future care problems of these patients must be confronted not only on an individual, but on a societal level. We should be prepared to care for these patients in the same way we care for spinal cord injury victims. Mr. B.'s condition leaves him unable to represent himself, but does not divest him of his right to medical care. His is exactly the type of case where our safeguards for ensuring care must be redoubled. As the question stands, both on the basis of personal autonomy and appropriate medical care, Mr. B. is a candidate for vigorous life-sustaining therapy.

10

"Make Me Live": Autonomy and Terminal Illness

M.G. was a sixty-two-year-old while female who had had a mastectomy for breast cancer. She received only three of a proposed six courses of adjuvant chemotherapy because of severe bone marrow suppression. Fourteen months later she was found to have bone and lung metastases. Her oncologist explained to M.G. and her family that her illness was terminal and suggested that she receive supportive care through Hospice. He advised that chemotherapy was not indicated because of the previous bone marrow suppression and history of congestive heart failure.

M.G. had always been in control of her life and became angry and depressed that she was losing her battle against cancer and could do nothing. Morphine was prescribed for pain relief. She was placed on home oxygen to relieve shortness of breath caused by lung metastases. M.G. was seen weekly by Hospice, but she did not respond well to the program. The hospice workers felt that she was denying the terminal nature of her illness. She insisted that she wanted the emergency squad called to attempt resuscitation if she arrested at home.

When M.G. returned for outpatient followup, she was in a wheel chair and extremely short of breath, and was described by her oncologist as being "in a panic" about her impending death. M.G. continued to ask about chemotherapy but her husband confided that he knew his wife was terminal and wanted her to be kept comfortable. The next day she became more short of breath and called paramedics who brought her to the Emergency Room. Repeated attempts at thoracentesis by the staff and the resident on the inpatient service were unsuccessful. The resident told M.G. that she had advanced cancer and that nothing could be done to reverse the course of her disease. M.G. reportedly told the resident "I want you to do everything possible to make me live."

The following morning the resident presented the case to her attending physician. She said that she had attempted to determine whether M.G. was aware of her prognosis but that M.G. either remained silent or accused the resident of being incompetent because she was unable to tap the pleural fluid in her chest. The resident planned to send M.G. to the radiology suite where a thoracentesis could be obtained under ultrasound guidance and suggested that the attending physician write a Do-Not-Resuscitate (DNR) order because M.G. might arrest during the procedure and be placed on a respirator and taken to the Intensive Care Unit. When the attending physician entered M.G.'s room he found her curled up in a fetal position. He asked if he could do anything to help her. M.G. responded "make me less short of breath" and again complained about the difficulty the staff had had in doing the thoracentesis, but she was not willing to discuss the nature of her illness or its prognosis. The attending physician conferred with the patient's oncologist who confirmed that M.G. had not tolerated previous chemotherapy and that further treatment would be futile.

Should the attending physician write a DNR order without informing the patient?

COMMENTARY
Robert I. Misbin

Discussions of terminal care are always difficult, even with a patient with whom one has a long-standing relationship. In this case the attending physician must make a decision about life-prolonging treatment in a patient he has never seen before and who has consistently dealt with her illness with anger and denial. What can the attending do to gain the trust and confidence of this patient? To talk of respirators and endotracheal tubes would do little but add to the patient's anxiety. Nevertheless, a decision must be made about a DNR order. Authoritative sources insist that the patient has the right to participate in this decision. What should a virtuous physician do?

Before analyzing the ethical issues, it is first necessary to be clear about the medical facts. I shall assume that this patient is indeed terminal and that no therapy exists that would alter the progression of her cancer. The patient's shortness of breath could potentially be relieved (at least temporarily) by removal of fluid from her pleural space. Several attempts at thoracentesis have failed, however, suggesting that either there is very little fluid in the pleural space or that it is inaccessible due to the large amount of tumor in the patient's chest. Either explanation would decrease the likelihood that thoracentesis would provide much relief and increase the likelihood of pneumothorax (accidentally nicking the lung while attempting to remove the fluid). Since the patient's respiratory status is already compromised, a pneumothorax would likely cause a respiratory arrest requiring that the patient be placed on a respirator and taken to the intensive care unit. Since nothing can be done to reverse progression of the cancer, the patient would remain on the respirator indefinitely until the tumor destroyed so much lung that it would technically be impossible to ventilate her.

Given the possibility of an impending respiratory arrest, it would be ethically unacceptable for the attending physician to proceed with thoracentesis without considering a DNR order. To subject M.G. to the violence of a resuscitation without her knowledge and consent would be completely wrong. Although most patients would prefer a quick death to a prolonged and agonizing one, this is not invariably the case. The religious convictions of some patients require maintenance of biological life as long as technically possible, while others believe that suffering the agonies of death leads to ultimate salvation. A few days of extra life, even on a respirator, may permit a patient to meet a desired goal such as disposal of personal property or knowledge of the birth of a grandchild. It is for the patient and not the physician to decide if achievement of these goals is worth suffering one's last days attached to a respirator. A patient's autonomous choice should be respected. However, autonomous choice means that the patient understands the nature of the therapy she is requesting and its likely consequences. For a dying patient to demand "Do everything to make me live" is panic, not autonomy. M.G. has never accepted her terminal illness and that the best that medicine could offer her was comfort care. An autonomous choice is also one made from available options. "Life," in a meaningful sense of the word, is regrettably not an option available to M.G.

The attending might be tempted to write a DNR order unilaterally on the grounds that resuscitation is futile and that he is acting as a beneficent physician by allowing his patient to die in peace. Indeed, until recently, it would have been considered unethical for a physician even to tell a dying patient that she is actually dying. This is the therapeutic privilege that can be traced back to Hippocratic writings and was firmly established by Percival in his *Medical Ethics* of 1803. Until recently, a physician could actually do little except to provide comfort, so whether patients understood the nature of their illnesses or not was irrelevant.

Now, meaningful choices can be made, so it is important that patients understand the nature of their illnesses and alternative therapies. The paternalism characteristic of the ethics of previous generations would never be tolerated by today's well-educated and consumer-oriented patients. Even with respect to writing a DNR order, we recognize that a patient has a "right to know."

What should the physician do? The attending physician must return to his patient and again attempt to engage her in a discussion of her care. He should explain gently, as the resident had previously, that they can do nothing to reverse her cancer but that they would attempt to relieve her shortness of breath by removing pleural fluid. He must assure M.G. that he will provide whatever is necessary to ease her anxiety and relieve her pain and ask her if she has any questions or has anything else on her mind that she wants to discuss. He should then step back and wait. He ought not to push the patient into a discussion of her impending death. A "right to know" does not mean a "duty to know." If M.G. remains silent, he should write the DNR order without further discussion. Not to do so would run the risk of subjecting the patient to an unwarranted resuscitation. To insist that this dying patient discuss the time and nature of her death simply for the sake of "autonomy" would be unspeakably cruel and contrary to the physician's primary directive of "do no harm."

COMMENTARY
David H. Miller

No, the attending physician should not write a DNR order without informing the patient. M.G.'s case displays some fundamental problems in decisionmaking when a patient and the responsible physician disagree on management approaches and invites reflection on whether the patient or the physician should be the final voice in resolving the controversy over issuing a DNR order.

Consent to a DNR order presents a unique situation in medicine whereby permission is requested to omit a procedure that physicians may feel is not indicated in the first place. DNR issues need to be treated in this unusual fashion given the emergency nature of the medical event that calls for resuscitation. Judgments about the worth of CPR should not be made when the cardiac arrest occurs, but should be carefully thought out and determined in advance. Lifesaving measures are expected to be provided unless clear instructions to the contrary have been established.

M.G. has responded to efforts to address the subject of resuscitation and the possible issuance of a DNR order with avoidance rather than outright refusal. The situation is complicated by the involvement of a hospital resident unfamiliar to the patient and not involved in her long-term care. One would think, and some evidence suggests, that long-standing physician-patient relationships enable decisions such as this to be made in a less confrontational fashion. Physicians who are well acquainted with their patients' personal and physical needs and patients who are well acquainted with their physicians' styles and approaches tend to share a more trusting relationship that allows easier decision making. Perhaps M.G.'s oncologist could have accepted a greater role in guiding her through this unfamiliar territory.

Fundamental to the bias toward the patient in resolving this problem is the underlying and legitimate right of patients to know about and be involved in decisions made about themselves. To have the option to refuse CPR, patients must be informed that CPR is a potential treatment option, and that it entails certain benefits and risks. Only then can an informed decision be made.

If decisions to withhold CPR are made without the patient's involvement, a cloak of secrecy develops, distancing the patient from the physician and disengaging the patient from the decision-making process. As a result the physician-patient relationship becomes weakened just when a strengthened relationship is needed.

But who really is best equipped to make the DNR decision—the patient or the physician? In addition to patients' underlying right to make decisions about their own care, they have an innate sense of their own well-being that is often overlooked. After all, M.G. has lengthy firsthand experience of the symptoms associated with metastatic breast cancer and is able to place those experiences in the perspective of her overall life achievements and expectations. Her fear of death may alternately be considered a will to live that could provide the wherewithal to sustain life longer than expected. Such attitudes can be driven by personal goals unknown to the physician—such as the need to support a spouse or a close relative, or the need to survive an important event. Why should a physician impose his or her own standards on the personal aspirations of the patient?

Physicians have been described as the appropriate decision makers because of their abilities to understand the extent of illness, the limitations of therapy, and the predictions about outcomes. But these abilities are not absolute. Prognosis determinations cannot be made with enough accuracy to warrant the physician assuming the dominant role in decision making. In the case of M.G., the gloom associated with the unrelenting nature of her illness might divert attention from potentially treatable and reversible causes of her symptoms, such as unrecognized infection, untapped fluid accumulations, and unopened airway obstructions.

Moreover, if the physician is right and all other therapeutic efforts are destined to fail, survival should be brief even if intubation and other resuscitation efforts are initiated. What then is the harm of attempting resuscitation in this setting? True, the patient may suffer more, the processes of dying will be lengthened, and the patient's agony may be prolonged rather than alleviated. But the patient is the best judge of what hardships can be endured and is often still capable of changing his or her decision about life-prolonging measures even after they have been initiated. By identifying an appropriate surrogate who is aware of the patient's attitudes toward therapeutic interventions, and by completing appropriate advance directives this patient's attitudes can be expressed even after her capacity to make decisions is lost.

There is also the harm that futile efforts to sustain M.G.'s life may mean that such efforts cannot be made available to a "more deserving patient." But such issues should not be subject to the individual whims of one attending physician and that physician's approach to the management of an individual patient. Rather, issues regarding the most appropriate utilization of limited resources should be reached through specific policy development, subject to review and scrutiny by appropriate supervisory bodies.

In the end these arguments substantiate the patient's right to prevail in the decision over whether to be resuscitated. In this case, protecting M.G.'s right to self-determination is paramount.

11

AIDS and a Duty to Protect

Mr. B., age twenty-eight, reported to the community health center of a large city teaching hospital for counseling after being confidentially informed that his blood test was positive for antibodies to the Human Immunodeficiency Virus (HIV), the virus that causes AIDS. The patient had no symptoms.

Dr. T. informed Mr. B. that although he did not have AIDS, there was between a five and thirty-five percent probability that he would develop the disease within the next five years. He was also told that he could probably infect others through sexual contact, by sharing needles, or by donating blood and blood products. He was counseled not to donate blood, and to engage in "safe sex," that is, sex that does not involve the exchange of bodily fluids such as semen.

Mr. B. then revealed that he was bisexual, and that he believed that he had contracted the infection during one of his homosexual encounters. He also said that he was engaged. Dr. T. advised him to inform his fiancée of his diagnosis. But Mr. B. refused to do so, saying that it would ruin his marriage plans.

Should Dr. T. inform her of his patient's test results, or should he protect the confidentiality of the therapeutic relationship?

COMMENTARY
Morton E. Winston

Dr. T. must weigh his duty to safeguard confidential information against a duty to protect his patient's fiancée, and any children the couple might conceive, from possible harm caused by Mr. B.'s infection.

The American College of Physicians Ethics Manual (1984) states that "the physician shall keep secret all that he knows about the patient and release no information without the patient's consent, unless required by the law or unless resulting harm to others outweighs his duty to his patient." The laws of most states require reporting of cases of sexually transmitted diseases such as syphilis, gonorrhea, and hepatitis B, to public health authorities.

At present, AIDS is a reportable disease in all states. However, only a few states, Colorado and Montana among them, presently require confidential reporting of persons who test positive for antibodies to HIV.

In this case, however, the relevant ethical question is not whether the physician should report the patient as being seropositive to public health authorities, but whether Dr. T. should warn his patient's fiancée that she may be at risk of developing AIDS.

Because the law is presently unclear regarding cases of this kind, physicians are exposed to uncertain legal risks: they may be sued by patients for wrongful disclosure and personal suffering that might result from such disclosure if they breach confidentiality; they may also be sued by their patient's sexual partners if they knowingly fail to protect them from preventable harm or risk of infection from their patient's illness.

In 1976 in the case of *Tarasoff v. Regents of the University of California*, the California Supreme Court ruled that therapists who know or should know that a patient poses a violent threat to an identifiable third party have an obligation to take reasonable steps to protect that person. It also noted that "a doctor is liable to persons infected by his patient if he negligently fails to diagnose a contagious disease, or having diagnosed the illness, fails to warn members of the patient's family."

However, the medical risks involved in the present case are different from those in diseases spread by casual, that is, nonsexual contact. Not all seropositive persons are viremic, that is, known to be producing virus, and some might not be infectious. There is evidence that male-to-female transmission of HIV occurs, but the efficiency of such transmission is unknown, though it may be high in some settings. Finally, the outcome of infection with HIV is not predictable with confidence, and not all infected persons will develop full-blown AIDS. These risks may vary for persons in different age, sex, and other groups, and our medical understanding of this disease is undergoing rapid change. These uncertainties argue strongly against instituting legal requirements mandating contact tracing for persons who have tested seropositive to HIV. The exceptional cases, such as this one, where patients refuse voluntarily to disclose their diagnosis to their sexual partners, are best handled on a case-by-case basis.

But then physicians must weigh carefully their responsibility to protect confidentiality against their duty to protect others who might be placed at risk by their patients' illnesses. While physicians should violate their prima facie obligations to protect confidentiality only with the greatest reluctance, it is morally permissible, and may sometimes be obligatory, for physicians to do so.

The *Tarasoff* decision is often incorrectly interpreted as creating a "duty to warn." In fact, it creates a duty to protect potential victims of violence that can be discharged in various ways. If a physician determines that a patient's illness poses a significant risk to others, he could have him arrested for being a danger to public health, or move to have him civilly committed. In either of these cases, the damage done to the patient's rights and civil liberties would be considerable. In the present case, such extreme measures would be unjustified. In general, the duty to protect should be discharged in the way that is least invasive of the patient's rights while still effectively serving to protect potential victims from harm and significant risk.

Dr. T. could best discharge his duty to protect by persuading Mr. B. to reveal his diagnosis to his fiancée himself, and by offering serologic testing and counseling to her through his patient. Given contemporary sexual mores, it is possible that the patient's fiancée may have already been exposed to the infection; she should still be informed of her risk of exposure, offered testing, and counseling, particularly concerning the risk of infecting any children she might conceive. Since the patient's fiancée is presumably not aware that she is a member of a high-risk group, it is unlikely that she would suspect that she may have been exposed.

If Mr. B. will not agree to voluntary disclosure, Dr. T. must seriously consider revealing the information himself. He should first discuss the case with appropriate legal, public health, and perhaps ethical authorities. If, after such consultation, he determines that the risk to his patient's fiancée is significant, and if all other means of persuading the patient to accept his moral responsibility have failed, then Dr. T. should attempt to contact her, either directly or through public health authorities.

COMMENTARY
Sheldon H. Landesman

The question posed in the case is whether a physician is obligated, that is, has a legal or ethical duty, to inform the sexual partner of an HIV-positive man that she may be at risk of acquiring AIDS through intercourse with him. Such a duty would appear to violate the principle of patient-physician confidentiality.

Medical confidentiality, however, has never been sacrosanct. The physician has always had the *option* of *not* maintaining patient-doctor confidentiality. Confidentiality can be breached when the patient's life is at stake and, in certain clear-cut situations, for society's benefit. The requirement to report communicable diseases and gunshot wounds, as well as suspected cases of child abuse, are clearly violations of confidentiality that are legally mandated and socially sanctioned.

The question can best be answered by looking at the broad societal problems associated with HIV infection. A central aspect in controlling the epidemic is counseling and testing the 1.5 to 2 million infected individuals in the U.S. Mandatory testing of the entire population is a logistically impossible and ethically unacceptable way of reaching infected persons. Encouragement of voluntary, confidential counseling and testing is more acceptable. The expectation is that many, if not most, people who discover they are infected will behave appropriately by informing their partners and practicing safer sex.

Any legally or socially sanctioned act that breaches confidentiality or imposes additional burdens (such as job loss or cancellation of insurance) acts as a disincentive to voluntary testing. Thus if all physicians were legally required to report HIV-positive persons to a health department or to inform sexual partners at risk from the HIV-positive person, no one would come forward for testing. This is especially true if the physician is known to treat many patients with AIDS and HIV infection. The public knowledge that such a physician has violated confidentiality would result (indeed, has resulted in several cases) in a sharp decline of potentially infected persons seeking counseling and testing. Consequently, a growing number of persons would remain ignorant of their infectiousness as would their sex partners.

Furthermore, which sexual partners might the physician inform? The spouse, the current girlfriend, the old boyfriend, the sexual partners not yet identified? As a general rule physicians should not be *legally* required to breach the confidentiality of an HIV-infected person for two reasons: it is ultimately counterproductive to the broader goal of encouraging voluntary testing and it is difficult to implement fairly.

The price of such a policy is high. The woman discussed in this case may pay the price; her future infection might have been prevented. For a Dr. T. to sit back and let such a scenario be played out is a painful, difficult thing to do. But his discomfort and the woman's infection may be the cost that society pays if it wishes to implement public health measures to minimize the spread of the virus.

Dr. T. does have room to maneuver. He can strongly urge Mr. B. to inform his fiancée, he can act as an information broker and make himself available to counsel the patient and the partner, or he can work with Mr. B. over weeks or months and gradually move him to a more reasonable position.

If all else fails, Dr. T. must review his own situation: he always has the *option* of informing the fiancée, although he should not do so without telling his patient of his intentions. If the physician is heavily involved with this epidemic; if he counsels, tests and treats many such patients, then violating confidentiality and informing the fiancée may ultimately result in more infected individuals. The breach of confidentiality will undoubtedly discourage others from being counseled and tested. If he does not have an "AIDS practice," it is easier to justify the violation of confidentiality.

The courts are the ultimate arbiter of the presence or absence of a legal duty to protect a sex partner from infection. In the absence of a clear legal mandate, the difficult ethical dilemma is one of balancing long-term societal benefits against short-term benefit to an individual. Although it is a difficult decision, and there may be exceptions to the rule, maintaining the patient's confidentiality ought to be the first principle.

12

A Duty to Warn, An Uncertain Danger

Ms. L., a twenty-eight-year-old, unmarried woman, is admitted to General Hospital to deliver her first child. In the past, she has been treated for pyromania and schizophrenia (paranoid type), and since the age of eighteen she has spent a total of five and a half years in a state mental hospital or in the inpatient unit of the local community mental health center in the suburban community where she lives. She has also been arrested for arson on three occasions. Each arrest led to a court referral for psychiatric care.

Mrs. D., the social worker on the Ob-Gyn service at General Hospital, is familiar with Ms. L.'s psychiatric history and arrest record because she was formerly employed by the community mental health center where Ms. L. had been a patient. During a pre-delivery conversation with Ms. L. about her plans, Mrs. D. discovers that Ms. L. has no current residence and spent the previous year drifting from shelter to shelter. Ms. L. informs Mrs. D. that after her baby's birth she is planning to move in temporarily with a local Rabbi and his family, who occasionally share their home with people in dire straits.

Mrs. D. immediately begins to wonder about warning the Rabbi, Rabbi P., about the possible danger to him, his wife, and young children. As a member of Rabbi P.'s congregation, Mrs. D. is aware that, on occasion, he opens his home to transients. She is very concerned about the welfare of Rabbi P.'s family, given Ms. L.'s documented history of arson. The next day, Mrs. D. asks Ms. L. for permission to talk with Rabbi P. about her housing needs and about the difficulties she has experienced over the years. Ms. L. refuses permission for such disclosures.

Is Mrs. D. obliged to warn Rabbi P. about Ms. L. and her history, despite Ms. L.'s refusal to consent? Is it relevant that Mrs. D. came upon the confidential information about Ms. L. serendipitously, as a result of her previous employment in the local community mental health center?

COMMENTARY
Frederic G. Reamer

The commitment to confidentiality in the various health and mental health professions is deep-seated. Codes of ethics routinely cite the professional's obligation to hold in confidence information that a client shares. The Code of Ethics of the National Association of Social Workers—which is pertinent to Mrs. D.'s predicament—is representative: "The social worker should respect the privacy of clients and hold in confidence all information obtained in the course of professional service."

Difficulties arise, of course, when there appear to be good reasons for revealing confidential information against a client's wishes. The circumstances surrounding Ms. L. are typical in this respect, and every profession can produce similar stories. Understandably, confusion exists about the circumstances that warrant a breach of confidentiality, especially when a threat to a third party is involved. Though every professional knows that there must be limits to guarantees of confidentiality, there is no consensus about where the line should be drawn.

Debates about professionals' duty to warn generally address several often conflicting rights and obligations: the client's right to privacy; the professional's duty to protect the client's interests, along with those of the general public; and the professional's right to avoid being held liable. Based on these considerations, a good case can be made that Mrs. D. has a duty to warn Rabbi P. and his family about Ms. L.'s history and, thus, has a right to reveal confidential information against Ms. L.'s wishes. As do many codes of ethics, the NASW code qualifies its principle on confidentiality with a statement that "the social worker should share with others confidences revealed by clients, without their consent, only for compelling professional reasons." Though this code does not define "compelling professional reasons," no doubt most would agree that the genuine threat of arson qualifies (especially since Mrs. D.'s information is based on law enforcement and mental health records, not hearsay).

This position is also supported by case law established by the California Supreme Court's well-known *Tarasoff* decision. *Tarasoff* held that when a therapist determines that a client presents a serious danger of violence to another person, the therapist incurs an obligation to use "reasonable care" to protect the potential victim from harm. This may require the therapist to warn the victim, notify the police, or take whatever other steps "are reasonably necessary under the circumstances." Though Ms. L. has not threatened to harm Rabbi P. and his family, the spirit of *Tarasoff* supports disclosure of confidential information in this case.

Is it relevant that Mrs. D. acquired her knowledge of Ms. L.'s past accidentally, by virtue of her previous employment? No. What matters is that Mrs. D. has become party to confidential information that may need to be revealed in order to protect a third party from serious harm. No victim would be consoled to learn that information about an impending threat was withheld because it was not acquired through ordinary channels. Though we would not want to advocate or condone the use of improper channels, we cannot afford to ignore compelling information that lands in our lap as a result of fortuitous circumstances.

It is not enough merely to conclude that Mrs. D. has a duty to warn. One must also ask what specific information ought to be shared. As a rule of thumb, professionals should reveal as little as possible, while ensuring that a potential victim has sufficient details to be able to react in an informed way. Professionals sometimes reveal more information than is necessary to warn a potential victim adequately. In this case, Mrs. D. should limit her disclosure to information about Ms. L.'s history that appears to pose some genuine risk to Rabbi P. and his family. If Ms. L. does not contact Rabbi P. no confidential information should be disclosed to him. Mrs. D. would do well to have a committee comprised of hospital colleagues and administrators review, critique, and authorize her plan, to protect both Ms. L.'s right to confidentiality and the right of Mrs. D. and the hospital to avoid being held liable.

How likely is it that Ms. L. will harm Rabbi P. and his family? Unfortunately, there is no way of knowing. The ability of mental health professionals to forecast dangerousness in such cases does not have an impressive track record. Our instinct to protect potential victims in these circumstances is a good one, however. Though professionals must take care to avoid gratutitous disclosure of confidential information, we cannot fail to acknowledge, as *Tarasoff* makes clear, that "the protective privilege ends where the public peril begins."

COMMENTARY
Sylvan J. Schaffer

The practitioner in this case faces a difficult choice: whether to preserve a confidence or to protect the safety of a generous cleric and his young children. In trying to resolve this dilemma it is important first to consider the purpose of the confidentiality rule and then to consider when it applies.

In social work, as in the other mental health professions, honoring confidentiality is a fundamental consideration in fostering a trusting relationship with the patient. Without the promise of privacy few people would be willing to trust relative strangers with their innermost thoughts, fears, and secrets. Thus, confidentiality allows the therapeutic relationship to develop and continue. It is difficult, if not impossible, to imagine psychotherapy without the guarantee of privacy.

Recognizing the importance of confidentiality to the psychotherapeutic process, some states have extended the right of privileged communication to mental health professionals. (While there may be some differences between statutes concerning psychiatrists, psychologists, and social workers, for the purposes of this article the professions will be treated as equal.) John H. Wigmore, a legal scholar, has delineated the criteria that warrant the recognition of confidential communications: the communication must originate in confidence; the confidence is vital to maintaining the relationship; the relationship is one that should be encouraged; and the detriment to the relationship through the fear of disclosure is greater than the benefit which would result from disclosure.

However, confidentiality is not absolute. There are circumstances under which a social worker would not be bound to keep a confidence. These include cases in which a patient has introduced his mental condition in a civil proceeding; or a judge has ordered a psychiatric examination and the patient is informed that confidentiality does not exist; or there is imminent physical danger to the patient or to a third party. This case is an example of the third type of exception. That exception provides the mental health professional with the most difficult choice since the standard of "imminent danger" is subjective and difficult to delineate.

The most influential source used by the courts and mental health professionals in dealing with the conflict of danger and the duty to warn is *Tarasoff v. Regents of the University of California*. In that case it was held that a psychotherapist whose client had indicated during a therapy session that he would kill a particular third party had a duty to warn that party. The ruling in *Tarasoff* indicates that, given the circumstances present in that case, a psychotherapist who is engaged in a therapeutic relationship with a patient who has threatened to do physical harm to a particular person has a duty to breach confidentiality and warn the intended victim.

It is not clear that the duty enunciated in *Tarasoff* would apply to this situation as significant differences distinguish the two cases. To begin with, the social worker is not engaged in a psychotherapeutic relationship with the client. This is important for two reasons: first, she does not have the type of detailed, intimate knowledge about Ms. L. that would enable her to make such a difficult judgment concerning her future behavior. Accurate prediction would be difficult even for a psychotherapist who knows a patient intimately; it seems an almost impossible task for a relative stranger. Second, the law generally does not impose an affirmative duty to control the behavior of another person or to warn of a threat. The duty in *Tarasoff* arose from the special relationship between the therapist and patient, which did impose an affirmative duty on the therapist. Mrs. D. did not have such a special relationship with Ms. L. Her familiarity with the patient was based solely on secondhand information. This is not the kind of relationship present in *Tarasoff*.

Second, the nature of the danger is different from that in *Tarasoff*. In *Tarasoff*, the patient made a definite threat against a specific identifiable person. In this case, Ms. L. has indicated no malice toward anyone. We do not know the nature of her arson arrests. Were they for fires in garbage pails? In abandoned buildings? For insurance? Is there any indication that she would do the same to people who were showing her a kindness, with her own newborn baby in the house? Also, to what degree can her past behavior be considered an accurate predictor of future behavior? Had her treatment for schizophrenia and pyromania been effective? In sum, does Ms. L. present a threat to the Rabbi and his family that justifies that breach of confidentiality? What will be the fate of the social worker if she erroneously breaches confidentiality when the patient presents no real danger? Is the social worker liable for malpractice? Defamation of character? Breach of fiduciary duty?

Third, even if there is an element of risk, is the breach of confidentiality necessary in order to warn Rabbi P? In *Tarasoff* the intended victim did not know of the potential risk. The Rabbi in this case had previously hosted transients and could reasonably be expected to have assessed the risk of allowing strangers to stay in his home. Thus he would not be a naive victim dependent solely on the warning of the social worker.

This last point raises the possibility of a third course of action—neither silence nor breach of confidentiality—an alternative that has its own advantages and perils. The social worker, who is a member of Rabbi P.'s congregation, and is aware of his work with transients through a nonprofessional source, could engage in a general conversation with him about the risks of such an activity without ever referring to her knowledge about a particular patient. In this way she could ensure that the Rabbi is aware of the possible risks posed by strangers, without ever mentioning Ms. L. or divulging any information about her. Admittedly, this alternative treads a fine line between breaching confidentiality and preserving it. Yet it would allow the social worker to alert Rabbi P. without defaming Ms. L. or disclosing confidential information. Given the paucity of guidelines and legal precedents dealing with such cases and the state of the art in predicting the future dangerousness of patients such dilemmas will continue to trouble conscientious mental health professionals.

13
"My Husband Won't Tell the Children"

Forsythe Archer, a successful scientist with exacting standards and a rigid personality, is being given palliative treatment for cancer. During the course of the relapses and remissions of the disease, Mr. Archer has steadfastly refused to discuss his illness with his two teenage children and has barely discussed it with his wife. He has made her promise to keep it a secret. His treatment program with its ups and downs has caused severe and unpredictable mood swings, which have exacerbated the children's emotional problems.

In an effort to help the children cope with their father's behavior, Mrs. Archer wants to break the promise and tell the children what is happening. However, when she suggests this to him he angrily rebuffs her. Mrs. Archer believes his refusal is causing undue distress and she fears for the emotional health of her children; one daughter in particular has been showing serious tendencies toward self-destructive behavior.

In desperation, she pleads with the family doctor to do whatever he can—even use coercion if necessary—to get her husband to "open up," lest his cancer destroy not only his life, but the life of one or more of his children. What should the physician do?

COMMENTARY
Nancy Neveloff Dubler

The physician-patient bond is forged by combining need and special skills. It is supported by tradition and by the much maligned and oft-disregarded doctrine of confidentiality.

The clear directive to a physician to protect the utterances of the patients— to hold privacy primary—has its roots in three sorts of ethical and legal developments. Ancient oaths contain exhortations to guard confidentiality. Modern state licensing statutes refer to these credos as a measure of ethical conduct and impose penalties for breach of the standard. Finally, the patient's utterance may be privileged, an issue which the patient may raise in a court of law.

Most patients do not consider it necessary to make explicit the implicit though fuzzy protections for their physical and emotional secrets; they assume it and hope that their wishes will be understood. But in this case the patient was quite explicit: he did not want his children told. He would not or could not discuss, consider, or confront the issue. Perhaps he even chose to remain silent out of perversity, anger, disregard, or conscious cruelty. Any of the above are possible; none justify disregarding his specific directive.

There is neither a direct danger to the population, which justifies breach of confidentiality for public health, nor an identifiable action that both threatens another and violates a legal and moral norm, as for example, an instance of child abuse. It may be argued that this behavior was in fact a sort of child abuse, that exclusion and silence will result in developmental disability or adult inability to function.

This assertion has a number of unconvincing aspects. First, child abuse reporting laws represent a required departure from the standard of professional behavior. Second, they challenge the usual prerogatives of adult caregivers in relation to their children. This last is most important. Parents may be charged and held to account for violence that oversteps understood societal limits. Clearly, spanking a two-year-old who runs in the street in front of an oncoming car is not child abuse. It may (or may not) be bad parenting. Beating that same child insensate or burning him with cigarettes to punish the same infraction is child abuse. The excessive and inappropriate physical battering of a child is the sort of action that requires professionals to speak and that shatters the privacy claims of parents.

This case presents no such immediate and recognizable danger. What if this same father—not ill—declared that he loved one of his children most and would thus finance college for that one child; all others could fend for themselves. Is that abuse? Does the physician want to enter the complex emotional web of interfamily relationships over this sort of issue? Is the danger any more quantifiable or direct in the case under discussion?

Many children suffer from the inept emotional responses of their parents. Many are limited in adulthood from bizarre or destructive parenting. Lacking more data, should the physician enter these marshes? Will the Archers' children suffer more than a child who has been "scape-goated," or deprived of a college experience, or forced to enter adulthood with stunted emotional skills? Our belief in parental prerogatives and physician limitations wisely decrees forebearance.

Furthermore, in this case there is another option. These children can be provided with outside counseling and support. Counseling may not make up for the withdrawal and loss of their father, but it may offer comfort and more. In contrast, Mr. Archer may feel lost if his wishes are disregarded. This physician is his support—directing his care, responding to his needs, and honoring his integrity. The failure to honor his clearly stated wishes may leave him feeling abandoned at the moment of greatest need.

Mrs. Archer has a clear problem—the sort of conflict in loyalty that often besets a parent. Parents differ in the skill and creativity with which they handle their children. Children seek to "divide and conquer," to capitalize on the differing approaches. Often a united front supports parenting. Sometimes the divisions must be acknowledged.

In this case the mother must take those measures necessary to protect her child. She must tell the child the truth and seek the professional assistance that is necessary to sustain her daughter through the present medical crisis and the death of a father. But she need not tell Mr. Archer. Withholding this information will require courage and thespian accomplishment but it need not threaten her relationship with her husband. Lying is not always a wrong when it prevents pain and suffering and alleviates danger. This mother may be paralyzed by fear, conflicts of loyalty, lack of courage, or despair. The physician must offer her support, which can permit her to act. As there is another route available to protect the children, the physician need not endanger his relationship to the primary patient—the father.

Physicians in family practice often negotiate intergenerational conflicts involving clashing personality and value systems. They often weigh the risks and benefits of sharing information imparted in confidence. The justifications for breach of confidentiality are narrow: direct and immediate danger with no alternatives. This family's situation does not qualify. This father has explicitly invoked the protections of confidentiality for the time surrounding his death. He is entitled to the physician's full support.

COMMENTARY
Lawrence J. Schneiderman

This case illustrates a potential conflict in duty facing the physician who cares for more than one member of a family. The patient's right to privacy is a powerful ethical warrant that runs from the Hippocratic tradition to the present. Of more recent vintage is a concept arising out of family therapy and family medicine, which views illness as not limited to an isolated person but rather as potentially involving a nexus of persons who are intimately connected. The latter concept logically requires that the physician's treatment decisions must weigh risks and benefits to all the Archer family members and indeed to the family structure itself on which their well-being depends.

A patient's right to privacy mandates that the physician resist any demands by third parties to violate confidentiality in the absence of rare justifiable exceptions. Is Mrs. Archer's claim such an exception? She pleads that Mr. Archer's failure to reveal and discuss his illness with his children is jeopardizing their health. Her claim might be difficult to evaluate and problematic if the physician were not caring for these children as well as for Mr. Archer. But the physician is professionally obligated to all of them.

Obviously, the thoughtful, experienced, sensitive physician will seek to use his or her skills in ways that will resolve the problem without causing conflict. Perhaps gentle persuasion, emotional support, and counseling will persuade Mr. Archer to "open up" and the family will benefit from the new level of intimacy and honesty achieved. But the possibility exists that Mr. Archer will adamantly refuse to alter his personal mode of coping with his illness. What then? Almost certainly the physician with the aforementioned attributes will also use his or her skills to counsel Mrs. Archer on ways in which to deal with this problem at home. After all, they are her children too. She must pursue ways to inform the children about her husband's condition and seek to open communication among them.

Chances are, however, the physician will inevitably be drawn into this process. The children may have questions a mother cannot answer, and will need emotional support beyond that which the mother can provide.

Can the physician, under these circumstances, refuse to recognize the needs of these other patients? Is Mr. Archer's right to privacy so inviolable? In my opinion, no. Admittedly, this view that the father's behavior is part of the illness that is affecting the children puts us on the notorious slippery slope. Would the physician feel entitled to intervene if Mr. Archer had capriciously excluded one child from his will—an act that surely could lead to unpleasant emotional consequences? How forceful should the physician be? Should the physician use threats to get a parent to stop smoking? Substantial evidence documents the adverse health consequences of smoking behavior on children. Lose weight? A shortened life span of the breadwinner has adverse implications for the dependents. Keep up life insurance and health insurance payments? It is notorious that unexpected health diasters have ruined family fortunes and prospects.

Obviously one has to draw a line. Where? One place to begin is that area of health care for which the physician was consulted. Within this circle, the physician must weigh the relative risks and benefits not just to one person but to all the parties to whom a duty is owed. Although the physician is not entitled to challenge privacy rights in matters of wills, life insurance payments, and so on, the physician would regard it as his or her ethical duty to take strong measures to warn and protect the other family members if Mr. Archer were harboring a serious contagious disease. It is not at all farfetched to extend the analogy to emotional disorders. Emotional illness in one family member can have severe impacts on the others.

How to weigh the risks and benefits? If the physician goes so far as to break confidence or attempt to coerce Mr. Archer into doing something he finds unacceptable, the physician puts the therapeutic relationship (and Mr. Archer's well-being) at risk. What would justify such an act? Surely, in my opinion, if the children's self-destructive behavior included threats of suicide. But also if the children's behavior had ominous implications for their futures, such as delinquency, drug use, or school problems.

From the family-oriented perspective, the patient's refusal is a manifestation of dysfunctional coping with his disease, which is not only harming him but harming others as well. The physician's duty is to ameliorate such harm. Thus I believe that in this situation Mr. Archer's wishes with respect to privacy may have lesser weight than the needs of the children for information and communication, benefits that potentially will influence long future lives.

The physician faced with this ethical dilemma cannot confine his or her duty to one person, thereby ignoring the extensiveness and complexity of the medical problem. In my opinion, the physician is forced off the ideological position of protecting privacy to the slippery slope of weighing risks and benefits. The physician's duty is to all the patients under his or her care.

14

The Price of Silence

John C. Fletcher and Dorothy C. Wertz

Mrs. S., at age forty-five, has just been told that she has Huntington disease, following a workup—including CAT scanning of the brain—after she developed abnormal body-jerking movements. Huntington disease (HD) is a disorder of genetic origin, appearing without warning between the ages of thirty and sixty. It causes irreversible mental and motor deterioration, leading to death after several years of intense suffering for both patient and family. There is no treatment. The disease is a Medelian dominant disorder: everyone who has inherited the gene will develop the disease and will also transmit it to half of his or her children. By the time its symptoms appear, most patients have completed their childbearing and may have transmitted the gene to another generation. Until recently, no tests could tell whether the children of a person with HD had inherited the gene. They had to wait for symptoms to appear. Sometimes, as in Mrs. S.'s family, there is no family history of HD because those who had the gene died before symptoms could appear.

Mrs. S. has three children, ages sixteen, nineteen, and twenty-four; her eldest daughter married last year. She also has three sisters and a brother, ages thirty-four, thirty-five, thirty-seven, and forty, who have eleven children ranging in age from two to twenty. None of her siblings has developed any symptoms of HD, nor do they suspect they are at risk. However, new developments in diagnostic technology make it possible, in some families, to test people for the presence of the HD gene before they develop symptoms. It is also possible to test fetuses.

Although both the genetic specialist and the family's doctor have tried to persuade Mrs. S. that it is her moral responsibility to tell her siblings and children of her diagnosis so that they can plan their lives with the knowledge that they are at 50 percent risk of developing HD, she refuses. Mrs. S. says she is ashamed of her condition and is afraid that her family will ostracize her or that her employer will fire her.

Unless members of Mrs. S.'s family know that they are at risk for HD, they will not be able to request the tests. Moreover, even if the doctors tell then that they are at risk, the relatives will still not be able to use the tests, because DNA testing requires a blood sample from a family member who has HD to identify the DNA markers for the gene specific to that particular family. Mrs. S. says that she will not cooperate in testing.

What should the doctors do? Should anyone besides Mrs. S. know the diagnosis and what it means for the family? Should the public health department require doctors to notify all persons at risk of developing the disease?

COMMENTARY
Abbyann Lynch

This scenario gives rise to at least four ethical dilemmas. Of immediate concern is the ethical balance to be achieved between repecting Mrs. S.'s autonomy (maintaining confidentiality in the matter of her illness) and providing appropriate care for her (organizing a coordinated, continuing support system as her illness progresses). Ideally, the latter activity will include her relatives, who will learn of her illness later, if not sooner. In the immediate case, the family physician must choose to care for Mrs. S. either as an individiual or as a family member.

In either situation both her family physician and the genetic counselor face conflicting eithical concerns regarding any communication with Mrs. S.'s relatives. To apprise them of the possibility of their risk for HD is at once to violate any desire they might have to remain ignorant of that risk. At the same time, granting that Mrs. S. has a claim of confidentiality, her family surely has some claim on the practitioners (and on Mrs. S.) that they be forewarned of any harm or injury Mrs. S. might cause they be reason of her progressing illness (for example, possible injury to passengers in her car, should she suddenly lose muscle control while driving the vehicle; possible mental anguish, if family members are subjected to illness-caused rage exhibited by Mrs. S.). In a similar vein, her relatives seem to have some legitimate claim to learn of Mrs. S.'s disease and thus have an opportunity to express their sympathy, love, and concern for her.

The genetic specialist will have a particular ethical dilemma here. Fidelity to confidentiality for Mrs. S. appears to inhibit fulfilling any professional responsibility to decrease the incidence of HD in the community. To achieve this latter end, Mrs. S.'s relatives need timely warning of their possible genetic risk, and counselling regarding the disease, with discussion of their reproductive options as required.

Finally, there will be ethical conflict for the practitioners regarding disclosure with Mrs. S.'s employer, should Mrs. S. not choose to initiate such discussion. Depending on her occupation, Mrs. S. could pose workplace risk to her fellow employees; it appears that her employer should be warned of these possibilities. The practitioners might also discuss Mrs. S.'s illness with her employer to ensure there is no misunderstanding about her work performance and no discrimination against her on the basis of her diagnosed illness. Such discussions could be a positive means toward securing a cooperative and suitable work regime for Mrs. S.; it might also involve planning long-term financial compensation for her when she is no longer able to work.

Any avowedly "Canadian discussion" of these issues must reflect at least three aspects of the current "Canadian scene."

First, there is ethical disarray among Canadian physicians regarding respect for patient confidentiality. Observing confidentiality with regard to "significant others" was recently questioned during a national meeting of the Canadian Medical Association (CMA). The CMA adoped a resolution noting that "...it is not unethical...to make discreet disclosure(regarding the AIDS status of a patient) to an appropriate (other) person with the patient's knowledge...when the public interest clearly outweighs the interest of the patient..."* Significant here is the fact that the CMA has professionally accepted *Code of Medical Ethics*, according to which the ethical physician is responsible to "keep in confidence" information derived from his patient, or from a colleague regarding a patient, or from a colleague regarding a patient, and divulge it only iwth the permission of the patient except when the law requires him to do so.** This *Code* is the basis for any official professional administered "disipline" regarding "professional misconduct," but disciplinary action is the responsibility

*P. Sullivan, "AIDS, Report on Elderly Dominate Annual Meeting," *Canadian Medical Association Journal*, 15 September 1987, 531–35.
**Canadian Medical Association (Ottawa, 1986), #6.

of the provincial (state) licensing body, not the CMA. In certain Canadian provinces, Ontario for example, the statutory definition of professional misconduct includes "giving information concerning a patient's condition or any professional services performed for a patient to any person other than the patient without the consent of the patient unless required to do so by law."* In the case of Mrs. S., then, while it might be "not ethical," professionally speaking, for Ontario physician to reveal her genetic status to her relatives, disclosure would still be considered "professioanl misconduct" and investigated by the Disciplinary Committee of the Ontario College of Physicians and Surgeons.

At this time, medical practitioners in Canada appear to have no clear "duty to warn" third parties who might be at risk of harm by reason of a patient's medical condition. True, in the public interest, certain Canadian laws require that physicians "report" named diseases to the Medical Officer of Health (for example, AIDS is reportable in Ontario) and in certain jurisdictions physicians must report their patients' medical conditions if these would cause possible impairment with regard to the operation of a motor vehicle.**

Finally, while there will be local differences in resolution of the dilemmas presented by Mrs. S.'s case, there is substantial Canadian experience that affirms preserving confidentiality for her as the accepted norm for Canadian practice. In defense of that position, it would be argued that they might not so wish to know of their genetic risk, but that they might not so wish; to "coerce" then in this matter might be to invade their (Canadian) "security of the person." Further, while Mrs. S. might believe her relatives or employer would abandon or ostracize her, they might not; both possibilities should be explored further. Given these uncertainties, the physician and the genetic specialist must thus begin with their ethical commitment to confidentiality regarding Mrs. S.'s illness. While honoring this commitment, they should attempt to discover the depth of Mrs. S.'s refusal to share the relevant information with her family or employer and advise her of the "price of being quiet"—that she might deprive herself of her relatives' love and support or that her employer might misunderstand her actions or nonactions in the absence of any information regarding them. Mrs. S. should be encouraged, not coerced, to share her knowledge of her condition, and reassured that the decisions are hers and that practitioners will unconditionally support her in her illness and preserve her confidentiality. Whatever the concern for claims of her relatives or employer, Mrs. S. must not be abandoned in her current need for medical care, which includes her current need for confidentiality. To take a contrary stance is to realize Mrs. S.'s worst-case scenario: to be a person with HD is to be doubly victimized.

---

*Health Disciplines Act R.S.O. 1980. c.196, s.60 with R.R.O. 1980, Reg. 448, s.27; O.Reg. 112/83, s.1; 334/85, s.4 at #22; HDA s.51 at k.

**Health Protection and Promotion Act R.S.O. 1983, c.10, s.25 and s.26; O.Reg. 162/84, s.1 at #1; Highway Traffic Act R.S.O. 1980, c.198, s.177.

COMMENTARY
Andrew Czeizel

A central principle of any medical oath is medical confidentiality. The Hippocratic oath states; "Whatsoever things I see or hear concerning the life of man in my attendance on the sick or even apart therefrom, which ought not to be noised abroad, I will keep silence thereon, counting such things to be as sacred secrets."

Current Hungarian practice is determined by, §77-78 of the Public Health Act that regulates the "Obligation of Confidentiality." According to Regulation No. 11/1972 (VI. 30):

> The obligation of confidentiality of the physician (medical institution) includes information regarding the health of any person examined by said physician (medical institution), ... as well as any other information concerning the circumstances of the disease and other facts disclosed by the examination.

This means that, in the course of genetic counseling, only the persons seeking advice may be informed about their own manifest or latent condition and about the extent of the risks their future offspring may face. In some cases, recognition of the genetic risks may indicate an increased genetic risk in their relatives, including their prospective offspring. We ask our clients to call their relatives' attention to the increased risk. If we are not sure that the client will comply with our request, we ask for permission to approach their relatives directly as permitted according to §23(1) of the Public Health Act. "The physician (medical institution)...is not bound by the obligation of confidentiality...if (d) the interested party authorizes him/her to disclose information." If clients refuse to give such permission as in the case of Mrs. S., Hungarian geneticists ought to maintain Mrs. S.'s confidentiality despite the fact that it renders genetic counseling impossible for her relatives and for their potential offspring.

In Mrs. S.'s case, consciously remaining silent may mean that adequate medical care is not provided, with grave consequences. Some further concrete examples occurring in our practice may illustrate this problem.

A couple with a six-month-old multimalformed child came to our Genetic Counseling Service. Chromosome examination disclosed a partial trisomy. Upon examining the parents, we found that the healthy father was the carrier of a balanced reciprocal "translocated" chromosome that resulted in his child's disorder. Chromosome analysis of the husband's parents showed that he inherited this translocation from his healthy mother. The man had five siblings, who could also be carriers of the translocation. The risk expected in their offspring is singificant, but intrauterine fetal chromosome tests are available to detect affected fetuses and the parent would have the option to terminate the pregnancy. The father was embarassed about the problem and did not consent to a consultation with his siblings or to informing them about the problem.

A divorced woman came to the Genetic Counseling Service before entering a new marriage. One of her brothers and her son suffered from and died of a severe form of hemophilia A, a disorder caused by a defective gene in the X chromosome that is manifested only in males. There is a 50 percent risk of hemophilia for any sons of her new marriage. In such cases we offer intrauterine determination of fetal sex or more recently, a DNA probe to identify affected fetuses. The woman listened to our information, but stated that she was not going to tell her husband-to-be about this problem. She had told him that her son's death had been an accident and was afraid that if the groom found out about the defective gene she carried and about the risk involved should they have a male child, her would refuse to marry her. Since her future husband was "crazy about children," she had no desire to risk her furture by the unforeseeable consequences of telling him the truth. This way, however, she carried the risk of recurrence of hemophilia in case of pregnancy with a male child, at a time when it was already possible to prevent it!

When keeping genetic risks secret precludes the possibility of preventing recurrence of genetic disorders, legally, ethically, and professionally the medical geneticist may inform a directly involved relative about the risk and the possibilities of prevention even without the patient's consent as part of that relative's right to health and to be born healthy. The Public Health Act provides that "In spite of protest by a legally competent patient, who is of legal age, the physician may inform the patient's relative only of the facts required for treatment" (24 [1]). In the above cases, however, the information in question would not aid treatment, but "only" prevention.

Obviously, the physician can be released from his obligation of confidentiality in such special cases only if it is permitted by the legal system of society and by the ethics of medicine. Yet, while it is important and necessary to know and observe the written and unwritten laws of a profession, there are no "final and unalterable" social and ethical rules. In certain cases life may force us to revise even the Hippocratic principles.

COMMENTARY
Francisco M. Salzano

Some special circumstances related to the present case must be stressed at the outset: there is no treatment for the disease; its symptoms appear in middle age; and diagnostic tests for carrier status rely not on products of the gene, but on linkage of markers closely associated to it. Therefore, results may be inconclusive due to lack of variation in these markers, a situation estimated to occur in about 4 percent of the population. An added complication is the possibility of recombination between them and the HD gene, which is of the order of 5 percent.

In such a context, should the patient's right ot confidentiality be preserved? If not, who should have access to this genetic information and in what way?

Recently Brazilian medical genticists were asked what they would do if confronted with a similar situation. Only three (9%) asserted that they would unconditionally respect the client's desire for confidentiality; the majority (17 of 29, or 59%) would disclose information *only* if it were requested.

The ethical problems raised here can be approached from two perspectives: the carriers' clinical symptoms and their right to plan their offspring to optimize health and happiness. HD does not differ markedly from other chronic degenerative diseases and the preeminent question is what should be considered that optimal life span in our species. The peak of physical vigor occurs in the twenties, and most of a scientist's decisive discoveries, for example, are made during the third and fourth decaded of his or her life. From a strict biological point of view, all energy expended after the time of reproduction is an unnecessary luxury. The usual explanation for the longevity of *Homo sapiens* is that elders become repositories of a society's cultural values; but this reasoning may become obsolete in an era of powerful computers.

Thus, in simple, evolutionary terms, there are no strong reasons why the HD gene should be eradicated from our gene pool. On the other hand, how can we balance the postitive and negative contributions of a person to his or her society? The benefits received during the productive years may far outweigh the burden produced by an incapacitating illness. The brilliant achievements of renowned Cambridge physicist Stephen Hawking, bravely fighting against the symptoms of amyotrophic lateral sclerosis that appeared in his later life, are an example. These considerations are pertinent to the decision a carrier and his or her spouse may make concerning their offspring, with the added complication that due to deficiencies of prenatal diagnostic procedures, abortion of an unaffected fetus may result.

The crucial issue, therefore, involves the dialectical relationship of the right to know and the right not to know. The essence of ethical action involves freedom to choose, and freedom implies knowledge. This is why most Brazilian medical geneticists, in a case like Mrs. S.'s would override the patient's demand for confidentiality. On the other hand, if our ultimate goal is the pursuit of happiness, would I be happier by the information that within a given period of time I will be afflicted by a degenerative disease? The answer is cerainly negative, but it is always possible that some people faced with this perspective may want to adequately plan their lives well in advance.

Two features of life in Brazil (and any underdeveloped country) may lead to decisions quite different than those in First World countries. Average life expectancy is lower in Brazil than in developed countries (an average 63 years for the overall population in 1985 compared to 75 years in the U.S., for example). And planning one's future may seem a strange concept in a nation where the annual inflation rate recently exceeded the one thousand mark and that is therefore plagued by economic and socal instability, poverty, and associated problems.

Should others be informed of Mrs. S.'s condition? Mr. S. will know, sooner or later, that his wife is deteriorating, so this will not really be an important dilemma. But I would strongly oppose notification of Mrs. S.'s relatives on grounds of their right not to know.

COMMENTARY
Kåre Berg

The most significant ethical issue in this case is the conflict between protecting the patient's confidentiality and other people's (the relatives') need to gain access to information that is of vital importance to them, their offspring, and other family members. There are many persons in this kindred with a very high risk (50% for each of Mrs. S.'s three children, three sisters, and brother; 25% for her eleven nieces and nephews, her future grandchildren, and future nieces and nephews) of contracting this very disabling disease and of transmitting its gene to offspring. The interest of all these relatives must be weighted against Mrs. S.'s concern about confidentiality.

Mrs. S.'s attitude is ethically questionable and at variance with most caring mothers' desire to do everything that would help their children. Her reaction to the information about her disease could have its basis in mental and emotional changes caused by the disease itself. Such changes may be subtle at an early stage, not constituting an adequate reason for legal action such as appointing a custodian for her. The problem of securing responsible actions in situations such as this is unresolved. Mrs. S.'s attitude could also reflect shock after receiving frustrating information that she has not yet been able to process. If so, time might resolve the problem. Mrs. S. may also not fully understand how important information about her disease is for her relatives. If so, adequate counseling may in itself solve the ethical dilemmas.

Mrs. S.'s attempt to conceal her disease could earn her little more than a delay. The involuntary movements, the dementia and personality changes characteristic of HD would probably soon be noticed and become sources of worry and problems at home, at work, and in many social situations. She could be considered bad-tempered and mischievous, or under the influence of alcohol. How much better would it not be for her if her loved ones were forewarned so that in due time they would know that the changes were caused by a merciless disease for which she had no responsibility?

Contracting a serious disease does not relieve a mentally healthy person of the duty not to cause harm to others. In my optinion, people from kindreds with severe genetic disorders have a moral duty to help limit disastrous consequences of the disease to other persons and families, as well as to help promote research that could reduce suffering and problems in future patients and families facing the same situation. In families with inherited disorders, one often experiences strong feelings of moral obligation to the families, and of solidarity with (future) individuals and families. The time may have come to formulate, together with spokesmen of patients and families with inherited disorders, an ethical principle of solidarity that may override principles of data protection, or of a claimed right not to know about one's own genetic health. In Huntington's chorea, the lay societies play an extremely important role. They encourage an attitude of honesty and openness and are a source of strength. In Norway, a person in Mrs. S.'s situation could have benefited greatly from contact with the Huntington's Chorea Society.

The needs of Mrs. S.'s family members originate from thier risk of themselves contracting the disease and of passing the gene on to their offspring and to future generations. It is a major tragedy when one's spouse, father, or mother succumbs to a cruel, degenerative, and long-lasting disease such as HD. The possibility of having unknowingly passed on the disease gene to children is an extremely difficult situation to handle. Many people who marry into families with Huntington's chorea are not informed about the threat to the health of spouse and children. A great many of such innocent third parties have expressed bitterness because the spouse, other family members, and physicians have concealed the disease problem, and several have stated that they would not have had children had they been informed about the genetic problems in the spouse's family.

With new developments in DNA analysis, specific genetic tests may be conducted to remove unfounded fear and to make exact gene diagnosis (even in fetuses). For people who work closely with Huntington's chorea families, their need in this area appears to have such a strength that it could form the basis for a *right*. It is then far from clear that Mrs. S.'s preferences should be respected at any cost. Strong competing needs go a long way to provide a right for relatives of a patient to acquire the minimum of risk information necessary to make rational and responsible decisions concerning family and life planning and to avoid putting third parties in an extremely difficult situation.

In Norway, as well as in several other Western European countries, the emphasis on data protection is at present so strong that an ethics committee confronted with the above problems could well decide that Mrs. S.'s condition should be kept secret, even from close relatives, for whom the information would have been of vital importance. Yet, withholding risk information does nothing but cause fear, suffering (even disease), and sorrow to *more* people (spouse, children), and the choice not to know would have the same effect. Where suffering and sorrow is unavoidable it seems logically and ethically indefensible to spread it to more people than necessary.

The most important data protection issue in cases such as this is to prevent insurance companies, empoyers, pension funds, the military, or educational institutions from using information about high risk for developing a serious disease to an individual's disadvantage.

Selected Bibliography

Part One: Health Care Professionals' Responsibilities and Patients' Rights

Annas, George J. *The Rights of Hospital Patients: The ACLU Guide to a Hospital Patient's Rights*, 2d ed. Clifton, NJ: Humana Press, 1992.

Benjamin, Martin, and Curtis, Joy. *Ethics in Nursing*, 3d ed. New York: Oxford University Press, 1992.

Bok, Sissela. *Lying: Moral Choice in Public and Private Life*. New York: Pantheon Press, 1978. Cassell, Eric J. *Talking with Patients*. 2 vols. Cambridge: MIT Press, 1985.

Childress, James F. *Who Should Decide? Paternalism in Health Care.* New York: Oxford University Press, 1982.

Faden, Ruth R., and Beauchamp, Tom L. *A History and Theory of Informed Consent.* New York: Oxford University Press, 1986.

Katz, Jay. *The Silent World of Doctor and Patient.* New York: Free Press, 1984.

May, William F. *The Physician's Covenant: Images of the Healer in Medical Ethics.* Philadelphia: Westminster, 1983.

Muyskens, James L. *Moral Problems in Nursing: A Philosophical Investigation.* Totowa, NJ: Rowman and Littlefield, 1982.

Pellegrino, Edmund D., and Thomasma, David C. *A Philosophical Basis of Medical Practice: Toward a Philosophy and Ethics of the Healing Profession.* New York: Oxford University Press, 1981.

President's Commission for the Study of Ethical Problems in Medicine and Biomedical and Behavioral Research: *Making Health Care Decisions,* 3 vols. Washington, DC: U.S. Government Printing Office, 1982.

Ramsey, Paul. *The Patient as Person.* New Haven: Yale University Press, 1970.

Veatch, Robert M. *The Patient-Physician Relationship: The Patient as Partner, Part 2.* Bloomington, IN, Indiana University Press, 1991.

Reproductive Rights and Technologies

INTRODUCTION

Louise Brown, Baby M, the seven frozen embryos created by Mary Sue and Junior Lewis Davis—although most children still come into the world by the traditional route, with increasing possibilities to intervene technologically in conception, pregnancy, and birth, human reproduction has taken a turn for the complex. And with new possibilities come new questions about the extent to which medicine should intervene in the process of seeking—or avoiding—parenthood.

The cases gathered here address questions in both areas. Those in the first section—"Reproductive Rights"—consider the new problematics of medically assisted conception, and physicians' responsibilities in assuring a healthy outcome for both mother and child now that it is technologically possible to look on the fetus as a separate patient. What challenges do the possibilities opened by in vitro fertilization and surrogate motherhood raise for our understanding of what it means to be a mother or father, child or sibling? What duties do pregnant women owe to the fetuses they carry? And should physicians or the state intervene to see that women fulfill those obligations?

The second section raises the troubled issue of terminating pregnancies. The cases in this section—"Abortion"—explore moral questions that remain deeply divisive in contemporary society. The discussions here presume that the matter of when abortion may be morally permissible is still open to debate. For example, can a mentally ill woman consent to or refuse an abortion? What are the duties of individual professionals or institutions to victims of rape? Are those duties compelling when for reasons of personal conscience or institutional policy caregivers decline to participate in abortions? And what are we to make of abortion as a "solution" to the problem of multiple pregnancies created by the very reproductive technologies that hold out hope of parenthood to infertile women and men?

Such cases illuminate the kinds of fundamental questions about human goods and societal values posed by modern medicine's ability to intervene in matters of reproduction.

15

When Baby's Mother Is Also Grandma—and Sister

David Fassler

Sally Morgan is forty-six years old and has been divorced for ten years. She has one child, a twenty-five-year-old daughter. Recently she married Frank Charlton, a forty-nine-year-old childless widower. They would like to start a family of their own, but she is now infertile.

Mrs. Charlton consults a university in vitro fertilization (IVF) program, where she is told that she is not a suitable candidate for the procedure. However, her husband's sperm could be used to fertilize an egg cell from an anonymous donor. The embryo could then be implanted in a surrogate mother and carried to term.

Since Mrs. Charlton would like her child to be genetically related, her daughter offers to donate the egg cell to be utilized in the in vitro fertilization process. Each of the daughter's cells contains 50 percent of her mother's genetic material; therefore the baby would have one-half of that amount, or 25 percent. In this manner, the child would be genetically related to Mrs. Charlton. Mrs. Charlton would be in the unusual position of being both mother and grandmother to the child; her daughter would be both its mother and sister.

Should the donation be approved?

COMMENTARY
Lori B. Andrews

This case adds a twist to the debate raised by the involvement of third parties in procreation by asking whether a daughter may serve as a gamete donor. Although the advantages and disadvantages of such a situation will differ markedly depending on the particular individuals involved, such an arrangement should be allowed.

The donation would allow Mrs. Charlton and her husband to have a child genetically related to both of them. It may be the only realistic opportunity for her husband to have a child within the marriage since anonymously donated eggs may be scarce and costly (particularly in comparison to donor sperm).

The donation could give the daughter the chance to express her altruism. The prospective child might gain by experiencing greater love and support as well as a more definite identity than if produced by an anonymous donor. And permitting the donation would reinforce the strong moral and legal protection of autonomy regarding decisions about how to create and raise a family.

Some may object to the procedure because it seems unnatural, contrary to traditional notions of family, or may present risks to the parties. In attempting to assess the ethical merit of the donation, professional practices and the law should follow the model used for determining the scientific merit of a new therapy. Under the best of circumstances, a medical innovation is adopted when it is anticipated to be an improvement over the existing treatment modalities and is unlikely to cause risks that outweigh its potential benefits. In this ideal situation, as the procedure is done more frequently, its effects are closely monitored to determine whether it should continue to be used.

All forms of parenting, including traditional reproduction, present potential physical and psychological harm to the participants; yet society is reluctant to interfere with procreative decisions. This is the backdrop against which the donation of an egg from a daughter to a mother must be judged. I do not think that the risks presented by a daughter's gamete donation are sufficiently different in type or greater in magnitude to warrant banning the procedure. Rather, such donations should be allowed and scrutinized for their actual, rather than possible effects.

The potential physical risks to the participants do not appear serious enough to preclude the procedure.

Since many women have undergone laparoscopies and pregnancies, the potential physical harm to the daughter and surrogate is readily quantifiable and can be explained during the informed consent process. When IVF first came into use, the potential physical risks to the child were unknown. Although there are still not enough births to assess whether IVF presents a slightly increased risk of anomalies in offspring (say, 5 percent), it is clear that IVF is generally safe and surely does not present the 25 percent risk of affected offspring that parents with a lethal recessive gene trait run when they choose to have children.

Although most of the human IVF births have involved pregnancies in which the embryo was implanted in the woman who provided the egg, the use of a surrogate should not present additional risks. Indeed, most of the animal IVF studies (showing no increase in anomalies) have involved transfers of the embryos to a surrogate.

Nor do the potential psychological ramifications for the participants seem a sufficient reason to ban the donation. Unlike the unknown risks presented by manipulations of embryos in the early attempts at IVF, the psychological harms can be predicted by analogy to existing situations, such as an adoption or a grandmother raising her daughter's child because of divorce or the daughter's young age.

In this case, three women and one man have an emotional investment in the creation of a child. The physician should discuss with the participants the ways in which the proposed donation arrangement might threaten their emotional well-being. This is in keeping with the approach taken by Great Britain's Warnock Committee and the Victoria, Australia legislation, which require careful counseling when an identifiable egg donor is used.

The discussions should not be a form of licensing for parenting. Since we do not prohibit forty-six-year-old women from conceiving, bearing, and raising children naturally, Mrs. Charlton should not be discouraged because of her age from entering this arrangement. Rather, the interviews should focus on how the participants will handle the unique aspects of this case—the severing of the maternal genetic relationship and the maternal rearing relationship, with the former being provided by the daughter and the latter being provided by the mother.

One of the principal potential hazards lies in the possibility that the daughter could be coerced into donating her egg. In attempting to assure that the daughter has given her voluntary informed consent, the physician should make sure she has thought through the many possible future ramifications of the procedure. How would she feel if she lost her ability to conceive (perhaps as a result of the laparoscopic surgery itself) and her mother's child was her only link to motherhood?

How will the parties deal with the impression, though not the reality, of incest? Currently, stepfather-stepdaughter sexual relationships are considered incestuous and subject to civil penalties in eleven states and criminal penalties in five states. Although fertilizing the daughter's egg with her stepfather's sperm in a petri dish does not violate these laws, the unusual relationship may make the parties uneasy or cause them difficulties in dealing with outsiders who feel they have violated a basic taboo.

The physician should also discuss with the participants whether or not they will tell the child that its sister is the genetic mother. Because of the emotional harm unplanned disclosure can cause the child, the possibility of being candid with the child should at least be raised. It will clearly be stressful for the family unit if the parties do not agree on how to handle this point.

Yet the practitioner's ethical responsibilities do not end with the application of appropriate policies and principles to this particular decision. Since the request for gamete donation between friends or relatives is likely to come up again, there is an ongoing responsibility to better inform the next decision. Just as a new medical procedure is monitored to collect information on the physical risks it presents, physicians and mental health professionals have a responsibility to research the psychological effects of the new reproductive technologies they introduce. The track record of the medical and psychiatric professions in conducting such studies is poor—witness the dearth of well-designed research about the psychological effects on the donor, recipient, recipient's spouse, and child of the century-old technique of artificial insemination by donor. But such studies are especially important where practitioners are helping to conceive a new individual in ways that give birth to new ethical dilemmas.

COMMENTARY
Hans O. Tiefel

A forty-six-year-old mother of a twenty-five-year-old daughter who wants to start parenting all over again, who will not be denied by nature, who will be sixty-two with a husband of sixty-five when the hoped-for child will reach the mature age of fifteen—such a woman must be extraordinarily optimistic about what it means to raise a child. One cannot help but wonder whether a child out of season meant to enhance the marriage may prove extraordinarily taxing to a couple who normally would welcome the visits, and the departures, of grandchildren. Yet such doubts seem condescending since both Mr. and Mrs. Charlton are old enough to know what they are doing. Foolishness need not be immoral. Therefore one should assume that they are willing to pay the price for wanting to start "a family."

But not any child will do. A handicapped child, an abandoned child, a racially mixed child are not mentioned. The offspring must be their own genetically. This genetic connection necessitates the circuitous route of in vitro fertilization and surrogate motherhood. Yet the value of genetic linkage should be questioned when it is pursued in such a complex manner, when it draws other agents into this marriage as contributing agents, and when it raises the possibility of harm to the offspring since sperm deteriorate with aging. Moreover, since genetic percentages seem to matter in this case, 25 percent of the genetic inheritance will come from Mrs. Charlton's divorced husband. One expects that neither Mrs. Charlton nor her husband Frank care much for this genetic interloper. But this unhappy link does offer an opportunity to ascribe any undesirable characteristics of the child-to-be to that man who is well gone but not gone completely.

The role of Mrs. Charlton as both mother and grandmother does not seem troubling; both roles are nurturing and many grandmothers take over the functions of mothers by default. More questionable in this case is the exact meaning of "mother." There are three contenders for that title: the genetic mother (the daughter who contributes the egg), the surrogate, and the social mother (Mrs. Charlton). Whom shall the child call "Mom"?

And if that seems a trivial question, who will be responsible for the care and nurture of the child when it turns out differently than expected? Would Mrs. Charlton still acknowledge the child as hers if it were born with a genetic defect, since her genetic contribution is half that of her daughter? Would she claim to be the real mother if the child were born with a handicap that could be directly attributed to the carelessness of the surrogate mother during pregnancy? Normally mother and child are bound to each other by birth, for better or worse. When these natural ties disappear, bonds of loyalty and care for offspring may also weaken.

More interesting than the combined role of mother and grandmother is the dual status of the daughter and egg donor as both mother and sister. The arrangement assumes that the genetic relationship, which is decisive to the couple, should be disregarded by the daughter. The child-to-be will be half hers, genetically speaking, but this is considered irrelevant once the child is conceived. The parties seem to have contradictory value judgments about genetic derivation.

The surrogate's role is also problematic. Surrogates have been known to become unexpectedly attached to the children they have borne for profit or love. Assuming that the child is carried for love rather than money, would love require her to undergo amniocentesis and, if that showed the presence of defects, an abortion? If she refused abortion out of love for the child-to-be, would the child become hers in every sense, including responsibility for its medical care and upbringing?

And what of the child-to-be itself? It is still too early to tell if in vitro fertilization and embryo transfer pose long-term risks to the child. Even if aspiring parents take that risk (not for themselves but for their offspring), other problems remain. If our self-identity is shaped largely by lineage, if it is important to whom we belong and who belongs to us, then the child may want to relate to all three mothers. The couple cannot expect the child to be indifferent to "the woman who is my flesh and blood" or to "the woman who brought me into the world."

Even naturally born children complain of not being loved enough and of not belonging. Won't triple motherhood create additional tensions and resentment? Will the child not seek refuge from real or imagined grievances with the most sympathetic, and therefore the "real," mother? One might reply that the risks of dispersed kinship ties will not outweigh the good of this child's existence. But that begs the question, since such a value cannot be invoked before the child has come into being.

We live in relationships. But this case reads as if complex begetting were a private matter, as if the issues pertain only to this particular case and as if the wishes of the couple should be decisive. The case reads true enough in times in which morality is reduced to private choice, legality, and consumer satisfaction. But it is also misleading, especially in regard to medical matters. Medical professionals play an indispensable yet deplorably passive role here: Just tell us what you want and we will make it possible. Happily this is counterfactual; no institution is yet quite so accommodating.

Should physicians demur, the couple could claim that its rights have been violated. For rights remain the only powerful and public tool in otherwise privatized ethics. True, no one has a right to interfere with claims to beget children. But such rights remain negative. They establish no corresponding duty on the part of the physician to facilitate reproduction, any more than my right to marry obligates any woman to marry me. Moreover, relying on rights is rather self-centered. Rights cannot guide us in deciding who we should be as spouses or parents or what we owe one another in love.

The loving decision in this case is not what Mrs. Charlton and her husband "would like." It is one that seeks the good of all who are part of these relationships, especially the child-to-be. And the good of this envisioned offspring is obstructed by the risk of harm, by contradictory values about genetic ties, by confusion over who may claim the child and who is responsible for it (and whom the child may claim and be responsible to), and by a need for personal selflessness on the part of the genetic mother that exceeds realistic expectations. In this case moral judgment supports common sense: this foolishness is also immoral.

16

When a Pregnant Woman Endangers Her Fetus

Janet M., in her early twenties, is pregnant for the third time. She has been an insulin-dependent diabetic since the age of twelve but has experienced no major complications of diabetes.

Dr. L. has repeatedly advised her of the risks that uncontrolled diabetes poses to her fetus. Congenital malformations are two to four times more common in infants of mothers whose diabetes is poorly controlled. Furthermore, uncontrolled diabetes can result in the birth of a premature, stillborn fetus.

He admits her at fifteen weeks gestation as an inpatient to treat her diabetes, but she discharges herself against his advice five days later before her diabetes has been satisfactorily controlled. Once home, she ignores pleas from Dr. L. and other physicians to obtain chemstrips or a dextrometer for monitoring blood sugar. In response, she tells them she "has no money" or "forgot."

At twenty-one weeks gestation she is hospitalized for a threatened abortion but quickly announces her intention to leave. Dr. L. decides that her behavior poses a clear risk to the well-being of her fetus. Unless she changes her mind, he says, he will seek a court order to keep her hospitalized.

Is his response justified?

COMMENTARY
Thomas B. Mackenzie and Theodore C. Nagel

Three generic questions can be posed in cases like this one. First, does the physician have an obligation to the fetus to ensure its well-being that cannot be abrogated by the parents? Second, is there sound scientific evidence of a relationship between the specific condition or behavior observed and fetal risk (or damage) to justify concern? And third, is there any way to control the condition that does not significantly endanger the physical health of the mother?

We believe that in order to justify legal action, the answer to all three questions must be yes.

Did this woman's physicians have an obligation to her fetus that superseded her wishes as expressed in her conversation and behavior? In answering this question one must consider two intertwined issues: abortion and viability. Present judicial doctrine clearly subordinates the physician's obligation to the fetus in favor of the woman's right to abort prior to fetal viability. Thus the intention to abort would waive any obligation to protect fetal well-being. But Janet M. gave no indication that this was her intention.

Whether the physician's obligation to the fetus (presuming an intention to carry to term) is the same before as it is after viability is a complex question. From an ethical point of view that demarcation is not compelling, since fetal conditions that require diagnosis and treatment can be identified prior to viability. Thus the fetus can be a patient independent of the mother in the sense that it is the sole possessor of a disease or condition. It is also clear that maternal behavior during early pregnancy may adversely affect the fetus and result in irreversible injury. Consequently the physician's ethical responsibility to the fetus prior to viability (or prior to the woman's decision to abort) is not different than it is at a later stage of pregnancy.

Whether the physician has a legal obligation prior to viability is less clear. While all American jurisdictions allow a child to recover for prenatal injuries negligently inflicted after viability, only some jurisdictions have abandoned the viability standard. Thus whether a physician could be sued by a child for malpractice regarding care given before viability depends on the state.

At the time when intervention was considered in this case, Janet M.'s fetus was not viable. However, we do not feel that the fetus's nonviability diminished the obligations of her attending physicians. The mother clearly had information about her pregnancy and the potential consequences of uncontrolled diabetes. Her behavior was not a result of ignorance. Her explanations for failing to obtain the equipment that was necessary to control her diabetes were inconsistent and vague. Overall her behavior indicated an unwillingness to manage her diabetes in a manner that minimized the risk to her fetus. Under these circumstances, we believe her physicians had an obligation to the fetus that could not be waived by the mother.

The second question asks whether there is sufficient certainty of a relationship between a recurrent behavior and damage to the fetus. In other words, a physician could not tyrannize the mother by holding her to frivolous or unproven standards in the name of fetal welfare. The answer to this question is yes. A clear relationship has been established between careful management of insulin-dependent diabetes mellitus and reduced incidence of stillbirth, intrauterine deaths, respiratory distress syndrome, macrosomia, and congenital malformations.

The final question asks: Can the threatening condition be reasonably controlled or reversed without significantly endangering the physical health of the mother? If the answer to this question is no, then positive responses to our first two standards would be immaterial. In the case at hand, effective control of diabetes during pregnancy appears well within reach. This may involve close surveillance in the hospital with three to four subcutaneous insulin injections per day. Hospitalization also permits early recognition of emerging complications in the last weeks of pregnancy. Alternatively, patients may monitor their diabetes at home using home blood glucose monitoring, with fetal monitoring done as an outpatient. The latter was offered to Mrs. M. but was not accepted. Thus the answer to the third question is yes.

Since we have answered all three questions in the affirmative, we would support the decision of Janet M.'s physicians to seek enforced hospitalization and treatment to protect and preserve the well-being of the fetus. After noting that protecting the fetus would involve violation of the mother (drawing blood and administering insulin), the court might well decide against the actions urged by the attending physician. Such an outcome would not indicate that her physician was overly zealous. It would reflect the growing capacity of medicine to observe, diagnose, and treat the developing fetus and the consequent conflict between the woman's freedom to control her own body and the potential adverse effects of her behavior on her unborn child.

COMMENTARY
Barbara Katz Rothman

Had this discussion been written twenty-five years ago, it might have read as follows:

> Janet M., a diabetic, refused her DES treatment, prescribed as especially important in the prevention of miscarriage among diabetics. Further, although she was eleven pounds overweight at the time of conception, she refused to limit her weight gain over the course of pregnancy to under thirteen pounds. She compounded the problem by not taking the diuretics prescribed, and twice refused to show up for scheduled x-rays, citing a distrust of medications and radiation. Her irrational refusal to comply with her doctor's advice, plus her unwillingness or inability to limit her weight gain, indicate fetal abuse. Should Dr. L. seek a court order ...?

And a potential scenario for twenty-five years from now:

> Mrs. M., suspecting pregnancy, engages the services of an attorney who specializes in family law, especially prenatal agreements. On her initial visit to the fetologist, Mrs. M. and her attorney will be informed of the conditions to which she must adhere throughout the pregnancy, and a second attorney will be appointed to act as fetal guardian. Violations of the prenatal contract will result in the state gaining custody of the fetus: either forcibly removing it to

an artificial womb, or putting Mrs. M. in one of the new high-security wings of the maternity hospital for the duration of her pregnancy.

These two scenarios, past and future, illustrate the two major problems I see with an obstetrician calling on the power of the state to control a pregnant woman's behavior in the interests of her fetus. First, obstetrics has too long a history of errors in management for us to be certain that obstetricians always *know* the best interests of the fetus. Each of the procedures cited above, recommended twenty-five years ago, has since been discarded as dangerous. It is too soon to be certain of the standing today's obstetrical practices will come to have in the future.

But even if one had perfect faith in obstetrical knowledge, a second and more serious problem remains: the costs to the civil liberties of pregnant women are too high. We are in danger of creating of pregnant women a second class of citizen, without basic legal rights of bodily integrity and self-determination. Competent adults in this society have the right to refuse medical treatment, even when it is believed to be life-saving. But as reproductive rights attorney Janet Gallagher has warned in a chapter from a forthcoming book, *Biology and Women's Policy*, "The law's concern for human dignity and self-determination all too readily yield to the recurrent temptations to view and treat pregnant women as vessels." It is wrong to allow obstetrics or the state to subsume the interests and the civil rights of pregnant women to those of the products of conception within them.

The basic ethical question in this case is: What are the obligations of obstetricians toward their patients? Or more precisely, who exactly is the patient of an obstetrician? A long-standing definition of obstetrics is "the branch of medicine concerning the care of women during pregnancy, labor and the puerperium." But that definition may no longer seem appropriate, as obstetricians such as Dr. L. increasingly define themselves as physicians to the fetus. The medical model of pregnancy, as an essentially parasitic and vaguely pathological relationship, encourages the physician to view the fetus and mother as two separate patients, and to see pregnancy as inherently a conflict of interests between the two. Where the fetus is highly valued, the effect is to reduce the woman to what current obstetrical language calls "the maternal environment."

A more appropriate and ultimately more useful perspective is to see the pregnant woman as a biological and social unit. With a more holistic view, Dr. L. might remember that Mrs. M. has controlled her diabetes for over half her life, and through two pregnancies. It may not be a matter of behaving "as she chooses." As a mother of two young children, Mrs. M. may have a variety of compelling reasons preventing her from staying for more than five days in the hospital, from returning for an indefinite period, or even from taking good care of herself at home. As *her* physician, Dr. L. might consider what *her* needs are—social and economic as well as medical—and how he might help her to meet those, rather than calling on the courts to control her.

17

Live Sperm, Dead Bodies

Kathleen Nolan

Bill K., a twenty-two-year-old man engaged to be married in four months, has just been diagnosed as brain-dead after a car accident. His father arrives and agrees to mulitple organ donations to be coordinated by a local organ procurement agency. Bill's father also makes an unusual request: can sperm be obtained and frozen for later use? Bill's fiancée is unavailable for consultation, but the father believes that she may be interested in conceiving Bill's child, so that "a part of him can live on." Sperm have been successfully harvested in similar circumstances in a few cases. Bill was his father's only son, and the father states that even if the financée is not interested in using the sperm, he would welcome the donation so that the family line could be continued in at least that fashion. Assuming that adequate technical means are available, should the sperm be retrieved?

COMMENTARY
Cappy Miles Rothman

Not only do technical means exist for post-morterm sperm recovery, but compelling ethical reasons as well. As a physician, my primary motivation is to relieve pain and suffering. Eleven years ago I harvested sperm from a young man who had sustained fatal head injuries. While the deceased was unmarried and without a fiancée, this man's father was consoled by knowing that viable sperm were stored. When I recovered sperm from another young man who had died of a gunshot wound, his parents followed me to the sperm bank and were comforted when they saw motile sperm from their son. Preserving "part of the deceased" let them identify with their lost son, and allowed the possibility of continuation of the partilineal heritage. To bestow such consolation at a time of grief and tragedy is clearly part of my role as a healer.

Thousands of children have been born from sperm stored for many years and some have been conceived after the death of their fathers. The most publicized case occurred in France when the National Sperm Bank refused to release sperm to a woman whose husband had recently died. Public opinion in her favor was so strong as to compel the release of the sperm to her. Such instances provide for individual rights, pose no harm to society, and allow for freedom of choice on an issue that, while unusual, is important to them.

Clearly there is a growing demand for information on post-mortem sperm recovery. National medical conferences, lay publications, radio, and television have all covered this issue. More and more instances occur where a wife requests recovery and stores the sperm from her recently deceased spouse.

At present, no legislation exists to restrict or regulate sperm retrieval. To date, no children have been born from sperm stored after such recovery, but the possibility exists; recent advances have enabled men with vas obstruction to have children by aspirating epididymal sperm. Such valuable and available technology should not be unnecessarily restricted. If parents can legally release their son's organs for transplantation, why should they not be able to store his sperm? And if a man can store sperm prior to an anticipated death, why shouldn't the wife of a man who dies an untimely death have the same opportunity?

Certainly situations could complicate what might seem a fairly straightforward issue. If Bill's fiancée, for example, objects to the use of his sperm, should his father or parents retain the rights to its use with another woman? What would be the rights of the offspring with regard to property and position? Who will establish informed consent for the woman who will carry this child and also have a genetic interest? (Perhaps Bill has genetic abnormalities that his fiancée is unaware of and that are not apparent during harvesting and storage. . . .) Who controls release of the stored sperm and for which purposes?

I can envision circumstances under which I would decline to retrieve sperm from a deceased—when there is clearly a conflict of interest between survivors as to the use of the sperm or when there are questions regarding the intent of the deceased to father children. But deciding whose rights prevail is not my role, lessening grief and offering alternatives remain my priorities.

Sperm harvesting requires immediate action to recover viable and motile sperm. At present, sperm recovery has been successfully performed because such immediate action can be taken based on the "best judgment" of the physician. If an ethics committee review were necessary for each procedure, would the sperm still be viable? If the committee ruled "yes," and the delay prevented successful retrieval, who would be liable? Unless a clearly adverse situation exists, recovery should proceed at once to enable well-considered decisions later.

COMMENTARY
Judith Wilson Ross

Is Bill, dead, simply bits and pieces that can be used to fulfill others' rational desires? Surely not. Sperm harvesting should not be permitted because persons should participate in a decision to beget a child and because children should be assured a relationship with their genetic parents based upon each parent's acceptance of the child's future existence.

The parallel implied by Mr. K.'s request is that, as he is legally and morally empowered to donate his dead son's heart, liver, etc., to save the life of another person in need, so also is he entitled to donate his dead son's sperm. Organ donation by proxy does not provide an appropriate parallel to "sperm harvesting," however. First, there is a great shortage of donated organs, but there is no shortage of donated sperm. While taking organs from those who have not consented in advance is justified by the recipient's great need, there is no comparable need in this case. Second, organ donation involves an existing person in need; sperm donation creates the possibility of a new person who would otherwise not exist. If we permit surrogates to consent to organ removal because society has a commitment to help identified individuals with life-threatening or debilitating illnesses, no such individuals exist in this case. Sperm harvesting creates new needs rather than fulfilling existing ones.

We might try to justify the sperm removal by speculating that Bill would want this done if he could be asked. However, in the absence of any indication that he has such wishes (a desire to become a parent when he was alive would not be sufficient), or that most people would have such a preference, this line of argument is not convincing.

Suppose Bill had not been killed in the car accident but had suffered significant brain injury resulting in permanent and severe mental incapacity. Though alive, he would not be able to experience parenthood in any meaningful way. He would not be able to express personal preferences. Under these circumstances, Mr. K., as Bill's guardian, might be able to donate Bill's kidney, but only if the donation would benefit Bill in some distinct manner. (Suppose it was his cousin who needed the kidney and she was Bill's caretaker.) It is difficult to see, however, how Bill could benefit in any comparable way from sperm harvesting. Indeed, such harvesting would constitute the use of Bill purely as a means to his father's or fiancée's desires. This would be morally unacceptable.

Does the fact that Bill is dead, rather than alive but lacking self-consciousness, make it acceptable to use him (or his body parts) in this way?

Because in our culture procreation represents a more direct kind of personal continuity than does organ donation, the fact that Bill is dead, rather than alive but unaware, should make no difference. Mr. K.'s desire to continue Bill through sperm harvesting appears to reduce Bill to his body parts. If Bill had said that, in the event of his sudden death, he wanted sperm harvested and made available to his fiancée or a sperm bank, such a wish could be honored (though it would not be obligatory), for it would represent Bill's desire to be a father, even if he could not fully realize that role. In the absence of such wishes, it is difficult to see how the proposed use of Bill's sperm would foster any central cultural values, in particular those of personal identity or of parent-child connection.

Parenthood, both in terms of *being* a parent and of *having* a parent, is integral to personal identity. Parenthood offers to child and adult a sense of continuity, of belonging, and of identification, resting as it does on the acknowledgment of the parent-child relationship. As parents, in intending or accepting a pregnancy, further define and discover themselves in acknowledging their relationship with the child-that-is-to-be (even if they do not accept the relationship), so the child-that-is begins to understand its own self through that parental acknowledgment and connection. Because this society places so much value on the individual's understanding and development of self, it behooves us to support every person's having that sense of continuity, belonging, and identification through acknowledged relationships. We can achieve this goal by keeping decisions to beget a child as closely connected as possible to those who are the parents-to-be. We acknowledge this value in our unwillingness to let procreation decisions be made for minors by parents, for metally disabled individuals by conservators, or for women by doctors.

Clearly, in the face of this sudden and tragic death, Mr. K. has a psychological need to extend Bill's life. But there are many ways of dealing with that need other than setting in motion the mechanistic manufacture of a child who cannot be acknowledged by the genetic father (and who can thus have no beneficial relationship with the memory of that father). If a decision to harvest the sperm represents Mr. K.'s desire to extend his own genetic line, then perhaps he should investigate the possibility of donating his own sperm — an act that would reach his goal more directly and with greater genetic integrity.

18

Maternal Rights, Fetal Harms

A twenty-two-year-old patient at the county obstetrics clinic received upsetting news when an ultrasound exam revealed that her fetus had hydrocephalus, an abnormal accumulation of cerebrospinal fluid within the ventricles of the brain. The fluid build-up can raise intracranial pressure and enlarge the head, making normal passage of the fetus through the birth canal impossible. If persistently high, the pressure destroys white matter and causes mental retardation. Serial ultrasounds showed progressive build-up of fluid and moderate head enlargement. In addition, a lumbar meningomyelocele was identified, but ultrasound exams revealed no other anomalies. Viral cultures of amniotic fluid and karyotyping revealed no infection or other anomalies. The gestational age of the fetus is thirty-four weeks, and tests show that the fetal lungs are mature.

Placement of a ventriculo-amniotic shunt *in utero* would be possible, bu this approach has had limited success. Given mature lungs, the balance of risk: and benefits for the fetus favors prompt delivery and postnatal shunting if needed, rather than the still-experimental intrauterine shunting.

A decision is needed concerning the method of delivery. Prompt delivery, by cesarean section if needed to avoid trauma to the fetal head, would permit assessment of the infant's condition and provision of treatments, including ventriculo-peritoneal shunt insertion if necessary. Recent reports suggest that among hydrocephalic fetuses for whom full treatment efforts are provided approximately 60 percent survive. Among survivors, about half are mentally retarded in varying degrees. This approach, however, exposes the woman to the various risks associated with surgical delivery, including infection, hemorrhage sufficient to require transfusion, and iatrogenic injury to the urinary tract.

An alternative approach would minimize the physical risks to the woman by avoiding cesarean section, permitting the pregnancy to continue until labor begins spontaneously. If the fetal head is too large to pass through the pelvis, a needle can be inserted into the cranium and cerebrospinal fluid extracted to reduce head size. However, this cephalocentesis almost always results in stillbirth or neonatal death within a few days, due to the rapid decompression of the head or needle-induced hemorrhage.

What recommendation, if any, should the physician make to the woman? Should he seek a court order for surgical delivery if the woman refuses cesarean section?

COMMENTARY
Carson Strong

The questions raised are of great concern to obstetricians detecting prenatal hydrocephalus, a common malformation. Cephalocentesis is ethically problematic for several reasons. First, if one knowingly performs an act that is highly likely to cause the death of another, and if the act causes the death, then it seems reasonable to say that one has killed the other. Even if the purpose is to prevent harm to the woman, and fetal death is not desired, the action would still be killing. Second, because the fetus is near term it deserves serious respect; causing death would then be a grave matter, regardless of whether it is the death of a neonate or of a fetus. Third, it can be argued that physicians have special role-related obligations to avoid causing death. Fourth, it is hardly ever plausible to claim that causing its death is in the interests of the hydrocephalic fetus, and certainly not in the case at hand.

Nevertheless, it can be argued that it is ethical for the obstetrician to decompress the fetal head when anomalies incompatible with long-term survival have been detected (such as trisomies 13 or 18), or there are anomalies that are not necessarily incompatible with long-term survival, but are highly likely to result in death or severe handicap (such as holoprosencephaly).

In the present case there are no detected anomalies that are certain or highly likely to cause death, and the physician should strive to avoid killing. If the woman prefers cesarean section, her choice should be strongly supported. If she appears to favor vaginal delivery or asks for a recommendation, the physician should recommend delivery that is atraumatic for the fetus. It is acceptable to attempt to persuade the mother to assume risks, within limits, for the sake of the fetus.

A firm refusal of cesarean section by the mother would create a dilemma. Such a case would challenge those who maintain that forced maternal treatment is never justified, for the likely alternative is the physician's causing the death of a neonate or fetus with serious moral standing. It has been argued that forced maternal treatment should always be avoided in part because of its adverse consequences, which could include brutalization of the physicians and other caregivers involved, weakening of the liberty of pregnant women generally, and disruption of physician-patient relationships. If these effects can occur, might not causing the deaths of infants or fetuses near term also have adverse consequences? A similar brutalizing effect might occur. Respect for life might generally be weakened. Patients might become less secure in their belief that physicians do not kill one patient for the sake of another, and this could adversely affect therapeutic relationships. Weighing the pros and cons in such a case involves a complex judgment.

A resolution of the dilemma exists if we consider the likelihood that cesarean section will benefit the fetus. Forced cesarean section would be justifiable only if, among other factors, there is a very high probability that it will significantly promote the fetus's well-being. Forcing the mother to undergo such an invasive procedure when there is a great chance that it will not significantly benefit the fetus seems unwarranted. Even in the present case there is too much uncertainty about survival to claim that there is a very high probability that cesarean section will make such a contribution. Our ability to detect anomalies *in utero* is limited, and associated life-threatening conditions still often go unnoted. As our technology improves and we are better able both to diagnose and care for handicapped newborns, arguments for forced intervention may become more persuasive. At present, however, we cannot predict that survival of a hydrocephalic fetus is very highly probable. It is justifiable, then, for the physician to perform cephalocentesis if the woman firmly states an informed, volunatary preference for vaginal delivery.

COMMENTARY
Kathy Kinlaw

Two broad issues are addressed by this case: (1) What is the ethically justified treatment recommendation to make to this pregnant woman? (2) Procedurally, who should decide and how should the decision be carried out?

Several medical facts are pertinent. A fetus with mature lungs at thirty-four weeks gestation has hydrocephalus with "moderate head enlargement" and a lumbar meningomyelocele of unknown extent. Neither anomaly is incompatible with survival. Indeed, the 60 percent survival rate given for hydrocephalus appears quite low. Morbidity varies widely with these combined anomalies once treated; shunting problems, infection, lower extremity motor and sensory deficits, and neurogenic bladder disturbances are possible. Normal IQ levels are relatively common for individuals with hydrocephalus secondary to meningomyelocele. In sum, this child-to-be is not at clear risk of either death or of severe cognitive/developmental deficits. Given the current state of technology this fetus is clearly "viable," having an excellent chance of being successfully delivered, surgically treated, and surviving.

Though not clearly indicated, we might assume that this woman desires this pregnancy, has some commitment to the fetus at least as a child-to-be, and is influenced in her decisionmaking by some consideration for the fetus and the fetus's health. This is a reasonable assumption given the advanced state of pregnancy and the physical intrusiveness she has accepted to this point. Given the high percentage of cesarean sections performed in this country—25 percent of all births—it is also quite possible that *this* method of delivery has been broached as a possibility in any case.

Due to the viability of the fetus, the potential for a relatively "good" fetal outcome, and a reasonable assumption of some level of commitment to the fetus, a recommendation for cesarean section to maximize fetal outcome appears ethically sound. Such a recommendation would incorporate supportive counseling about the anomalies diagnosed as well as the increased risks of the procedure to the woman. These risks are apparently medically "reasonable" risks as cesarean sections are regularly recommended by the medical team and accepted by expectant parents in order to promote the health and safety of the woman and fetus.

One might also propose a slightly different alternative. Depending on the actual meaning of "moderate head enlargement," induction of labor *now* with the hope of vaginal delivery might be possible to promote fetal outcome *and* minimize any risk to the woman. The physician would inform the woman that every attempt at vaginal delivery would be made, but that a cesarean section would be resorted to should there be a determination of risk to the woman or fetus. The mother would thus need to agree to the cesarean section as an acceptable option *prior* to induction of labor.

If this pregnant woman is hesitant about any possibility of cesarean section, one might determine whether her desire to await spontaneous vaginal delivery and cephalocentesis is motivated primarily by (1) the perceived risks of cesarean section to her own health, or (2) her desire not to have to deliver and make caretaking decisions about an affected child. The woman's concerns are real in either case but would be interpreted differently by the ethical concept of double effect. In the first case the woman desires to avoid self-harm and does not primarily intend the death of the fetus or newborn. Here the burden is on the medical team to make sure that the woman is fully informed about the true risks of the procedure and the anticipated fetal or newborn death by cephalocentesis. In the second case a morally objectionable effect—the death of the fetus or newborn—is intended and is the means to the morally acceptable end of respecting the woman's autonomy and avoiding any increased risk of harm to her. An objective assessment of the risks of cesarean section as weighed against some "claim" to respect for the fetus and thus the promotion of a good fetal outcome supports the position of giving this fetus a chance.

Though judicial precedents do not ethics make, the clear intention of the *Roe v. Wade* decision is to allow some protection of the state's interest in preserving viable fetal life. This interest is outweighed if the life or health of the pregnant woman is in danger. Yet the woman is not the sole judge of when her health is endangered. Such a decision is, rather, based on much medical information and experience. Just as there are some increased risks with a cesarean section, the continuation of the pregnancy entails risks (such as risk of a ruptured uterus as fetal head size increases). Such increased risks should be assessed by the woman in conjunction with the medical team.

No woman gives up her rights when she becomes pregnant, but there is a sense in which her rights and concurrent responsibilities are enlarged. Having accepted this pregnancy to the thirty-fourth week, she must carefully consider what effects her decisions have on herself, her fetus, and her relationship to other significant people in her life. An ethics of responsibility evolves which suggests that the "self" deserving of respect in autonomous decision making has been enlarged in some meaningful ways.

Given all of this "reasonable" discussion, what should be the medical team's response in the event this pregnant woman still refuses any possibility of a timely cesarean section? Given the potential for a relatively good fetal outcome, cephalocentesis, which leads inevitably to fetal or neonatal death, is difficult to defend. Should this fetus have had anencephaly or perhaps a trisomy condition that anticipated infant death, the ethical interest in promoting a good fetal outcome would carry little weight against the desire to respect the woman's wishes and to maximize her own good. But the current case justifies some respect for the fetus that the direct harm of cephalocentesis does not permit. Respect for the woman's wishes to avoid the risks associated with a cesarean section (*if* needed) should not lead to the positive obligation of a physician to conduct a procedure at the point of live delivery that will lead to the death of the fetus at birth or of the infant shortly after. In this situation respect for autonomy is not without limits. The woman is not reduced to a "fetal container" merely because other interests are recognized.

In the current legal / judical atmosphere, a physician who believed that a cesarean section might be necessary would be unwise not to seek a court order to support this decision. However, the adversarial nature of the court system makes this a less than desirable body for intervention into the decision. The idea of forcing a woman to undergo any procedure against her will is ethically repugnant and the gross instrument of a public policy that required such intervention in every instance is odious. The ethics committee as an avenue for communication may be a better intermediary process to encourage consensus between the woman and medical team as the decision makers in the case. Without such consensus, the physician who would not perform cephalocentesis has two options: (1) assist in finding the woman another physician who could accept the woman's wishes, or (2) be compelled to obtain a court order and perform the cesarean section in order to give the fetus a chance and not allow the woman to die in vaginal delivery. Neither respect for individual autonomy nor a desire for maintaining the integrity of the physician-patient relationship calls for health care givers to abandon their personal or professional values.

ABORTION

19

When a Mentally Ill Woman Refuses Abortion

Ann Brown is a twenty-seven-year-old woman with a diagnosis of chronic paranoid schizophrenia. She has a history of prolonged institutionalization, with intermittent attempts at independent living. Presently living in a mental hospital, Ann Brown is now twelve weeks pregnant. She has firmly indicated her desire to continue the pregnancy and to keep the child. Abortion, she declares, "is against my principles." The father is unknown.

While Ann's psychiatrist does not consider her capable of responsible parenthood, he does think that she is capable, at times at least, of meaningful moral decisions. Her schizophrenia and medication taken early in pregnancy slightly increase the possibility of fetal defect.

Ann Brown's mother wants her to have an abortion, and has secured legal custody of her daughter in order to effect that result. She feels that the experience of pregnancy and the trauma of labor and delivery will worsen Ann's mental state. Moreover, she herself is unable to care for the child and fears that Ann will suffer further if she is forced to give up the child to strangers.

The hospital attorney has indicated that she will oppose Ann's mother's request for an abortion. She will argue that it cannot be performed without consent.

There is little likelihood that Ann Brown would be allowed to care for her child. However, because of the ambiguity surrounding parental consent, the child would probably be placed in foster care rather than with adoptive parents.

Should the abortion be performed? Who should decide?

COMMENTARY
Mary Mahowald

Among the diverse ethical and legal issues raised by this case, I would like to address two: the moral status of incompetent adults, as well as fetuses; and the relationship between the hospital and the courts.

"Informed consent" is generally viewed as essential to legal and moral justification for medical procedures. There is also general agreement that informed consent entails three factors: competence, understanding, and voluntariness. The same factors are present in proxy or substitute consent, which is neither legally nor morally as strong a basis for medical intervention as informed consent. Accordingly, parents' refusal of treatment for their offspring is less binding on practitioners than is their refusal of treatment for themselves. Proxy dissent may be overruled on grounds that it violates the best interests of the person for whom consent is refused.

In securing legal custody of her daughter, Ann Brown's mother has assumed certain rights and responsibilities regarding her, but these do not necessarily imply either Ann's incapability for informed consent or her mother's right to choose abortion for her pregnant daughter. A court judgment would have to be obtained to warrant overriding Ann's refusal of the procedure.

In requesting such an order, Ann's mother could argue that it is in her daughter's best interest to have an abortion, because continuing the pregnancy, experiencing labor and delivery, and probably delivery of the child into another's custody would together entail a burden greater than the abortion. Against that argument stands the fact that Ann has clearly indicated a desire to continue the pregnancy, and that most second-trimester abortions entail the experience of labor and delivery. (Alternatives to labor are available for either childbirth or abortion.) Moreover, the possibility that Ann's sense of "wrongness" about abortion might impose an added psychological burden needs to be considered in evaluating her best interests.

As the psychiatrist apparently recognizes, even legally incompetent individuals may be capable of moral decisions. In addition to mental illness, youth is often a criterion for denying a legal right to choose or refuse medical care. Yet most adolescents, and many younger children, are morally responsible for some of their acts, even as adults may be legally competent while morally incompetent. Moreover, a sophisticated understanding of complicated medical procedures is not requisite to informed consent. The crucial cognitive component of a moral decision is recognition of the cause-effect relationship between election of a procedure and its results. If Ann has a basic understanding of what abortion entails, and what continuation of her pregnancy entails, that cognitive requirement is satisfied.

While ambiguity may remain about whether Ann has made a moral decision in this instance, the moral standing of the fetus tips the scale in favor of respecting her refusal. Moral standing does not imply personhood; it merely means that an individual has some moral claim on others, for example, a prima facie right to, or interest in, continued existence. In this case, the probability that the child will be normal, and live a life that is better than death, argues that the interests of the fetus coincide with Ann's desire to continue the pregnancy.

Nonetheless, since *Roe v. Wade* (1973) there is no legal requirement to consider the interests of a nonviable fetus. Therefore, a legal determination of Ann's competence to dissent or consent to an abortion is crucial. This might be provided through a court decision, based on psychiatric evaluation of Ann's competence.

The possibility that Ann is incompetent both legally and morally suggests an important criticism of the popular "pro-choice" view of abortion. Some women who are pregnant are clearly incapable of autonomous decisions (for example, those who are unconscious or profoundly retarded). Others, particularly minors, are questionably competent. Exclusive emphasis on autonomy undercuts the principles of beneficence and nonmaleficence, which remain applicable in such cases.

COMMENTARY
Virginia Abernethy

There is little question that the hospital attorney would prevail in a court of law and that the abortion would not be performed over her and Ann Brown's objections. But although the case will be decided in Ann's favor, I maintain that this is an absurd outcome based on a fallacious understanding of liberty.

Ann's objection will be honored because abortion is a medical procedure and a competent person has the nearly unqualified right to refuse any unwanted health care intervention. However, this right to refuse apparently does not overwhelm a state interest in protecting *others*, so limited coercion is permitted in issues of immunization or quarantine, or where refusal of blood transfusion endangers a third-trimester fetus. Even when the patient's own life is at issue, if the refusal is "ambivalently" given and the intervention is not major (as in blood transfusion), a patient's refusal may be overridden. Ordinarily, however, a competent person's right to refuse is respected even when the decision appears life-threatening and is "irrational" in terms of others' thinking and values. Legal precedents affirming the person's right not to be touched without personal consent derive both from the common law and from the constitutional guarantee of privacy.

The question thus turns on whether Ann Brown is competent. It is relevant here that competence is presumed and the burden of proof is on those who challenge it; that schizophrenia is not conclusive evidence of incompetence to refuse a medical procedure; that Ann has the capacity to understand the procedure and its meaning to her (that is, abortion means no baby, and no abortion means she will probably deliver); and that the psychiatrist declares "she is capable, at times at least, of meaningful moral decisions." If Ann wanted to have the baby even after being forewarned that, since she was psychiatrically ill and institutionalized, she would never be entrusted with her child, that would constitute telling evidence of her incompetence. But to support the conclusion of incompetency, one might still have to argue that denying those facts because of *hoping for recovery* from schizophrenia is so unrealistic as to be, in itself, grounds for judging a person to be incompetent.

I am unwilling to agree that hoping for recovery is a sign of incompetence. I also doubt that a court of law would find Ann incompetent on the totality of evidence. If she is competent, she can refuse the abortion. End of case.

Unfortunately, this leads to an absurd outcome—so absurd that one must search for an underlying fallacy. The outcome is absurd because Ann Brown does not want the pregnancy and childbirth as ends in themselves; she wants the resulting child. But it is acknowledged by all (except Ann, presumably) that she cannot care for the child, her mother cannot care for the child, and so the child will be taken from her for indefinite foster home placement. No one's good is served: not Ann's and not society's, because society will be burdened with the cost of foster care. All this happens because society will take away Ann's child but cannot prevent or take away Ann's pregnancy.

The fallacy, in my view, is in assuming that Ann has the right to bear a child. This is a wrong-headed belief into which we have muddled because of overemphasis on rights and privileges and neglect of duties and responsibilities.

A well-functioning, stable society matches every right to a responsibility. A "person" in either the philosophic or social sense has both rights and responsibilities. There is a correspondence between them. This suggests that Ann's right to procreate might be compromised by her very limited capacity to be responsible as a parent.

If no one felt obliged to care for the child it would be different; the child would die and Ann's "right" would be nullified. But our society *does* feel obliged; this is not Dickensian England. Since children are thought to create a responsibility, perhaps there should not be a right to procreate by those unable to assume that responsibility.

No right is so broad that, morally, it can extend to harming others. Thus, there is a public right to use water, but not to pollute it. Industry has rights to free conduct of their business, but not to destroy the environment for others. Your right to swing your fist ends where my nose begins. Ann's right to procreate ends where the responsibility to raise her child becomes mine—ours—society's.

Acceptance of the underlying principle would raise questions for others who are arguably deficient as parents: for example, the severely retarded, ambulatory schizophrenics, the socially maladjusted, people who have proven to be "poor parents" in the past and had their children taken from them. Possible extensions of a principle of reciprocal rights and responsibilities are disquieting and raise questions about how due process would develop in order to prevent abuse.

Nevertheless, since the present rules seem seriously flawed I do not withdraw my proposal. Since Ann's pregnancy is leading to a child for which she cannot be responsible, a child for which society will be responsible, her right to privacy does not extend to refusing an abortion. The right to procreate should be limited by the capacity to take responsibility for the result. Ann's right to bring forth ends where my duty to care for her child begins.

20

The Hospital's Duty and Rape Victims

Dr. Maria DeCicco is Chief of Emergency Care at St. Mary's Hospital in a large southern city. She has been put in a difficult situation by the passage of a state Rape Victim's Emergency Treatment Act and recent amendments to the municipal code mandating certain services for rape victims. The state law requires hospitals to collect evidence for the police. Kits are provided for this purpose at no expense to the hospital. Hospitals must also provide, with the patient's consent, minimum treatment including an emergency room examination, counseling, and advice about possible infection or pregnancy.

The city's municipal code specifies the treatment in greater detail and creates the real problem for Dr. DeCicco. The treatment required by the code includes, with the patient's consent, medication against conception and venereal disease. Dr. DeCicco has, as a matter of conscience, always tried to use her medical skills to preserve life. She feels that abortion is morally wrong and went to great lengths to find a position where she could practice medicine without having to provide such services. That is why she joined the staff of St. Mary's. Their policy against abortion was firm and well known. Patients in the community would normally not come to St. Mary's if they were considering abortion.

The new municipal code appears to require that she and her staff provide not only emergency medical services, which she is happy to do, but also medical intervention to interrupt any pregnancy that may result. Although the cells to be destroyed by the "morning after" pill are newly fertilized, to her their destruction is the moral equivalent of an abortion.

Dr. DeCicco recognizes that the ethical issues are a matter of substantial controversy. She is not seeking to impose moral judgments on anyone else. She only wants to practice medicine as her conscience dictates, yet the new state and municipal mandates seem to require her to participate in what she believes is a morally objectionable practice in order to protect the rights of the rape victim.

She has talked with the administrator of the hospital. He strongly agrees that the hospital should not be forced to provide medical intervention to stop any potential pregnancy. He proposes that they ask the municipal authorities for an exemption from the requirement if they would pledge to provide counseling to rape victims coming to their emergency room including information to the effect that the hospital does not provide any services that could lead to an interruption of any possible pregnancy. This would leave the patient free to seek such service elsewhere.

Dr. DeCicco is not satisfied with the suggestion because she objects to being put in a position where she would have to counsel patients or refer patients to services where the end result was possibly going to be an interruption of a pregnancy. She is beginning to feel that she can no longer practice what she considers responsible medicine without violating the law. Should society provide some escape for Dr. DeCicco? If not, should she violate a law that she objects to so strongly?

COMMENTARY
J. David Bleich

Much of the current debate concerning abortion practices is clouded by a failure to distinguish between the legal and moral issues involved. *Roe v. Wade*, the Supreme Court decision governing abortion statutes, established a "right to privacy" insofar as performance of abortions is concerned and serves to prevent governmental authorities from prohibiting such procedures. There is absolutely nothing in that decision that *requires* a physician to perform an abortion. The physician retains freedom of conscience and freedom of religious practice either to perform or not to perform an abortion. The physician, no less than the mother, enjoys a constitutional "right to privacy." Any municipal ordinance *mandating* that the physician destroy a fetus upon the demand of the mother would probably be held unconstitutional by the courts.

A municipal ordinance requiring that a rape victim be informed of the medical options available to her and be provided with information concerning availability of abortion services is an entirely different matter both legally and morally. Legally, failure to provide such information, even in the absence of a legal requirement to do so, may constitute malpractice. As such, the rape victim may have a cause of action to recover damages from the physician. That, however, is a civil matter upon which the legality of the municipal ordinance has no bearing. Morally there is a conflict between the patient's moral autonomy, which can be exercised only if she has an informed awareness of the viable options available to her, and the physician's conscientious objection to providing information which, from his or her moral vantage point, can be used only in an immoral manner.

There may be a way to escape from between the horns of this dilemma. Although, by virtue of the tenets of her faith, Dr. DeCicco cannot refer patients to another medical institution for interruption of pregnancy she may well be able to provide information with regard to the options available. While I am certainly not qualified to pass upon matters of canon law, it would appear that merely providing information constitutes no more than "remote material assistance" to an immoral act which, from the vantage point of Catholic morality, is justified when "serious cause" exists for doing so. Loss of one's profession is recognized as constituting not merely "serious cause" but "grave cause."

Moreover, the prospect of St. Mary's Hospital being forced to close its emergency care department—with all that such a step would imply in terms of availability of treatment in life-threatening situations—is certainly "proportionate reason" for rendering what is no more than "remote material assistance." Whether civil authorities have a moral (or legal) right to require even remote assistance to an act perceived as immoral by some citizens is an entirely different question.

More significantly, the ethical problem posed in this case study may be more apparent than real. Assuredly, if such is her conviction, the physician, as a moral agent, is obligated not only to refrain from destroying the fetus but also to urge her patient not to seek an abortion elsewhere. Surely, any intelligent person living in our society should consider it not only likely but also highly probable that the rape victim will leave the emergency room of St. Mary's and proceed to seek aid in terminating her pregnancy elsewhere. Under such circumstances, it would be no more than proper for the physician to present the moral case mitigating against such a course of action. In the very act of offering moral counsel—which the physician should feel morally compelled to do even in the absence of a legal requirement—the physician will have provided the legally required information.

But let us assume that there is no way for the physician to provide this information without violating her moral principles. Such convictions deserve the respect of both society and the law. Any attempt to compel compliance with a law perceived by a responsible segment of society to be inconsistent with the moral code to which it subscribes, regardless of the goal which such a law seeks to further, is an attack upon morality itself. Violation of conscience very quickly leads to a breakdown of conscience—and surely there are few goals, if any, whose benefits outweigh the societal benefits of preservation of a sense of moral conscience.

Instead of tampering with Dr. DeCicco's conscience the municipal authorities would be better advised to embark upon a public information program designed to provide all citizens with pertinent information regarding available health care facilities and the policies adhered to by the various medical institutions in the community. They would also do well to provide information in an objective, dispassionate manner with regard to the moral perspective upon which the policies of such institutions are grounded. Indeed, it would be wise—and fair—to require St. Mary's Hospital to post a notice in a conspicuous place in the emergency room which would inform patients of the hospital's policy with regard to services leading to termination of pregnancy.

Should a conflict between law and morality remain, there is no question that Dr. DeCicco's duty to conscience is such that she cannot act in a manner which the law prescribes. The only options available to her are civil disobedience or abandonment of the practice of medicine. Under the circumstances I believe disobedience of the law would be morally defensible. One must remember that, for Dr. DeCicco, feticide is indistinguishable from homicide. Who would be unsympathetic to disobedience of a legal requirement to counsel homicide?

Indeed, the constitutionality of an ordinance requiring a physician to provide such information is open to question. Enforcement of such a requirement under these circumstances would require the demonstration of a "compelling state interest." It is not at all certain that such an interest exists. I would therefore urge Dr. DeCicco to pursue the matter in the courts. It may readily be argued that she has a moral obligation to do so. Historically, the courts have been extremely reluctant to permit the law to tamper with religious or moral convictions. May they have the good judicial sense to refuse to do so in this case as well.

COMMENTARY
Carol A. Tauer

Dr. DeCicco believes that the law requires her to participate in a morally objectionable practice in order to protect the rights of the rape victim. The rape victim's rights have already been gravely violated by an invasion of her body about which she had no choice. After the rape, it is essential that her right to choose be restored to her, that she be given the opportunity to decide how she will deal with the actual and potential consequences of the rape and with the weighty moral issues involved.

Beyond emergency care, the rape victim's primary right at this time is self-determination. But in order to exercise this right, she needs information about the options that are open to her. This information is standard scientific and medical knowledge. It is well-known to those who are educated and advantaged in our society. By providing the information to all rape victims, a doctor or hospital is simply equalizing opportunity, the opportunity of all rape victims to make an informed choice.

Dr. DeCicco is not being asked to convince the victim to take the "morning-after" pill. In providing information, she is in the position of a teacher who must clearly outline the scientific aspects of biomedical procedures that raise ethical questions. It is appropriate for either the teacher or the doctor to express her own moral or value judgment. But she cannot make this judgment for others. And in depriving the rape victim of information, the doctor is attempting to prevent the victim from making a particular choice, thus depriving her of moral freedom.

Although the hospital and doctor ought to provide the information the law requires, if they have serious moral objections to prescribing the "morning-after" pill, this should not be required of them. The hospital has a clearly stated position against abortion, and it regards intervention in the period between conception and implantation to be morally equivalent to abortion. In taking this position, the hospital has the support of the Ethical and Religious Directives for Catholic Health Facilities issued by the National Conference of Catholic Bishops. It should therefore be possible for the hospital to obtain an exemption from the specific requirement of providing the "morning-after" pill.

If Dr. DeCicco cannot bring herself to give the information and counseling required by the law and approved by the administrator, she should ask to be removed from her present position and assigned elsewhere in the hospital.

Beyond these immediate decisions, however, both Dr. DeCicco and the administrator should recognize that they may be wrong in their moral evaluation of the "morning-after" pill. For at least ten years, numerous Catholic theologians have been questioning the inviolability of the embryo during the first two or three weeks after fertilization. They respect it as nascent human life, but believe that it does not require all the protections given to an individual human being. For a serious reason, for example, the prevention of pregnancy due to rape, the early embryo could be deprived of the environment it would need for continued development. Dr. DeCicco and the administrator have the obligation to become familiar with this theological literature in order to inform their own moral judgments.

Another point for them to consider is the phrase "morally equivalent." In what sense is use of the "morning-after" pill morally equivalent to a sixth-month abortion? We may say that the energy crisis is the moral equivalent of war, and that chain smoking is the moral equivalent of suicide. Such expressions are at least partly figurative, and to take them literally leads to moral confusion. Catholic adolescents of my generation experienced this confusion on being taught that any deliberate sexual arousal was morally equivalent to premarital sexual intercourse. Sorting actions into large, all-encompassing categories is not a good way of making moral judgments. *Is* taking the "morning-after" pill in case of rape truly as great an evil as obtaining an abortion at six months? To say *yes* seems to indicate a rigid adherence to set rules and categories without regard for the morally relevant distinction that obtains.

If Dr. DeCicco and the hospital recognize that there is a moral distinction, that even if both acts are evil, one is a lesser evil than the other, then they ought to be interested in preventing the greater evil. Almost any woman who becomes pregnant after a rape will at least consider the possibility of having an abortion. Unless she is sexually ignorant, she will be thinking about the possibility of pregnancy and abortion when she is in the hospital emergency room. Dr. DeCicco claims that she does not want to be part of any practice where the end result might be an abortion. But in not allowing the patient to choose the "morning-after" pill, the doctor is limiting the patient's options so that the end result may well be a direct abortion. If the patient does not want to go through with a pregnancy, the doctor ought to counsel the least evil way of terminating pregnancy, and the more immediate the intervention, the better: physically, psychologically, and morally.

21

Selective Termination of Pregnancy

Ms. Q. is a thirty-year-old woman who is pregnant for the first time, having spent several years in a local infertility program. She had been treated previously with clomiphene citrate, a fertility drug that increases the incidence of multiple births among those who subsequently become pregnant from 1 percent to 8 percent. Dr. G., the physician who prescribed the drug, had indicated to the patient that its use involved "some risk of multiple gestation."

At nine weeks gestation, ultrasound reveals the presence of triplets. After discussion with her husband, Ms. Q. asks Dr. G. to terminate two of the fetuses. She says she really wants to have a child and "be a good mother," but doesn't feel capable of caring for more than one child at a time. Even though all three fetuses appear healthy, her preference is to abort all rather than have triplets.

A technique similar to amniocentesis (in which the uterine cavity is entered) has been used to terminate selectively a defective fetus, when a serious fetal anomaly, such as Down syndrome, occurs in a multiple gestation. This technique could be used to terminate two of the triplets, but it entails an incremental risk of miscarriage. Legally, Dr. G. could: (1) terminate the pregnancy through a standard method of abortion; (2) selectively terminate the gestation of two of the triplets; (3) refuse to terminate the pregnancy, with transfer of care to a physician who is willing to do so . Should Dr. G. acquiesce in Ms. Q.'s request? Is this request morally valid?

COMMENTARY
Angela R. Holder

The central question in this case is, "What are the limits of a physician's duty to do what the patient wants?" No physician is legally obliged to provide treatment he or she deems unwise, dangerous, or not indicated simply because a patient wants it. Dr. Q. is no more required to abort one, some, or all of Ms.. Q.'s fetuses than a physician is to give human growth hormone to a normal-sized child whose parents want a basketball star. The legal doctrine of informed consent means that a patient has the right to choose among reasonable medical alternatives; it does not mean that the physician must perform the chosen procedure if he or she thinks it is ill-advised. In case of necessary medical care, the physician may have a duty to refer the patient to someone who will comply with the patient's requests, but the condition of "necessary" would not apply to Ms. Q.'s situation.

Under normal circumstances, Ms. Q. would have no trouble finding a physician who would perform a standard abortion, and, at this stage in the pregnancy, she has every legal right to decide to have one. (Since family finances have apparently presented no impediment to several years of infertility treatment, presumably she can afford this procedure.)

However, the procedure for selective abortion presents about a 45 percent risk of loss of all fetuses. There is also a risk that triplets will be sufficiently premature to have serious difficulties—many are born at thirty weeks gestation. While some obstetricians might be willing to abort one fetus with a severe disorder, not many would agree to undertake a procedure still in its developmental stage only because a woman decided she was incapable of being a good mother to three children.

Ms. Q. had been in the infertility program for several years. That experience surely should have presented opportunity for adequate counseling about the possibility of multiple births, since they cannot be predicted or prevented when fertility drugs are used, and what such a possibility would mean in terms of expenditure of energy and finances. In advance of her pregnancy, Ms. Q.

should have been able to think through for herself whether she could cope with this eventuality. Did she really want a baby, or was she in this program to satisfy the desires of other people—her husband, for example, or her parents who wanted a grandchild? Does she have any idea how much energy one baby requires? Several years of treatment should have provided Ms. Q. with better counseling, rather than leaving her in this dilemma, since it was a reasonably foreseeable result of doing what she wanted to do.

Dr. G. should attempt to mobilize family and child care resources (including her husband, who presumably can learn to change diapers as well as she can) and facilitate contacts with mothers of triplets to find out how they cope with three children the same age. Perhaps Ms. Q. will discover that the situation is not as difficult as she assumes and continue the pregnancy.

As Oscar Wilde wrote, "In this world, there are only two tragedies. One is not getting what one wants, and the other is getting it."

COMMENTARY
Mary Sue Henifin

Unlike the "old woman who lived in a shoe, she had so many children she didn't know what to do," Ms. Q. has requested an available medical intervention as a solution. The question of whether Dr. G. should acquiesce in her request for partial termination of her multiple pregnancy is one that tests the limits of a physician's obligation to respect patient autonomy.

Self-determination and autonomy apply to a patient's "negative" right to refuse as well as her "positive' right to choose among beneficial procedures, yet these principles do not guarantee the right to demand nonbeneficial or harmful treatment. Before providing a requested treatment, the physician should determine whether the patient can define a recognizable problem that medical treatment may benefit. If a requested treatment is beneficial, it should be among the options offered to the patient.

In this case, triplet pregnancy presents many recognizable problems to which partial termination is one solution. Once a benefit can be identified, the pregnant woman is in the best position to weigh the alternatives. Each woman brings her own ethical principles to decisions about her pregnancy based on her own life circumstances.

In an ideal relationship, physician and patient share their mutual knowledge and perspectives until they arrive at an agreed upon course of treatment *prior* to commencing therapy. In the case of inducing ovulation with clomiphene citrate, the discussion should include the eightfold increase in the risks of multiple gestation and accompanying maternal and fetal complications, not merely the vague warning provided by Dr. G. that there is "some risk."

What information does Ms. Q. need to make an autonomous decision? First, the physician must present those options that can provide benefit and discuss their risks. Three options could benefit Ms. Q.: carrying the fetuses to term, complete abortion, or partial termination. A triplet pregnancy is by definition high risk, with stillbirth rates three times higher than for singleton pregnancy and perinatal morality rates almost twenty times higher. Multiple gestation increases the strain on the pregnant woman's circulatory, renal, and endocrine systems, and she is more likely to suffer from hypertension, anemia, respiratory distress, preeclampsia, placenta previa, and placenta abrupta.

The fetuses are also at increased risk. The majority of multiple births are preterm; and intrauterine growth retardation is the rule, caused by placental insufficiency and crowding. Labor and delivery are particularly risky. Moreover, children born of multiple gestation have higher rates of congenital disabilities and development problems after birth.

Finally, multiple gestation severely disrupts the life of the pregnant woman and her family. Bedrest is usually prescribed beginning in the third trimester and lengthy hospital stays may be required for both mother and newborns. Depression and, in rare cases, suicide have been reported to accompany multiple births as families try to cope with the caretaking, social, and economic pressures. Although support groups exist, such as The Triplet Connection in California and Central New Jersey Mothers of Multiples, reproductive choice may be circumscribed by inadequate access to medical coverage, housing, child care, and other necessities.

Once risks have been identified, the physician should avoid paternalism and respect the patient's evaluation of her own unique circumstances. Just as it would be unethical for Dr. G. to pressure Ms Q. to abort because of the *known* risks of multiple gestation, it would be wrong to try and pressure her to forgo partial termination because of alternative risks. Ms. Q.'s constitutionally protected right to privacy, including the right to make procreative decisions, supports her right to weigh the available options and their outcomes in selecting a course of treatment. Even when more accurate data are available on the relative risks of multiple gestation, abortion, and partial termination, privacy and procreative liberty must extend to protect the pregnant woman's choices. Dr. G. should either respect Ms. Q.'s decision or transfer her care to a competent physician who is willing to do so.

Ms. Q.'s case illustrates how the development of new reproductive techniques leads to technological imperatives: If a technology exists it will be used. The critical focus is usually on the morality of "consumer demand." A more direct approach would examine the moral responsibility of researchers who develop and promote new reproductive technologies like selective termination.

Selected Bibliography

Part Two: Reproductive Rights and Technologies

Andrews, Lori B. *New Conceptions: A Consumer's Guide to the Newest Infertility Treatments*, revised. New York: Ballantine Books, 1985.
Bayles, Michael D. *Reproductive Ethics*. Englewood Cliffs, NJ: Prentice-Hall, 1984.
Callahan, Sidney, and Callahan, Daniel. *Abortion: Understanding Differences*. New York: Plenum Press, 1984.

Cohen, Sherrill, and Taub, Nadine, eds. *Reproductive Laws for the 1990s*. Cliffton, NJ: Humana Press, 1989.

Elias, Sherman, and Annas, George J. *Reproductive Genetics and the Law*. Chicago: Year Book Medical Publishers, 1987.

Gostin, Larry, ed. *Surrogate Motherhood: Politics and Privacy*. Bloomington, IN: Indiana University Press, 1990.

Kass, Leon R. *Toward a More Natural Science: Biology and Human Affairs*. New York: Free Press, 1985.

Mattingly, Susan S. "The Maternal-Fetal Dyad: Exploring the Two-Patient Obstetric Model," *Hastings Center Report* 22, no.1 (1992): 13–18.

McCormick, Richard A. *How Brave a New World? Dilemmas in Bioethics*. New York: Doubleday, 1981.

Noonan, John T., Jr., ed. *The Morality of Abortion*. Cambridge: Harvard University Press, 1970.

Rothman, Barbara Katz. *The Tentative Pregnancy: Prenatal Diagnosis and the Future of Motherhood*. New York: Viking, 1986.

Steinbock, Bonnie."The Relevance of Illegality," *Hastings Center Report* 22, no.1 (1922): 19–22.

Thomson, Judith Jarvis."A Defense of Abortion," *Philosophy and Public Affairs* 1, no.1 (Fall 1971): 47–66.

Walters, LeRoy. "Human In Vitro Fertilization: A Review of the Ethical Literature," *Hastings Center Report* 9, no. 4 (August 1979): 23–43.

Warnock, Mary A. *A Question of Life: The Warnock Report on Human Fertilisation and Embryology*. Oxford: Basil Blackwell, 1985.

Death and Dying

INTRODUCTION

Among the most significant questions we face are those concerning our own death—its time, and place, and manner. Advances in scientific medicine have made it possible to prolong life significantly, but they may exact a great cost as well. Decisions either to withhold potentially life-sustaining treatments or to withdraw treatment once it has been started are among the most difficult that patients, their families, and their physicians must confront. Like decisions at the beginning of life, those at its end raise questions of personal values and goals well beyond concerns about what *can* be done clinically.

The cases in section one—"Decisions about Death"—explore tensions that can arise when patients, families, and caregivers must choose among treatment alternatives that they value differently, for different reasons. Thus, patients or their families may press doctors to give treatment that physicians judge to be clinically inappropriate, such as cardiopulmonary resuscitation (CPR) for a very ill elderly patient whose heart has stopped beating. How should we resolve dilemmas when patients, concerned about the quality of their remaining lives, choose to forgo life-sustaining treatment their loved ones would have them accept? Are parents helped or hindered as decision makers by being able to hold and nurture their severely ill newborn? Are decisions to commit suicide always irrational; should emergency room staff always intervene to save the life of someone who has attempted suicide?

In section two—"Refusal of Life-Sustaining Treatment and Euthanasia"—cases delve into patients' requests to be allowed to "die with dignity." When there is hope that continued treatment will enable a patient to have a reasonable quality of life, for example, how should caregivers respond to his request that painful therapy be stopped? How can we be sure that demands to be allowed to die express patients' sincere, considered decisions and not outside influences—subtle or otherwise—brought to bear? For example, when a gay man with AIDS says he does not "deserve" to take up a bed in the hospital, can we be sure that his altruism is not motivated by guilt about a lifestyle of which many disapprove?

Cultural factors shape decisions in other ways too: while respirators and feeding tubes may be considered "ordinary" care in the United States, they may be seen as "extraordinary" in the United Kingdom, with very different consequences for decision making. So too, family members in China, with its strong cultural tradition of filial devotion, may be very hesitant not to treat a loved one, even when the patient would refuse care, or the available treatment would ultimately be of little benefit. Finally, when dying is prolonged and painful ought physicians ever to be permitted to practice euthanasia, actively to hasten death?

Questions of how, and when, we die are becoming more acute precisely as medicine opens new choices to us as individuals and as a society. The answers we find are at the heart of our medical ethics and the moral community we share.

22
Does "Doing Everything"Include CPR?

Fred Walker, ninety years old and retired since 1955, was admitted to a community hospital with bronchial pneumonia, advanced pulmonary edema, urinary tract infection, and anemia. Mr. Walker responded to treatment initially but then his condition worsened. Mrs. Walker asked the attending physician to do "everything possible" for her husband and assured him that they were able to pay for the costs of treatment not covered by Medicare.

On the morning of the fourteenth day in the hospital, Mr. Walker's physician visited him and found his condition unchanged. Although he was not improving, Mr. Walker was alert and asked, "Am I all right, doctor?" Fifteen minutes later a nurse entered the room and found that Mr. Walker was not breathing and that all vital signs were absent. She summoned the doctor, who immediately decided not to attempt to resuscitate Mr. Walker. The cause of death was recorded as ventricular fibrillation.

According to hospital officials it is the institution's policy to make an all-out effort to revive all unresponsive patients. Like other hospitals, this one has a "code"—usually a series of numbers or a color—for summoning staff members with portable defibrillators and other resuscitation equipment to the bedside of a patient in cardiac arrest. "Code Blue"—as it is called at this hospital—is known only to insiders and can thus be called without alarming other patients and visitors. But physicians may also issue "no code" orders. That is, in certain circumstances they may direct staff not to resuscitate a patient should cardiac arrest occur. Patients, however, are usually not told about coding. "It would make already anxious patients and relatives even more fearful," one official explained. "They don't need to know about it. They will be coded anyway. People should assume whatever care is needed is going to be given."

Mr. Walker's physician and the hospital officials maintained that Mr. Walker was coded, but both conceded that "code blue" was not called. Mr. Walker's physician argued, "Doing 'everything' for a patient in my mind does not include cardiopulmonary resuscitation (CPR). In Mr. Walker's case it might mean doing nothing." According to the physician, Mr. Walker was not sent to the intensive care unit (ICU) for two reasons. There was a shortage of beds in the unit and Mr. Walker "didn't seem like he belonged there" because he was not acutely ill. "When it comes to resuscitating, it's reasonable for a man in his fifties or sixties, but criminal to try to resuscitate in [Mr. Walker's] age group to prolong life a week at the most, given his condition. I don't see any sense in calling code blue with a ninety-year-old man who has no future to look forward to. That's doing him a disservice and increasing his hospital costs."

Mrs. Walker disagreed. Upon being informed that no emergency measures were taken in her husband's case, Mrs. Walker said that that decision was against her wishes. "Doing everything," she said, "is the difference between life and death. The doctor was playing God when he decided he should not try to save my husband. You're not playing God when you've tried everything and exhausted all methods. All I wanted was for them to try. My husband knew how to love and be loved. That was his quality of life. That suited him and it suited me."

Should patients and their families be informed about coding policies? Did Mr. Walker's doctor act ethically in going against Mrs. Walker's wishes?

COMMENTARY
Ronald A. Carson

The routine introduction of life-prolonging technologies into medical care raises questions about the morality of extending life at all costs. Physicians are aware, as perhaps never before, of the centrality of values in clinical judgment and of the need to acknowledge and resolve conflicts in values that arise in medical practice. This is, in the main, a laudable development. But it may, on occasion, have unfortunate consequences, as in this case.

There is no reason not to assume good faith on the part of Mr. Walker's physician. My impression is that he was benevolently motivated when, upon being summoned by the nurse, he decided not to attempt to resuscitate Mr. Walker. Considerations of social worth may have entered into his decision. A young or middle-aged person would almost certainly have been resuscitated in similar circumstances, even in view of the possibility that irreversible brain damage had been sustained. Whether such considerations should enter a decision in cases like these can be debated. What is clear, however, is that to act contrary to the expressed wishes of a competent adult who was speaking on her husband's behalf, is to act immorally.

The physician's reasons for not putting Mr. Walker in an ICU prior to the final acute incident do not bear up under close scrutiny. Three reasons are mentioned. The first—that "doing everything" might mean "doing nothing"— is patently absurd. The second—that Mr. Walker was not acutely ill—is difficult to assess on the basis of the information given but, at the least, this assertion is inconsistent with the claim that, following an initial rally, Mr. Walker's condition worsened. The third reason—that it would have been "criminal" to try to resuscitate Mr. Walker—is the most confused.

The physician cites several factors in support of this last claim: the patient's age, his physical condition, the quality of his life, and hospital costs. But Mr. Walker's advanced age did not make him less worthy of care. His debilitated condition was of central importance in selecting a course of treatment but is not in itself sufficient to justify withholding treatment. Judgments about the quality of Mr. Walker's life were, as Mrs. Walker said, his (and hers) to make. Hospital costs, while inevitably entering into decisions of this sort, appear not to be at issue here since the Walkers were able to pay for services.(Conceivably, Mrs. Walker had an exaggerated notion of what could reasonably be done for her husband, as evidenced by her desire that the doctor "exhaust all methods," but that merely indicates the deep disparity between her expectations and those of the physician.)

There is irony (and perhaps some mean-spiritedness) in the hospital official's statement that entering patients should not be bothered with the details of resuscitation policy but should assume that they will be well cared for and coded if necessary. Mrs. Walker made that assumption. To say that her husband was coded but that the code was not called is a fine distinction—or a mincing of words. Mr. Walker was a victim of reverse moral discrimination motivated, I presume, by the wish not to prolong the dying of a very sick old man. The old man, however, wanted to live and expected to be treated and apparently his wife was not made aware that he was dying. A decision to resuscitate might have prolonged his life, or at least spared his wife unnecessary anguish.

COMMENTARY
Mark Siegler

Should health professionals perform CPR on every patient who is about to die in a hospital? This approach—equal CPR for all regardless of medical condition or patient preference—is indefensible, counterintuitive, and unethical, and would signal the ultimate transformation of medicine from an art based upon clinical discretion into an unthinking, unfeeling bureaucratic system.

Preserving or prolonging life is one, perhaps even a central goal of medicine. But it it not the only goal. In the case of the terminally ill, many physicians and patients often prefer alternative, attainable goals such as the relief of symptoms and the preservation of function. Which particular goals are preferred from a medical encounter (a value matter) should be determined jointly by the physician and the patient, but it is important to note that preferences and desires will be constrained by the medical-scientific realities (a factual matter) of what can be achieved. If dying without being accorded the full ritual of a CPR effort is regarded as the ultimate horror (the twentieth-century equivalent of the morbid nineteenth-century fear of being buried alive, as in Poe's *The Cask of Amontillado*), health professionals might have an obligation to explore any chance, however remote, of saving patients from such a fate. But I believe the existence of a medical technique does not and should not mandate its use in every case, nor should it necessarily generate a presumption favoring its use.

CPR is a relatively new emergency medical technique, developed originally to prevent sudden and unexpected death in the life-threatening situation of cardiac arrest. The standards for CPR issued by a 1980 national conference support this view (*JAMA* 1980: 244:453). It is the physician's responsibility to decide which patients can possibly be treated with which medical techniques, and it is the joint responsibility of the physician and patient to decide which should be so treated. CPR decisions should be examined in this context. For example, I believe that CPR is often not indicated in patients for whom vigorous intensive therapy has not been successful. It is unlikely that a final *pro forma* pounding on the chest or administration of one or several electrical shocks will reverse their progressive downhill course. Even if CPR is temporarily successful, such patients rarely regain consciousness and usually suffer a second arrest.

The principal ethical grounds for making a decision not to resuscitate a patient should be the sound medical judgment that the patient's death from the primary disease is imminent and that further treatment for the primary disease is futile. Although the medical details in this case are sketchy, the principal factor in the physician's decision not to perform CPR seemed to be Mr. Walker's deteriorating clinical condition. After Mr. Walker died, the physician invoked many reasons (some extraneous and some downright inappropriate) to defend his decision not to perform CPR, but this seems to be his central point: "When it comes to resuscitating, it's reasonable for a man in his fifties or sixties, but criminal to try to resuscitate in that age group *to prolong life a week at most, given his condition*" (italics added).

If Mr. Walker's chances for survival were poor prior to the arrest, they were infinitesimal afterwards. I am not aware of a single case report of a successful resuscitation in a patient such as Mr. Walker (i.e., unwitnessed arrest in a ninety-year-old person with multiple serious underlying medical problems).

A second and independent reason to decide not to resuscitate a patient would be if this were the stated preference of an autonomous, self-determining, competent adult. Unfortunately, we know very little about Mr. Walker's wishes or whether, in the face of serious illness, he retained the capacity to process information and to make choices concerning his care.

We know considerably more about Mrs. Walker's wishes. Her motto was: "Do everything!" The question arises: how much legal and ethical weight should be placed on the statements of the angry widow or on her preferences before her husband died? Family members have no legal authority to make decisions on behalf of patients unable to make decisions for themselves, unless such family members have been granted guardianship powers by a judge or by a legislative statute (only three states—Maine, Idaho, and North Carolina—have such a statute).* However, the statements of family members may be ethically important for two reasons. First, they may (but do not necessarily) reflect the personal preferences of the patient who is unable to express them. Second, the common practice of turning to family members acknowledges that we exist in communities of concern and that those who care most about us ought to have a special moral authority to assist in making decisions about us when we are no longer able to do so for ourselves. I sense that Mrs. Walker's statements,

---

*The situation has changed dramatically in recent years; at least sixteen states and the District of Columbia have now enacted legislation empowering family members as surrogate decision-makers.

however, reflect her personal wishes and preferences and not necessarily her husband's. Further, she appeared to be ignorant of medicine's limitations and nourished unrealistic expectations regarding CPR.

Perhaps the physician could be faulted for not having raised the issue of CPR directly or tangentially with Mr. or Mrs. Walker when he first believed the patient's condition was deteriorating and was likely to terminate in a cardiac arrest. Presumably, he could have used the occasion to gently inform them of the prognosis and instruct them on medicine's limitations (including, but not restricted to, CPR technology).

On reflection, however, *perhaps* the physician acted rightly in not raising this matter with Mr. Walker (even if Mr. Walker were competent). If the physician knew (within limits of uncertainty that characterize all medical knowledge) that CPR offered Mr. Walker no possible benefit, the patient's preferences would not have been germane.

Our CPR policies are enmeshed in rules, regulations, and procedures that minimize discretion and maximize bureaucratic bumbling. Some believe that placing the burden for such decisions on patients by invoking autonomy and self-determination will resolve the matter, but let me assure such legalists that the resolution will exist only on paper and not on hospital wards. This arena demands clinical discretion, a discerning judgment reached by the patient and physician after due consideration of all the patient's life (and death) circumstances.

In Mr. Walker's case, the decision not to resuscitate was made by his personal physician who came to his bedside immediately upon being summoned, and discovered that his patient was pulseless and without respiration and might have been so for a period of up to fifteen minutes. In these circumstances, who would have been in a better position to decide on whether to resuscitate? Surely not a code team, or the nurse, or Mr. Walker, or Mr. Walker's wife! The physician acted in the best traditions of equity—with reasonableness and responsiveness—in reaching a judgment based upon discretion not to resuscitate.

23
Surgical Risks and Advance Directives

Mrs. P. is a seventy-six-year-old woman with osteoporosis and a failed left hip prosthesis. In addition, she has severe chronic asthmatic bronchitis. The management of her lung disease has been hampered by her allergy to theophylline, which is one of the mainstays of treatment. As a result, she has had increasing difficulty walking and confinement to a wheelchair is imminent.

When surgery to replace the prosthesis was recommended, Mrs. P. expressed concern about the possibility of ending up after the operation dependent on a ventilator, possibly comatose. She feared that her resources would be depleted for medical expenses. Little or nothing would be left to pass on to her children.

She was willing to have an operation only if she could prepare a legal document that, in the event of prolonged ventilator dependence, would require her physician to remove her from the ventilator after a specified time (for example, two weeks). Should the surgeon agree to be bound by Mrs. P.'s instructions, or should he refuse her request even if doing so means that she will not have the surgery that might prevent increasing disability?

COMMENTARY
Daniel H. Lederer

In agreeing to surgery, a patient, while hoping for a favorable outcome, must accept the risk of a spectrum of adverse effects. These can range from a lack of benefit at one end to permanent disability or death at the other. The surgeon must also accept an element of risk, for the price he pays for failure may include an unhappy, angry patient; colleagues to whom he must explain major complications or death; and, possibly, malpractice litigation with its personal and professional penalties.

In this case the patient is unwilling to accept the risk of an unlikely but possible event, specifically that she may become dependent on a ventilator after surgery. Her attempted solution is to prepare a legally binding document that requires the surgeon to discontinue the treatment after a specified interval. Were the surgeon to accept such an agreement, the patient presumably would be willing to proceed with the operation. But such an agreement does not eliminate the risk; rather, it transfers it to the surgeon, who in accepting it may be placing himself in legal jeopardy. Of course, the patient's signed document may protect the surgeon should the issue come to court, but it cannot prevent the initiation of legal action by those who might interpret the surgeon's actions as collusion in suicide.

Beyond the legal considerations, such an agreement undermines basic principles that should guide every doctor-patient encounter. The first is the dictum of nonmaleficence, *primum non nocere*. With this patient, the risk of prolonged respiratory failure requiring mechanical support of breathing is low, but should it occur, one cannot predict *in advance* the point at which the likelihood of reversibility will seem unacceptably small to either the surgeon or the patient. In other words, a judgment regarding a patient's potential for recovery requires an assessment at that point, not days or weeks ahead.

Nor can one be sure what the patient would have wanted. If Mrs. P. does become ventilator-dependent, it will still be difficult to know whether she would have followed her own directive once a hypothetical scenario becomes reality. In this case, to discontinue ventilator support when the patient's respiratory failure may still be reversible must be considered a harmful act.

The importance of the principle of reverence for life is perhaps self-evident. Although a physician is not required to prolong life at all costs regardless of circumstances, it is the physician's obligation to try to preserve life as long as such efforts, in his or her judgment, are in the patient's best interests. Many factors, including the emotional and financial costs to the patient as well as the patient's projected quality of life, must be considered. For the surgeon to agree to accept a document as a substitute for this delicate judgment is potentially to convert his role from protector to executioner.

The agreement proposed by the patient disregards a third principle, more subtle but equally important, that of mutual trust. It implies that the patient does not trust the surgeon to determine appropriately when treatment is no longer beneficial and then to act accordingly. And the surgeon, by agreeing to the document, contributes to an atmosphere of mistrust by saying, again by implication, that the patient or her family cannot be trusted to make a reasonable judgment regarding prolongation of treatment during the postoperative period. The presence of mutual trust *per se* does not guarantee a successful outcome of surgery, nor does its absence preclude such a result, but without a sense of mutual trust a patient would be ill-advised to embark on any dangerous diagnostic or therapeutic procedure.

For all these reasons the surgeon should refuse the patient's request. This refusal will not be without consequences. The patient will be deprived of an operation that would probably have been successful and the surgeon must wonder whether he has been needlessly rigid and authoritarian in denying the patient some control over her own treatment. But respect for patient autonomy has limits. Although from her own perspective the patient may only be asking to exercise her autonomy, in this case she is asking too much.

COMMENTARY
Dan W. Brock

It is now widely accepted that a competent patient is morally entitled to refuse any medical treatment, including life-sustaining treatment, that he or she judges to be unduly burdensome. Why then should the surgeon be reluctant to make an agreement with Mrs. P. that ventilator treatment will not be continued beyond a specified time?

One reason may be that the surgeon, like many physicians, is reluctant to be bound even by a patient's competent request due to fear of legal liability (criminal or civil) for stopping life-sustaining treatment. Court decisions and advance-directive legislation around the country, however, increasingly support the legal permissibility of physicians carrying out patients' decisions to stop life support.* Such fears could also be allayed if hospitals and other health care institutions develop clear policies for making and carrying out decisions to withdraw life-sustaining treatments.

*The U.S. Supreme Court recognized the right to refuse life-sustaining treatment in *Cruzan v. Director, Missouri Department of Health*, 497 U.S. 261 (1991).

The surgeon's concern in this case may not be legal, but moral. Many physicians believe that although it is morally permissible for patients to decide not to initiate life-sustaining treatment, it is not morally permissible to stop it once it has begun, or at least that stopping it is a graver matter requiring weightier reasons to be justified. While still common, this view is increasingly rejected, quite correctly I believe, by physicians, patients, and their families.

What should ultimately be determinative of whether any form of life-sustaining treatment is initiated *or* continued is the competent, informed, and voluntary decision of the patient.

Even if there is no important moral difference between not starting and stopping life support, physicians and others who must make or carry out such decisions commonly *feel* more responsible for the patient's death when forms of life support such as mechanical ventilation are stopped. As a result, they often find it psychologically harder to stop life support than not to start it.

The most obvious bad effect of the reluctance to stop life support once begun is overtreatment. The case of Mrs. P., however, dramatically illustrates another bad effect. For fear of indefinitely continuing, patients and others may be reluctant or unwilling to accept any treatment. That can result in denying patients treatment that may prove beneficial—either life support itself or other beneficial treatment, such as replacement of the hip prosthesis, without which Mrs. P. is doomed to live disabled.

This is a case in which physicians should be much more willing to agree to—indeed to recommend—time-limited trials of various forms of life support. Such an agreement would allay Mrs. P.'s fears and might reduce or eliminate the uncertainty about whether, and to what extent, the treatment will prove beneficial.

One final issue that this case raises is whether agreeing to be bound by the patient's instructions would unduly infringe on the surgeon's responsibility to exercise his professional judgment. Physicians are not obliged to act in ways that would violate their own moral or professional integrity just because their patients want them to do so. Nonetheless, physicians should be flexible regarding the alternative treatments they are willing to offer. In Mrs. P.'s case she seeks an agreement with her physician only that treatment will not be *imposed* on her in circumstances in which she does not wish to have it.

The surgeon may be concerned that the agreement Mrs. P. seeks could commit him later to stopping life-sustaining treatment when he judges that doing so is not in the patient's best interests. It would be reasonable, even desirable, for the surgeon to seek an agreement that puts not only a time limit on the use of mechanical ventilation, but that also, or even instead, specifies in some detail the circumstances in which life-sustaining treatment will be withdrawn.

Since one of Mrs. P.'s fears is being left on a respirator indefinitely in a co-matose state, it could be made a part of the agreement that respirator treatment will be withdrawn if she has suffered an irreversible lose of consciousness and is in a persistent vegetative state. If she so desired, the agreement might further stipulate that other forms of life support such as nutrition and hydration will be discontinued in those circumstances. The agreement should insure both that the physician's expertise and the patient's values are brought to bear on decisions. Mrs. P.'s desire for such an agreement need not be seen as displaying a lack of trust in the surgeon, but only a desire to insure that her own values will guide later decisions.

This is a case in which an advance directive from the patient is appropriate about her care, and/or about who will act as her surrogate decision maker should she be incompetent to decide for herself. A number of states, like my own Rhode Island, have enacted legislation to enable persons to appoint a so-called Durable Power of Attorney for Health Care. Encouraging advance planning by patients about their health care is desirable public policy and squarely within medicine's long tradition of serving patients' well-being.

24

Nurturing a Defective Newborn

Baby Girl S. was born at a small community hospital, four weeks prematurely, after an uncomplicated pregnancy. At birth the baby breathed spontaneously, but shortly thereafter had an apneic episode in which respiration stopped, and oxygen was required. She also had unusual face and hands and showed little spontaneous motor activity. For these reasons she was transferred to a neonatal intensive care unit. Physical examination showed findings consistent with trisomy 18, a serious genetic defect. The infant continued to have occasional episodes of apnea which over the next twenty-four hours became sufficiently severe so that respirator assistance was considered. A heart murmur was noted and signs of early heart failure (normally treated with a variety of medications) became evident.

Mr. and Mrs. S. came to the center thirty-six hours after the birth, having been told that Baby S. had multiple birth defects. They met with the pediatrician and geneticist caring for the baby. The infant's primary problem was explained (a chromosomal "accident" resulting in extra genetic material in all of the infant's cells, with diverse manifestations), the immediate difficulties outlined (short periods where the infant "forgot" to breathe, and a heart defect which was probably an opening between the major artery to the body and the large artery to the lungs, with resultant heart failure), the child's abnormal features described (small size, unusual facial features, and deformed hands), and the long-term outlook explored (profound retardation with very high probability of death within the first year).

Within the next day or two decisions will need to be made:

1. Should resuscitative efforts be continued when the baby "forgets" to breathe?

2. Should a respirator be used if that becomes necessary to maintain the baby's life?

3. Should medication to control the potentially life-threatening heart failure be instituted?
4. Should other routine care be given?
Before these decisions are made, should the parents see the baby? Should the physician encourage or discourage them in touching and holding the baby?

COMMENTARY
Richard M. Pauli

Questions about resuscitation, medication, and allowing to die seem appropriate questions to ask in the case of Baby S. This baby has, with any treatment a very limited life expectancy; should it survive, it has very little likelihood of evidencing even the most minimal level of "personhood" (that is, affective interaction with other persons). Since the parents should have primary responsibility for deciding about Baby S., they must be given accurate information about diagnosis and prognosis as well as predictions about the results of alternative courses of action. But another way of "knowing" about their baby is to see and touch her. This information, like the other pieces of data, must be made available to them by others. Therefore the attitude of the physician-counselor about nurturing will inevitably influence their own decision.

The physician-counselor may already have decided what medical care decisions are "preferred." Based on this judgment, he could opt for or against the parents seeing and touching the baby depending on which action he viewed as being most likely to result in accord with his "preferred" decision. That, of course, would be paternalism and deceit. But even if the physician-knows-best strategy is rejected, one is left with a difficult question. Does nurturing or non-nurturing, in itself, determine what decision the parents will make about resuscitation and medical support?

One could posit that all parents who first held and touched their infant would be *unable* to *ever* allow it to die. I don't think this is true for most parents. For example, decisions about adult incompetents are often made by family with a nurturing commitment of many years duration, and this is held to be the best way of "assuring loving solicitude for the patient" (the Quinlan case is a good example).

On the other hand, the horror of physical deformity might be anticipated to produce the opposite effect. The loving care evidenced by families with surviving but severely defective children indicates that this need not be an inevitable consequence.

The tension for the physician-counselor in the case of Baby S. is the conflict between an active and compassionate concern to minimize the suffering (through overwhelming guilt) of the parents, and the more passive responsibility to allow them to act autonomously. The physician's goal of minimizing parental suffering may be misplaced. Given the opportunity to nurture their defective child, parents will need to be supported through the guilt and grieving following a decision to withhold care, just as a family who elects to treat such a baby will require personal and community support. But attempts to allay their suffering by discouraging or refusing to let them see their baby is to engage in another form of paternalistic deception.

An informed decision requires accurate information, which we may assume the parents received in the case described. Does a knowledgeable decision require more than accurate information? Perhaps a well-considered choice *requires* experiential nurturing and a special kind of caring.

I think this other way of "knowing" is beneficial in making truly informed decisions, is a parental right, and is the best safeguard against arbitrary or frivolous decisions. The physician-counselor's role, then, is to encourage independence and autonomy. He should allow the parents themselves to decide whether to touch and hold the baby, but should encourage them to do so. Our aim should not be easy choices, but real ones.

COMMENTARY
Eric J. Cassell

The birth of this child is a tragedy. No matter what decision is made, or whether the child lives or dies, sorrow and suffering will follow. Therefore, there are two immediate problems: first, to make a decision about treatment and second, to minimize pain and suffering, because such relief is a necessary and legitimate object of medicine.

There are two alternative decisions to be made about her care. Either the infant should be permitted to die from the complications of her genetic defect and given care that will comfort her and relieve her suffering; or she should be kept alive until, beyond the limits of technological rescue, she ultimately dies, usually, we are told, within a year. If she is to be kept alive, the tools to be used—respirators, cardiac drugs, resuscitation—are merely technical details.

The case offers four alternative treatment levels, suggesting some ambivalence in the medical staff. Physicians may say, for example, "I believe she should be kept alive, but only if resuscitation for apnea is sufficient," or "only if therapy for heart failure is sufficient." This ambivalence makes the baby's failure to survive beyond a certain level of technological support the factor that determines outcome. Such decisions merely extend the wheel of fortune from conception into the neonatal intensive care unit and seemingly remove human agency—an understandable strategy, but an illusion nonetheless.

The parents have two choices. Either life is to be saved at all costs, or the decision to treat the baby is based on the infant's individual characteristics. If the parents believe life must be preserved at all costs, then their decision to treat is obvious. We would all sympathize with them and should do what is necessary to minimize their pain whether the infant survives or dies.

But if the decision is to be made on the basis of what the infant will become—her quality of life, her ultimate length of survival, economics, their ideas about parenthood, the effect on siblings or other family members, and future childbearing—then clear thinking and as much information as possible will be necessary. Clear thinking is the ability to weigh the evidence and the sets of competing needs and feelings as objectively as possible—to sort out wishes and desires from the facts of this infant's existence now and in the future.

This kind of thinking may be difficult for the mother who has given birth, just three days earlier, to a child that probably bitterly disappoints her nine months of dreams and wishes. Clear thinking will be made even harder by the inevitable feelings of guilt that accompany such a birth. The mother will wonder whether she did something to bring on the defects. Indeed, it is often easier to accept blame and guilt than to accept one's helplessness in the face of a capricious fate.

Now we come to the more pernicious question. Should the parents be encouraged to nurture the child—to touch her and to hold her—before making their decision?

If their decision is to save her life at all costs, what harm could come from *not* nurturing? The child will not lack such attention in the intensive care unit where nurses will hold and fondle her without the aversion that the inexperienced first feel with a defective child. What good would come from the physician *encouraging* the parents to hold and touch the infant before making the decision? They could ask to do so if they wished.

If the decision is to be based on a careful weighing of the baby's individual characteristics and the therapeutic possibilities, I cannot conceive how nurturing would clarify the mother's painful thinking or provide her with more "information." If the child lives there will be time enough for nurturance.

And if the child dies? Recent research confirms what even the most primitive people know: the bonding of parent and child occurs through the mother's nurturance and the child's response. If an infant is adopted at birth and after a period the biological mother wants the child returned, we feel sympathy for the adopting parents. Why? Because nurturing experience has formed a bond between the parents and their adopted child, so that the loss of the child is not merely the loss of a desirable object, but the loss of a loved one.

Why do pediatricians sometimes *want* the parents with newborns like Baby S. to nurture the child? Does the physician wish to teach them, starting here, how to be good parents? Or is there possibly something punitive in encouraging the parent to touch and hold? Does the staff share the magical beliefs on which the parents' feelings of guilt are based? Nurturing this infant will not change her defects or the conditions upon which a decision must be based. But nurturance and the establishment of a bond may make a decision to save the life a selfish one based on the parents' unwillingness to lose a loved one. Furthermore, nurturance will only add to the parents' suffering after her death. Is either a selfish decision or further suffering desirable?

25

A Suicide Attempt and Emergency Room Ethics

Michael Jellinek

After the car that he is driving at high speed hits a telephone pole, Mr. D. is brought to the hospital emergency room in serious condition. The physicians who examine him recommend surgery to repair a major internal hemorrhage. But the sixty-eight-year-old man refuses, saying that he wants to be "left alone to die." The physicians also learn that three weeks earlier Mr. D. was diagnosed as having carcinoma of the tongue. He has refused surgery for the lesion and has asked his own physician not to tell his wife that he has a fatal disease.

The hospital physicians believe that Mr. D. will die without surgery for the hemorrhage, and they call a psychiatric resident to evaluate the patient. Dr. M. interviews Mr. D. and finds him coherent, rational, and alert. Mr. D. describes himself as a man who values independence. He feels he has had a good professional life as an engineer, and a good personal life with his wife and two children. He expresses some sadness at his situation, but says, "I have had a good full life and now it's over."

Dr. M. suggests, and Mr. D. does not deny, that the automobile accident was a deliberate suicide attempt. What should Dr. M. recommend? That the patient's treatment refusal for immediate surgery be accepted as the act of a rational person? That the refusal not be honored, and a court order sought on the grounds that a presumed suicide attempt is per se evidence of mental illness?

COMMENTARY
Richard B. Brandt

The prevailing law governing the requirement of consent for surgery was stated by Justice Cardozo in 1914: "Every human being of adult years and sound mind has a right to determine what shall be done with his own body; and a surgeon who performs an operation without his patient's consent commits an assault.... This is true except in cases of emergency, where the patient is unconscious...." (*Schloendorff v. Society of New York Hospital*, 211 N.Y. 125, 129, 105 N.E. 92, 93).

There may, however, be exceptions if the patient's decision conflicts with overriding "state interests" in the preservation of life, the protection of the interests of innocent third parties, and the prevention of suicide. A refusal to accept treatment may not be suicide, since the patient himself does not set into operation a chain of causes leading to his death; but in this case the patient did (it appears) produce the injury for which surgery is contemplated. It is also unclear whether there could be a state interest in prolonging his life, in view of his disease, although another person's killing him would clearly be murder.

Further, some psychologists might claim that his sudden death in these circumstances could be psychologically damaging to his children, so there is a question about the impact on innocent third parties. Both the physician and court might wonder whether he had given careful thought to this potential damage. So it is not self-evident that a court would refuse to issue an order requiring the surgery. However, the specific question raised about this case is a limited one: whether the requirement of consent fails because the patient is not of sound mind.

In this case it would be sound legal practice, and seemingly morally unobjectionable and perhaps morally desirable, for the physician to seek a court order for surgery. The court order would provide a decision on some of these issues, and in any event it would clear the doctor and hospital of responsibility should questions arise later about failure to treat the patient.

Ought the physician/court to decide that a person's having made a suicide attempt is sufficient reason to judge him of unsound mind? Is a suicide attempt evidence of irrationality?

Let us consider some senses in which a person might show himself to be irrational:

1. If his objective is *manifestly* to *injure* himself, irrationality might be presumed (other things being equal, for example, if he is not attempting to help others by self-injury); but it is not manifestly a self-injury to attempt to shorten life in order to avoid the pain of death from tongue cancer. Evidently the present patient has decided that such action would not be self-injury.

2. A person is not rational if he fails to see the connection of means and ends, and refuses to take the means that are essential for his ends. The present patient is not in that condition; he sees precisely the consequences of his actions, and is acting so as to realize his end.

3. A person might be said to be irrational if his end is one he would not pursue if he knew, or anyway visualized clearly, what kind of thing his objective would be if realized. The patient appears not to be in this position. Tongue cancer is normally terminal, at least when not treated (it is so assumed in the description of the case), and a death from this cause is highly unpleasant to the patient and family.

4. A person might be said to be irrational if his end is one he would not pursue if he were not drunk, or seriously disoriented mentally, or in a highly emotional frame of mind. There is no evidence that the patient is in one of these conditions.

A judgment, then, that the patient is incompetent must rest on a conclusion about (1), that it is self-injury to shorten one's life in order to escape pain. It might be argued that the courts should try to prolong life no matter what. But courts have recently been more explicit in affirming what already seems to be public opinion: some treatment refusals are acceptable. (It is unlikely that any rational person would prefer to live fifteen minutes longer, in order to be burned to death, rather than shorten his life by taking a cyanide capsule, except on grounds of some moral conviction.)

Otherwise conservative philosophers such as Philippa Foot hold that life is not worth living in a situation of extreme senility or of intense pain ("Euthanasia," 6 *Philosophy and Public Affairs*, 1977, 85–112). It is true that courts have generally tried to avoid qualitative judgments of this sort. In the present case, however, the patient himself has made a qualitative judgment after careful deliberation to the effect that the kind of life that lies ahead of him, if his life is prolonged, is not what he wants. If the court declares him incompetent, it is, in effect, substituting for his view its own about what kind of life is worth living.

The moral issue might be put in broader terms: would society be better off in the long run if physicians and courts did what is in their power to do, require people to undergo a painful termination of their lives when they do not wish to and when there is no evidence of irrationality beyond the very fact that they have made a decision not to live longer? It is not easy to see what would be the gain. On the contrary, there is the loss of needless suffering by the patient, not to mention his family: and the individual is deprived of assurance that he is in control of his own destiny in matters of most importance to him and which affect others only in an incidental way.

COMMENTARY
Robert E. Litman

Dr. M., the psychiatric resident, should take action as follows:

1. He should notify Mrs. D., the patient's wife, and his children of the emergency. They should be interviewed by telephone and asked to come to the hospital;

2. Dr. M. should get in touch with a senior staff psychiatrist, preferably the chief of the service, and request an immediate consultation;

3. Dr. M. should initiate the legal process for a court order authorizing surgery.

If the patient demands his release from the hospital, the psychiatrist should be prepared to place him on a "hold" order for observation for mental disorder, because he is a danger to himself and to others. Another such suicide attempt might result in injury to a pedestrian.

Meanwhile, there should be a surgical consultation. If the surgeons find the patient's condition immediately life-threatening, then there is no time available for further persuasive efforts to obtain Mr. D.'s cooperation, nor sufficient time to obtain a court order. Given these emergency circumstances, the surgeons should proceed, trusting in the group consensus as a substitute for the consent of the patient, the family, and the court.

The hospital has an ethical and legal obligation to prevent further damage to Mr. D.'s life and health, and the patient has no ethical or moral right to demand that the emergency room doctors cooperate in his suicide efforts. By placing himself in the position of requiring emergency medical help to save his life, Mr. D. has forfeited his autonomy for the time being. In the emergency room, the doctors are properly immersed in, and bound by, the ethic of saving lives; and these physicians, together with the other emergency personnel, simply do not have the time or the training to challenge this ethic in order to make exceptions for individual cases.

This is true in general for suicide attempters, and it is true in particular for Mr. D. The scant data we have strongly suggests that Mr. D.'s recent behavior has not been rational. I would not be inclined to accept his statement, "I have had a good full life and now it's over," as a rational self-evaluation in the given context; but instead, I would suspect that the statement probably represents a delusion of hopelessness, the direct result of depressive mental illness. It is quite likely that the physicians will learn from the patient's wife that there was a noticeable change in the patient's attitude several months ago, a change possibly connected with one of life's important transitions, for example, forced retirement from his job. And his refusal to allow treatment for carcinoma of the tongue because it is a "fatal disease" is another sign of his irrational hopelessness.

Clinical experience suggests that with appropriate psychiatric treatment, including a combination of antidepressive drugs and psychotherapy, the patient will feel much more hopeful in a month.

We can expect that within a month or two, this patient will have regained his full autonomy. At that point, if he chose to commit suicide, he might still do so, choosing, I hope, a method with less potential danger to other persons. Suicide is fairly common in the United States. In California, 2 percent of all deaths are by suicide. A person who is rational and relatively unambivalent about committing suicide can usually find a decisive and effective method for ending his life. Mr. D., on the other hand, chose a suicide method that is unusual, even bizarre, suggesting a great deal of ambivalence on his part. Given this degree of ambivalence, quite typical of suicidal persons, and the excellent treatment for depression that is now available, it is reasonable to expect that the hospital personnel take appropriate action to preserve Mr. D. from further harm.

In principle, however, paternalistic action by physicians should be limited to emergencies, exceptional situations, and situations in which the use of authority is justified by the extreme difference in outcome that can be predicted from action versus inaction. For example, if a person has cut his or her wrists, and refuses remedial surgery, and the person's life is not in danger, I do not think that the surgeons are justified in immediately performing the reparative surgery on the grounds that a presumed suicide attempt is per se evidence of mental illness.

In summary, how Dr. M. should proceed depends on how acute the emergency is (i.e., how many hours will elapse before the threat to the patient's life becomes irreversible). If Dr. M. has time, he is urged to consult with the family and with other more senior psychiatrists and to use whatever time is available to persuade the patient to accept treatment, and failing this, to obtain court approval for emergency treatment. If there is no time, then doctors must proceed to remedial surgery with confidence in their own emergency room ethics. Although the patient's autonomy and self-determination is an important ethical value, Mr. D. has sacrificed his autonomy temporarily by placing himself in life-jeopardy in the emergency room, an eventuality which could reasonably have been predicted when he drove his car into a pole. If it turns out that there is no treatable mental illness, he will, at a later date, regain his autonomy and his capability of disposing of his life as he chooses.

REFUSAL OF LIFE-SUSTAINING TREATMENT AND EUTHANASIA

26

A Demand to Die

Two months after being discharged from three years of military service as a jet pilot, the world of Donald C. exploded in a flash of burning gas. He was then twenty-six years old, unmarried, and a college graduate. An athlete in high school, he loved sports and the outdoors. Rodeos were his special interest, and he performed in them with skill. Upon leaving the military in May, 1973, Donald joined his father's successful real estate business. The two of them had always had a close and warm relationship. On July 25, 1973, they were together, appraising farm land. Without realizing it, they parked their car near a large propane gas transmission line; the line was leaking. Later, when they started their automobile, the ignition of the motor set off a severe and unexpected explosion. Donald, his father, and the surrounding countryside were enveloped in fire. The father died on the way to the hospital, and Donald was admitted in a critical but conscious state. He sustained second- and third-degree burns over sixty-eight percent of his body—mostly third-degree burns. Both eyes were blinded by corneal damage, his ears were mostly destroyed, and he sustained severe burns to his face, upper extremities, body, and legs.

During the next nine months, Donald underwent repeated skin grafting, enucleation of his right eye, and amputation of the distal parts of the fingers on both hands. The left eye was surgically closed in order to protect it from the danger of infection; the cornea was badly scarred and the retina was partially detached. His hands, deformed by contractures, were useless, unsightly stubs. When admitted to the University of Texas Medical Branch Hospitals in April, 1974, the patient had many infected areas on his body and legs. He had to be bathed daily in the Hubbard tank to control infection.

From the day of the accident onward, Donald persistently stated that he did not want to live. Nonetheless, he had continued to accept treatment. Two days after admission to the University hospital, however, he refused to give permission for further corrective surgery on his hands. He became adamant in his insistence that he be allowed to leave the hospital and return home to die—a certain consequence of leaving since only daily tanking could prevent overwhelming infection. The tankings were continued despite his protests. His mother, a thoughtful and courageous woman, was frantic; his surgeons were frustrated and perplexed.

Although calm and rational most of the time, the patient had frequent periods of childlike rage, fear, and tearfulness. He engaged his mother by the hour in arguments regarding his demand to leave the hospital—which, of

118

course, he was physically incapable of doing unless she agreed to take him home by ambulance.

At this juncture, Dr. Robert B. White was asked to see the patient as a psychiatric consultant. Prior to seeing the patient he was given the impression that Donald was irrationally depressed and probably needed to be declared mentally incompetent so that a legal guardian could be appointed to give the necessary permission for further surgery and other treatments. The patient's mother was understandably in favor of his remaining in the hospital. She was deeply concerned about her son's welfare, and the prospect of taking him home to die from pus-covered sores on his body was more than she could bear. She was a deeply religious woman and was also concerned lest her son die without re-accepting the church which he had left some time prior to his burns.

Donald was the eldest of three children. By his family's account, he was an active, assertive, and determined person, who since childhood had tended to set his own course in life. What or whom he liked, he stuck to with loyalty and persistence; what or whom he disliked, he opposed with tenacity. His mother stated, "He always wanted to do things for himself and in his own way." Dr. White soon concluded that the mother's summary was apt. In the course of the first few interviews it was apparent that Donald was a very stubborn and determined man; he was also bright, articulate, logical, and coherent — not by any criterion mentally incompetent. He summarized his position with the statement, "I do not want to go on as a blind and crippled person." Arguments that surgery could restore some degree of useful function to his hands, and perhaps some useful vision to his remaining eye, were of no avail. His determination to leave the hospital was unshakable, and he demanded to see his attorney in order to obtain his release by court order if necessary.

COMMENTARY
Robert B. White

Donald's wish seemed in great measure logical and rational; as my psychiatric duties brought me to know him well, I could not escape the thought that if I were in his position I would feel as he did. I asked two other psychiatric colleagues to see the patient, and they came to the same conclusion. *Should his demand to die be respected?* I found myself in sympathy with his wish to put an end to his pathetic plight. On the other hand, the burden on his mother would be unthinkable if he left the hospital, and none of us who were responsible for his care could bring ourselves to say, "You're discharged; go home and die."

Another question occurred to me as I watched this blind, maimed, and totally helpless man defy and baffle everyone: could his adamant stand be the only way available for him to regain his independence after such a prolonged period of helplessness and total dependence?

Consequently, I decided to assist him in the one area where he did want help — obtaining legal assistance. He obviously had the right to legal recourse, and I told him I would help him obtain it. I also told him that I and the other doctors involved could not accede immediately to his demand to leave; we could not participate in his suicide. Furthermore, he was, I said, in no condition to leave unless his mother took him home, and that was an unfair burden to place on her. I urged him to have the surgery; then, when he was able to be up and about, he could take his own life if he wished without forcing others to arrange his death.

But Donald remained adamant, and the patient, his attorney, and I had several conferences. Finally, the attorney reluctantly agreed to represent the patient in court. The patient and I agreed that if the court ruled that he had the right to refuse further treatment, the life-sustaining daily trips to the Hubbard tank and all other life-sustaining treatment would be stopped. If he wished, he could remain in the hospital in order to be kept as free of pain as possible until he died.

Had Donald been burned a few years ago, before our increasingly exquisite medical and surgical technology became available, none of the moral, humanitarian, medical, or legal questions his case raised would have had time to occur; he would simply have died. But Donald lived, and never lost his courage or tenacity. He has imposed upon us the responsibility to explore the questions he has asked. On one occasion Donald put the matter very bluntly: "What gives a physician the right to keep alive a patient who wants to die?"

As we increase our ability to sustain life in a wrecked body we must find ways to assess the wishes of the person in that body as accurately as we assess the viability of his organs. We can no longer blindly hold to our instinctive tendency to regard death as an adversary to be defeated at any price. Nor must we accept immediately and at face value a patient's demand to be allowed to die. That demand may often be his only way to assert his will in the face of our unyielding determination to defeat death. The problem is relatively simple when brain death has occurred or when a patient refuses surgery for cancer. But what of the patient who has entered willingly on a prolonged and difficult course of treatment, and then, at the point at which he will obviously survive if the treatment is continued, decides that he does not want further treatment because he cannot tolerate the kind of future life that his injuries or illness will impose upon him?

The outcome of Donald's case does not resolve these questions but it should add to the depth of our reflections. Having won his point, having asserted his will, having thus found a way to counteract his months of total helplessness, Donald suddenly agreed to continue the treatment and to have the surgery on his hands. He remained in the hospital for five more months until medically ready to return home. In the six months since he left, Donald has regained a considerable measure of self-sufficiency. Although still blind, he will soon have surgery on his eye, and it is hoped some degree of useful vision will be restored. He feeds himself, can walk as far as half a mile, and has become an enthusiastic operator of a citizens' band radio. When I told him of my wish to publish this case report, he agreed, and stated that he had been thinking of writing a paper about his remarkable experiences.

COMMENTARY
H. Tristram Engelhardt Jr.

This case raises a fundamental moral issue: how can one treat another person as free while still looking out for his best interests (even over his objections)? The issue is one of the bounds and legitimacy of paternalism. Paternalistic interventions are fairly commonplace in society: motorcyclists are required to wear helmets, no one may sell himself into slavery, and so forth. In such cases society chooses to intervene to maintain the moral agency of individuals so that their agency will not be terminated in death or in slavery. Society chooses in the purported best interest (i.e., to preserve the condition of self-determination itself—freedom) of the would-be reckless motorcyclist or slave. Or, in the paradigmatic case of paternalism, the choice by parents for their children is justifiable in that at a future time as adults, the children will say that their parents chose in their best interests (as opposed to the parents simply using their children for their own interests). That is, the paternalism involved in surrogate consent can be justified if the individual himself cannot choose, and one chooses in that individual's best interest so that if that person were (or is in the future) able to choose, he or she would (will) agree with the choice that has been made in his or her behalf.

Thus, one can justify treating a burned patient when first admitted even if that person protested: one might argue that the individual was not able to choose freely because of the pain and serious impact of the circumstances, and that by treating initially one gave the individual a reasonable chance to choose freely in the future. One would interpret the patient to be temporarily incompetent and have someone decide in his behalf. But once that initial time has passed, and once the patient is reasonably able to choose, should one respect a patient's request to refuse life-saving therapy even if one has good reason to believe that later the patient might change his or her mind? This is the problem that this case presents.

Yet, what are the alternatives which are morally open: (1) to compel treatment, (2) at once to cease treatment, or (3) to try to convince the patient to persist, but if the patient does not agree, then to stop therapy. Simply to compel treatment is not to acknowledge the patient as a free agent (i.e., to vitiate the concept of *consent* itself), and simply to stop therapy at once may abandon the patient to the exigencies of unjustified despair. The third alternative recognizes the two values to be preserved in this situation: the freedom of the patient and the physician's commitment to preserve the life of persons.

But in the end, individuals, when able, must be allowed to decide their own destiny, even that of death. When the patient decides that the future quality of life open to him is not worth the investment of pain and suffering to attain that future quality of life, that is a decision proper to the patient. Such is the case *even if* one had good reasons to believe that once the patient attained that future state he would be content to live; one would have unjustifiably forced an investment of pain that was not agreed to. Of course, there are no easy answers. Physicians should not abandon patients when momentarily pain overwhelms them; physicians should seek to gain consent for therapy. But when the patient who is able to give free consent does not, the moral issue is over. A society that will allow persons to climb dangerous mountains or do daredevil stunts with cars has no consistent grounds for paternalistic intervention here. Further, unlike the case of the motorcyclist or the would-be slave, in this case one would force unchosen pain and suffering on another in the name of his best interests, but in circumstances where his best interests are far from clear. That is, even if such paternalistic intervention may be justifiable in some cases (an issue which is different from the paternalism of surrogate decision making, and which I will not contest at this point), it is dubious here, for the patient's choice is not a capricious risking of the basis of free action, but a deliberate choice to avoid considerable hardship. Further, it is a uniquely intimate choice concerning the quality of life: the amount of pain which is worth suffering for a goal. Moreover, it is, unlike the would-be slave's choice, a choice which affirms freedom on a substantial point—the quality of one's life.

In short, one must be willing, as a price for recognizing the freedom of others, to live with the consequences of that freedom: some persons will make choices that they would regret were they to live longer. But humans are not only free beings, but temporal beings, and the freedom that is actual is that of the present. Competent adults should be allowed to make tragic decisions, if nowhere else, at least concerning what quality of life justifies the pain and suffering of continued living. It is not medicine's responsibility to prevent tragedies by denying freedom, for that would be the greater tragedy.

27

Family Wishes and Patient Autonomy

Ralph Watkins, a seventy-five-year-old married man, was admitted to the intensive care unit of a university hospital in acute respiratory distress. He was anxious but fully alert and gasping for help. A retired laborer, Mr. Watkins had been suffering from a chronic pulmonary disease for the past fifteen years. For the past five years he had become progressively debilitated. Prior to admission he had been confined to his home and depended on his wife for the most basic of care: without her assistance he could not dress or feed himself. He had been a fiercely independent man and still enjoyed ordering people around. His wife and married son were totally devoted to him.

The diagnosis was bilateral pneumonia, and Mr. Watkins was given antibiotics and put on a mechanical respirator with supplemental oxygen. Within two weeks the pneumonia was largely cleared and Sarah Radburn, his physician, began attempts to wean him from the respirator. Unfortunately, he had become "respirator-dependent" as a result of a combination of poor nutrition, possible new damage to his lungs, weakened respiratory muscles, and fear of breathing on his own. Despite a slow, cautious approach with much reassurance, the weaning attempts repeatedly failed. Mr. Watkins, short of breath and terrified, would demand to be placed back on the respirator.

Dr. Radburn rated the ultimate chance for successful weaning as "maybe 20 percent." The patient became more and more discouraged with his lack of progress and the frequent painful medical procedures (constant intravenous feeding, frequent needle punctures for arterial blood gases, suctioning, and so on). After three weeks of unsuccessful efforts, Mr. Watkins refused to cooperate with further attempts at weaning. His wife and son became concerned that he had given up the "will to live." They begged the medical staff to "do something to save him." Although he had become less communicative, he remained alert and aware and, in the opinion of the staff, was fully competent. He told Dr. Radburn he wanted the respirator disconnected. "I want to die," he said.

What is the physician's responsibility in this case? Should the physician honor the patient's request? If we assume the patient is legally competent to make medical decisions, on what basis, if any, can the physician refuse or postpone acting on the request to stop life support? How much weight should be given the family's wish to "save" the patient?

COMMENTARY
Stuart J. Youngner and David L. Jackson

This case illustrates the often confusing and conflicting responsibilities that confront physicians in today's modern, high-technology medical environment. To preserve life, relieve suffering, do no harm, and respect the autonomy of this alert, competent man is no simple task. If Mr. Watkins were comatose or delirious, he could be declared incompetent and the family or a court-appointed guardian would make the decision. Confronted with the realities in this case, however, one could "solve" the problem most simply by taking one of two courses—both of which, we feel, are wrong.

First, one could insist that Dr. Radburn's primary responsibility is to try for the 20 percent chance of saving his life. After all, the patient placed himself in her care, and she can dismiss his wish "to die" as irrational, although not incompetent, and press on. This course is unacceptable because it violates the patient's autonomy. It also ignores the great degree of suffering and the small chance of regaining a "meaningful" life.

Equally simplistic, and in our view unacceptable, would be to respond to his expressed wish to die by immediately disconnecting the respirator, while piously proclaiming respect for patient autonomy.

It is noteworthy that both these courses (relentlessly pursuing treatment or rigidly following the patient's request) allow the physician to avoid a time-consuming and potentially painful dialogue with the patient and family. We suggest that before the respirator is disconnected and the irrevocable decision made to let the patient die, the physician must evaluate with the patient and family the following:

1. Does the wish "to die" represent a temporary depression in reaction to pain or a sleepless night? If the depression passes or is adequately treated, the patient may well retract the wish to die. Of course, depression may be a realistic and consistent response to a situation of great suffering and little hope.

2. The patient's request may be a reaction of fear based on misperception or misinformation. Before stopping treatment the physician should identify any fears underlying a refusal of treatment and explore their source with the patient. Fear may be appropriate to many situations, and a reasonable basis for refusing treatment.

3. In similar intensive care units, we have seen several cases in which patients have exhibited true ambivalence about stopping treatment. If adequate dialogue is not established, the physician may hear only that side of the ambivalence with which he or she agrees. Acting on such half-truths is hardly honoring the principle of patient autonomy.

4. A patient's request to have treatment stopped may be a symbolic attempt to regain control in a situation in which he has none. A critically ill, machine-dependent patient has little autonomy in the most mundane and basic aspects of his life such as sleeping, elimination, eating, and privacy. He is totally at the mercy of others. The request for termination of treatment may be a desperate effort by a helpless patient to get the attention of his family and caregivers and to assert his independence. Thoughtful investigation may discover alternative measures that restore the patient's sense of autonomy and with it a revival of the wish to pursue life vigorously.

5. An apparent clash between the wishes of the family and patient may identify underlying problems of communication between them. The physician must clarify with the family the meaning of their cry "to save" the patient. Are they acting out of guilt? Can they distinguish their own needs from those of the patient? A meeting with patient and family together may be the only means of clarifying the apparent disagreement. If the issue cannot be resolved the patient must have the ultimate input to the decision-making process. The physician's contract is with him and ultimately it is his fate being decided.

The possible interventions and evaluations we have suggested will postpone acting on a patient's request to stop treatment. In doing so we could be accused of "paternalism" and violating the patient's autonomy. However, as Eric Cassell (*Hastings Center Report*, December 1977, pp. 16–19) has pointed out, a sick person is not simply a well person with an illness appended. Life-threatening illness, dependence on machines, and the ensuing physical and psychological regression make the concept of autonomy much more difficult to apply. By postponing an irreversible decision until important issues can be clarified, physicians may not be violating the true autonomy of their patients. Reflex acquiescence to patients' wishes that treatment be stopped may be a way for physicians to avoid close dialogue with fellow beings in their hour of greatest need. If the dialogue is completed and the patient's wish to die remains, there is almost always time to withdraw life supports.

COMMENTARY
William Ruddick

In order to sharpen a single issue I shall assume that the courts, the hospital's regulations, and the physicians' professional and moral principles do allow patients in such circumstances to refuse life-saving treatment. Nevertheless in this case as sketched, Dr. Radburn should first explore the conflicting requests. Her first responsibility is to make sure that the patient's request expresses an informed, autonomous, and resolute desire to die and is not merely a show of "fierce independence."

Suppose that various inquiries convince the physician, staff, and consultants that the patient means what he says for reasons appropriate to his age, condition, character, and other circumstances. His pain is tolerable, but his increasing and irreversible debilitation and dependence are not. Even ordering people around has ceased to relieve his "burdensome" life. Despite his family's pleas, he wants to die—even if he can still be weaned from the respirator.

His wife and son want him kept alive, even if he cannot be weaned. They realize they have no legal means to prevent the physician's termination of treatment, but if the physician refuses the patient's request, they trust that he will be too weak to enlist legal aid (or to turn off his own respirator). For reasons of affection, shame, and "philosophy of life and death," they prefer his forced survival to his death by what they perceive as suicide.

These elaborations simplify the case:

1. The probability of weaning becomes irrelevant: the patient wants to die, even if weaned; his family wants him kept alive, even if respirator-dependent.

2. The direct conflict of their desires shows that the patient is not influenced by self-serving family suggestion or fear that he has become a resented burden.

3. Free of all other opposition to terminating treatment, the physician must base any refusal or further delay solely on the family's desire.

What then are the physician's professional and more general moral responsibilities? Should the family's desire, or considerations of their welfare, deter her from "honoring the patient's request"? I think not. The family are not her patient, nor the patient's proxies. Nor does his decision or welfare depend on their own. A physician often has a derivative responsibility for the welfare of family members who can provide a patient with hope, courage, nursing or financial aid, or legally required representation. But she has no such derivative professional responsibility for the family's welfare here. Indeed, to the extent that she shares her patient's belief that he would be "better off dead" or would die better now than later, she must oppose those who would forcibly continue treatment. A family's welfare does not compete with, let alone overrule, a patient's welfare in a physician's deliberations.

Though not professionally responsible *for* the family, Dr. Radburn is nonetheless responsible *to* them in at least two ways. Given their concern and past care for the patient, they are owed a thoughtful account of the decision to terminate treatment. Whether or not they are employing her, the physician must answer to them for the proposed course of action. Moreover, benevolence requires her to try to reconcile the family to her decision. If their religious principles cannot be interpreted to permit termination, she may only be able to prepare them for the patient's death. Even if the patient is being selfish in his distress, the physician should take concern for those he is (excusably?) ignoring and harming. And even if he is acting "within his rights," benevolence requires the physician to moderate the avoidable suffering produced. The demands of virtue cannot block the exercise of rights (otherwise rights would lose their force), but they can delimit the manner in which others facilitate the exercise of those rights.

In summary, the physician has two grounds for delaying, but none (as the case is elaborated) for denying the patient's request. Time is needed for: (1) making sure that the patient's request expresses a deliberate, resolute desire; and (2) trying to lessen the suffering of the family whose plea she professionally should reject but morally must respond to with compassionate attention. The first delay involves a paternalistic defense of a patient against undue influence by haste, pain, drugs, or others whose desires and welfare are not an integral part of the patient's own concerns. (This "subject paternalism" appeals to a patient's *characteristic* desires, not to his or her "best interests.") The second delay is justified by the coordination of rights with virtues that limit the manner of their exercise, especially with regard to the cooperation of the physician and the suffering of the family. Like any right to life, any right to die must be located in a context of virtues, as well as of other rights. Contrary to current slogans, people do not die alone.

28

"If I Have AIDS, Then Let Me Die Now!"

Dr. Lois Dorsey, a psychiatry resident, was paged by an intern from the Medical Intensive Care Unit (MICU) for an emergency psychiatric consultation. Gary Davidson, a twenty-eight-year-old gay man, had been hospitalized eleven days before for a first episode of *Pneumocystis carinii* pneumonia (PCP). One week earlier he had been told that the presumptive diagnosis for his illness was Acquired Immunodeficiency Syndrome (AIDS).

On the day Dr. Dorsey was called, the medical team discussed with Mr. Davidson the need for a Swann-Ganz catheter, which would be inserted in his pulmonary artery. Mr. Davidson refused permission for placement of the catheter, and requested that medical treatment be stopped. "Take the tubes away and let me die with dignity," he declared.

The medical team discussed in detail with Mr. Davidson, his lover, and his parents and sister his clinical status and prognosis; Mr. Davidson had, they believed, a 50 percent chance of surviving the current illness. However, people with AIDS rarely survive more than two years and Mr. Davidson could expect several bouts of severe illness during his remaining lifespan. They also pointed out that rapid advances were being made in understanding the pathophysiology of AIDS and offered the prospect for a future treatment as a result of current research efforts.

With the support of his lover and family, Mr. Davidson continued to insist on cessation of treatment, citing as his reasons "quality of life" and the "right to die with dignity." In the presence of witnesses he signed a living will and statement of competency. The legal formalities were carried out; however, for "legal reasons" and "completeness," before complying with the patient's request, the medical team was waiting for a psychiatric assessment.

Dr. Dorsey reviewed Mr. Davidson's records and interviewed him. Mr. Davidson reaffirmed his belief that quality of life was more important than quantity of life and that he wished to die with dignity. He admitted that he was feeling pain, fear, loss of control, extreme discomfort on the respirator, and sleeplessness. He added that he was distressed by his inability to eat (on the respirator). When Dr. Dorsey asked how he might feel should he recover from the pneumonia, the patient noted that he knew he had AIDS and that he would die within one or two years. Therefore, he said, he did not deserve to take up a bed in the hospital and continue to receive medical treatment that could better benefit another patient.

The patient had no psychiatric history and had never attempted suicide. He had never had any personal experience with death or dying among family or friends. He could not speak because of the respirator tubes but he communicated by writing notes and nodding his head. He was alert, not disoriented, wrote clearly and logically, and initiated his own statements and topics for the interview. He was not tearful but appeared anxious. In his own eyes he did not want to commit suicide but wanted to be allowed to die.

Dr. Dorsey concluded that the patient showed no evidence of confusion, psychosis, or delusional thinking, but that he did show symptoms consistent with depression, probably secondary to his underlying medical condition.

Mr. Davidson, then, was legally competent, understood the consequences of his decision to refuse treatment, and had the support of those closest to him. Yet, because of his age and depression, the availability of treatment for his current illness, and the possibility that some treatment for AIDS may become available within the next few years, Dr. Dorsey hesitated. Should Mr. Davidson's treatment be stopped as he wished?

COMMENTARY
Sophia Vinogradov and Joe E. Thornton

Dr. Dorsey's conflicting feelings summarize the essentials of the dilemma. On the one hand, her impulse is to evaluate and treat the underlying disease; on the other, she wishes to promote Mr. Davidson's autonomy and sense of control. Hence her hesitation. She agrees that a legally competent patient has the right to refuse treatment, and yet she wonders: when does the patient's right to refuse treatment encroach on the physician's responsibility to work in the patient's best interest? Or to do no harm? When does the physician have the right to impose treatment on competent patients?

Mr. Davidson was suffering from the discomfort of difficult breathing, from the pain of a respirator tube, and the effects of having been drugged and deprived of sleep for over a week—all reversible physical states. He was suffering from this extreme physical duress when his physicians sought his permission to inflict more pain by inserting a Swann-Ganz catheter.

His primary physical illness also led to secondary psychosocial effects of depression, isolation, loss of self-esteem, and altered body image—all reversible mental states. But patients may initially pass through stages of denial or despair and reject medical treatment that later they may be willing to accept. It is here, then, that the physician must seize the prerogative and help the patient adapt to his or her illness before permitting an irreversible or impulsive decision regarding treatment.

The notion of thoughtful decision making, of the reversible vs. the irreversible, of preparedness vs. impulsiveness, is the touchstone of this case. Refusal of treatment here implied cessation of life support therapy followed by immediate and certain death. Faced with a treatable illness that is imminently life-threatening, the physician must obey the injunction to "do no harm." At least in the interim while longer term strategies are being devised, she must work to support life and encourage thoughtful decision making. In the presence of reversible physical or mental states the physician has the right to impose treatment on competent patients in order to prevent irreversible decisions.

It is also possible that Mr. Davidson was being influenced by subtle external pressures. In a period of scarce resources, a vulnerable and distressed patient who is labeled as nonproductive or deviant by society may feel that he does not deserve life-sustaining medical treatment. If Dr. Dorsey recognizes those external pressures, she should resist them by imposing treatment on her initially unwilling patient.

We may appear to be saying "the ends" (life) "justify the means" (violating a person's free will). We are not. We are arguing for "informed refusal." Just as a person under physical or psychological duress cannot give informed consent, neither can a person under physical or psychological duress give informed refusal. As Dr. Randall Weingarten has pointed out to us, physicians have the right to impose treatment on competent patients when the patient is not capable of giving informed refusal.

Far from being antithetical to the right of a patient to decide his own fate, these conditions complement that prerogative. If Mr. Davidson is to make a truly informed decision regarding his illness, health, future treatment, and perhaps ultimately his death, that decision must be made under circumstances that are as free as possible from psychological and physical duress.

It is thus Dr. Dorsey's right to buy Mr. Davidson a little time, to allow him to recover from his initial sense of hopelessness and shock. Even more, she has a duty to permit Mr. Davidson to adapt to his altered circumstances, and to guide and comfort him through the fear and pain of invasive procedures and diagnostic uncertainty. Only then will he be fully free to accept or refuse treatment, free to say... "Let me die with dignity."

COMMENTARY
A-J Rock Levinson

Gary Davidson is a competent, rational adult and hence cannot be subjected to invasive medical procedures without his consent. That is a basic human right and the law of the land. Dr. Dorsey has found that Mr. Davidson knows the nature of his condition(s), has been informed of his options, and is aware of the consequences of his decision. He is "alert, not disoriented, clear and logical in his thinking."

Dr. Dorsey's reasons for hesitating are good ones: Mr. Davidson is depressed, has a potential life of several months even if no new developments are discovered for reversal of AIDS, and has a fifty-fifty chance of surviving his immediate life-threatening condition. However, none of these is reason enough to impose her perception of his situation upon his own perception of that situation.

Time is the crucial element. If Mr. Davidson's death is imminent, Dr. Dorsey could declare the patient incompetent—thus setting into motion the legal process for overriding his decision or declaring him "competent" and able to refuse the procedure. But if a court declares Gary Davidson to be "incompetent," from whom would the medical team get the required consent for the procedure? Those closest to him—therefore the ones best qualified to make a substituted judgment—have already declared their support for Mr. Davidson's decision. Why would a judge be better able to make such a personal decision?

If there is time for further consultation, Dr. Dorsey should talk with the parents, sister, and lover independently to try to elicit the rationale behind what appears to be their too facile acquiescence to Gary Davidson's demand to be allowed to die. Is the family reacting to new knowledge of his homosexuality? Are they all afraid that Mr. Davidson's recovery from this crisis will create for them the burden and threat of caring for an AIDS victim? If his family and lover knew more about AIDS, the evidence about transmission, and the training and supports available to help them care for him, would they try to change his mind?

Dr. Dorsey should also explore with Mr. Davidson his own feelings of abandonment, guilt, fear, shame, loss, despair, and anger. So far, he has had only a discussion of his clinical status and prognosis and an earnest but transparent prediction that research efforts might extend his life-expectancy beyond two years. If he could be reassured of his parents', sister's, lover's, medical team's, and society's wish to have him survive—even for a short time—perhaps his assessment of his situation would be different.

If time does not permit, however, Mr. Davidson must be considered the best judge of his own situation and treatment must be stopped. To do otherwise would exemplify the ultimate in medical paternalism and could have serious legal consequences.

This case raises other, more general questions:

Why was Dr. Dorsey not asked to consult with the patient and family as soon as AIDS was diagnosed? A suicidal reaction to such information is predictable and earlier psychiatric intervention might well have prevented the crisis.

If Gary Davidson had consented to the insertion of the catheter, would there have been "legal reasons" for "competence" to be assessed? Would Dr. Dorsey have been asked to evaluate his psychological condition or was she asked to intervene solely because his decision was contrary to the medical team's evaluation of his needs? (At a time when society—and even the medical profession—is discussing the abandonment of the psychiatric defense for violent crime, it is ironic that the psychiatrist is called in when we want to "preserve" the life of someone who has made an "informed," "competent" decision to relinquish it.)

Who is Dr. Dorsey's client? Is she serving Mr. Davidson's best interest (in which case she will work with him and his family and support whatever conclusion he reaches), or is she serving the medical team who want her to provide "completeness"?

If Mr. Davidson were in his seventies, suffering from terminal cancer but facing a procedure that might (or might not) provide a few more months of life, would the medical team respond differently?

All these questions need to be thoroughly examined by any medical team assessing a situation of this kind. However, their conclusions should not affect the outcome in this or any other case. Decisions made by an informed, competent adult must be respected.

COMMENTARY
Michael L. Callen

Choosing death can, under some circumstances, clearly be a rational decision that ought to be honored. Less clear are the criteria by which an individual can be judged sufficiently competent to make such a momentous decision. The facts presented convince me that Mr. Davidson is almost certainly competent to decide to refuse life-sustaining treatments. I would argue, however, that before affirming Mr. Davidson's competence, Dr. Dorsey has an ethical obligation to test his apparent resolve.

While Mr. Davidson may truly prefer to die, it is also possible that he has taken his dramatic position to see if his lover, family, and/or friends will attempt to dissuade him. Surprisingly, neither Mr. Davidson's lover nor his parents or sister disagrees with his decision. It would be useful and appropriate for Dr. Dorsey to interview each privately to ensure that support for Mr. Davidson's decision is indeed unanimous and genuine.

Should Dr. Dorsey discover that one or more of Mr. Davidson's significant others have misgivings about this decision, she should encourage that individual to share those misgivings with him. The intent here is not to badger Mr. Davidson, but to confirm that he is committed to his position. If the individual is hesitant or unwilling to share his or her misgivings with Mr. Davidson, Dr. Dorsey might offer to discuss their concerns with Mr. Davidson in a general sense—without mentioning which of his significant others expressed misgivings. Obviously, Dr. Dorsey would have to proceed very cautiously.

Dr. Dorsey would also be justified in testing the validity of Mr. Davidson's stated altruism. Mr. Davidson's statement that he does not "deserve to take up a bed in the hospital and continue to receive medical treatment that could better benefit another patient" is worthy of more careful exploration. "Deserve" is a loaded word; many gay men who develop AIDS harbor feelings of guilt about sexual promiscuity and its obvious connection to the development of AIDS in gay men. It would be tragic if such inappropriate "guilt" were playing any role in Mr. Davidson's decision to refuse life-sustaining treatment. Dr. Dorsey could point out the erroneousness of Mr. Davidson's belief that a decision to accept treatment would mean that others would have to be denied a hospital bed or care.

However, assuming that (1) Mr. Davidson's significant others do genuinely and unanimously support his decision; or (2) doubts expressed by his significant others do not persuade Mr. Davidson to change his decision; and (3) Dr. Dorsey has concluded that inappropriate "guilt" and/or altruistic misconceptions are not determining Mr. Davidson's decision, then only one additional test remains.

I believe that Dr. Dorsey *herself* has a professional and, indeed, an ethical obligation to encourage Mr. Davidson to reconsider. She should begin by challenging the presumption that everyone dies from AIDS. It is more appropriate to discuss mortality rates in terms of specific opportunistic infections. Although PCP accounts for a large portion of AIDS fatalities, some individuals have survived discrete bouts of PCP and remained free of further life-threatening illnesses for a year or more. Since Mr. Davidson has expressed a preference for "quality of life" rather than "quantity," he should be informed that many who have survived these periods of illness spend whatever time they have left living life quite fully. Some travel to places they always wanted to visit; others begin or finish pet projects; some resolve differences with enemies; and most spend precious time with loved ones.

AIDS is another "closet." Realization of one's gayness can initiate confusion, anxiety, and a sense of isolation; a diagnosis of AIDS can create similar feelings. It is Dr. Dorsey's duty to alert Mr. Davidson to methods and resources for dealing with such feelngs.

There have been some innovative responses to the stigma, misinformation, and emotional upheaval that often attend a diagnosis of AIDS. Persons with AIDS in various cities have formed their own support groups and I would strongly encourage mental health care providers to investigate these unique resources.

At a minimum, Dr. Dorsey should tell Mr. Davidson that support groups exist which include people with AIDS who have experienced the crisis he is facing. It could be extremely useful if Dr. Dorsey could arrange for Mr. Davidson to meet face to face with someone with AIDS who has had PCP and *accepted* life-sustaining treatments. In this regard, plans are underway to create a toll-free number so that people with AIDS can contact others diagnosed with AIDS during periods of crisis. Attempts will be made to match those with common opportunistic diseases.

The importance of such supportive networking cannot be overstated. I have personally experienced—and witnessed in others—how this process of sharing common experiences can radically alter initial perceptions of helplessness and hopelessness.

If Mr. Davidson declines to speak with another person with AIDS who has had a similar experience or if he objects to the idea of support networking, then I believe Dr. Dorsey should sign the necessary forms. If every reasonable effort made to test Mr. Davidson's resolve has failed to change his mind, I believe that his choice of "death with dignity" should be respected.

29

Whether "No" Means "No"

Dr. D. is an emergency physician in a large urban hospital. One relatively quiet evening Mr. R., a thirty-two-year-old male, presents to the emergency department complaining of shortness of breath. The problem, as it develops, is a depressingly familiar one to Dr. D. Mr. R., known to be HIV positive, turns out to be having his first episode of pneumocystis pneumonia, an often fatal disease of AIDS patients. The episode, fortunately, appears at present to be a relatively mild one; his blood test shows his lung function is only moderately impaired.

When Dr. D. begins to explain this, Mr. R. insists that his friend Mr. U. be brought into the emergency department to listen to the doctor. Dr. D. goes over the condition and describes the appropriate treatment: IV antibiotics. When asked, Mr. R. denies any drug allergies.

As they grapple with the news that Mr. R. has now changed from being a patient with HIV to one with AIDS, Mr. R. and Mr. U. produce a living will and durable health care proxy form designating Mr. U. as responsible for decision making if Mr. R. becomes incompetent. The living will forbids cardiopulmonary resuscitation and prohibits under any circumstances endotracheal intubation and respirator ventilation, along with numerous other measures.

Dr. D. believes strongly in patient autonomy. He therefore assures Mr. R. and Mr. U. that Mr. R.'s wishes, as clearly expressed, will be respected. After arranging for the papers to be copied and placed in the chart, he goes to admit Mr. R. and Mr. U. leaves.

While a bed is being readied, Dr. D orders a dose of the appropriate antibiotic to be given to Mr. R. and goes to see the next patient. Upon starting the antibiotic and leaving the room for a few minutes, the nurse returns to find Mr. R. unresponsive, with a bright red rash and severe trouble breathing. Immediately recognizing a life-threatening allergic reaction, she stops the antibiotic and calls for the doctor.

Mr. R. is in anaphylactic shock. Quickly ordering the four appropriate medications, Dr. D opens his mouth to ask for an endotracheal tube and respirator and realizes he has a problem.

Mr. R. will die as his airway closes up if patency is not immediately ensured by placement of a tube. Indeed, in a case like this, placement often requires cutting the patient's throat to maintain the rapidly narrowing airway. Seconds, quite literally, count. The good news is that this is a time-limited condition. With immediate aggressive action, only a few hours or days of ventilator support should be necessary and there should be absolutely no long-term sequelae. Of course, it is possible that Mr. R.'s pneumonia will acutely worsen. He might then be unable to be weaned off the respirator. An emergency physician with no experience in the long-term management of either pneumocystis pneumonia or anaphylaxis, he is unsure of the chances of that.

What should Dr. D. do?

COMMENTARY
Lewis Silverman and Manette Dennis

Realistically it is hard to imagine anyone planning his medical treatment better than Mr. R. Having either seen or, at least, heard of patients being tortured by medical management gone wild, he is apparently determined to avoid that for himself. Despite his careful planning, he is now at risk for exactly the fate he feared as worse than death itself, due to an unforeseen bit of bad luck.

Mr. R. made it as clear as he possibly could that "under no circumstances" should he be intubated and put on a ventilator. If we truly believe in patient autonomy, that would seem to settle it. No means no; let him go. Some would argue that only a rank paternalist would ignore this patient's cogently expressed desires. But Dr. D. does not appear to be motivated by paternalism.

He "believes strongly in patient autonomy." Can he then justify treating Mr. R. with intubation on any other basis?

It seems to us that he can and must. Common sense rather than literal interpretation must be used to guide action in this case. Let us suppose you hire a babysitter to sit with your infant. Since it is raining outside you give strict instructions: "Don't leave the house with the baby." Five minutes after you leave, the house catches fire. Would you expect the baby sitter to keep the baby in the house? Of course not!

Even in law, performance under a formal contract can be excused if unanticipated events frustrate the purpose of one or both parties. While we unfortunately (especially given Mr. U.'s absence) can only guess as to intent, it seems reasonable to assume that Mr. R.'s purpose was to avoid uncomfortable, life-prolonging procedures while still accepting routine medical treatment. Otherwise, why should he bother to come to the hospital? Mr. R. clearly does not wish to be kept alive artificially while dying from a terminal illness, but as evidenced by his acceptance of antibiotic therapy, he is not refusing treatment for nonterminal, generally reversible conditions. This is the agreement he wished to reach with his medical team through the means of his living will and his durable health care proxy. Dr. D will not be frustrating Mr. R.'s goals and purposes by intubation, as long as the intubation can end should Mr. R.'s condition change from a short-term crisis and turn into the long-term, hopeless situation that Mr. R. so consciously and deliberately sought to avoid.

In general, intubation and mechanical ventilation are certainly more invasive, uncomfortable, and onerous procedures than blood tests, IVs, and other routine modalities of diagnosis and treatment. In this instance, however, this is simply not true.

Dr. D. should intubate Mr. R. and place him on a ventilator. Immediately after stabilizing his patient, he should call Mr. U. and abide by his decision to extubate him or to maintain the respiratory support on a continuously reassessed basis.

COMMENTARY
Fenella Rouse and David A. Smith

The case study describes a critical failure in communication. Mr. R. had taken particular care to appoint someone who could speak for him as a proxy and to complete a living will that describes his wishes in certain specific circumstances. His living will, however, is far from standard. Most living wills describe what the person wants when his condition is incurable or irreversible, sometimes using expressions like "terminal" or "permanently unconscious" to trigger the effectiveness of the document. It is very rare, although not unheard of, for someone to state that he does not want cardiopulmonary resuscitation, endotracheal intubation, or respirator ventilation "under any circumstances." Most people, clearly, do want these forms of treatment if they will be restored to what is, to them, an acceptable quality of life. When people do refuse specified treatment "under any circumstances" it is usually because the person who makes that choice has thought long and hard about it and has special reasons for making it. In addition, if Mr. R.'s living will contained expressions such as "endotracheal intubation," it is very likely that he discussed his document with someone with medical expertise. It is unusual for a lay person to use technical medical terms in a living will unless detailed medical advice has been taken.

Mr. R.'s living will should thus have immediately raised questions in Dr. D.'s mind, particularly as Dr. D. is a strong supporter of patient autonomy and has presumably seen living wills before. But the case describes Dr. D. as assuring Mr. R and his proxy that the wishes are clearly expressed and will be carried out. What did Dr. D. think Mr. R.'s wishes were? Presumably, Dr. D. did not ask Mr. R. what "under any circumstances" meant. If he had, he would not have been uncertain about what to do later.

Similarly, he apparently did not ask why Mr. R. had such strong feelings about the treatment listed. Did he have a particular horror of the treatments described in his living will because they are more invasive? Did he believe, perhaps wrongly, that once respirator support was begun there would never be a circumstance in which he could be weaned? This was a vital conversation that needed to take place. Unlike some emergency situations, Dr. D. had the golden opportunity of a competent, conscious patient, a proxy, and even time (on this "relatively quiet evening") to explore why Mr. R. had expressed his wishes in this way. Dr. D. was wrong to assure Mr. R. and his proxy that his wishes would be carried out when he had not fully thought through or understood what those wishes were.

If Dr. D. is correct in assuming that Mr. R. wanted to refuse respirator support only if his condition were irreversible there would really be no dilemma. Of course he should treat, until it is clear whether the condition can be reversed. If it cannot be reversed, the ventilator will be withdrawn, allowing Mr. R. to die as he wished.

On the other hand, it is possible that Mr. R. was prepared to accept antibiotics but would not accept the treatments listed in his living will. Some people do have living wills in which they state that they do not want any treatment under *any* circumstances. Some people even have "do not defibrillate" symbols tattooed on their chests. Some people with AIDS choose to welcome an infection that would allow death to occur. It is very unlikely that Mr. R. is one of this group because he willingly allows antibiotic treatment for the pneumocystis pneumonia, but without discussing his wishes with him or his proxy, Dr. D. cannot be sure. Because Dr. D. didn't talk to Mr. R. about the meaning of his living will and because Mr. U. is not currently there, Dr. D. is left to proceed on his own unexplored and unverified interpretation. He must treat because he failed to talk to his patient.

The lesson of the case is clear: it is critical that the medical team be alert to ambiguities in advance directives. The pressures of emergency medicine sometimes make this difficult, but in this case there was time and opportunity, and the physician involved was informed and had relevant experience, making the failure to have the discussion inexcusable. The case points up the fact that advance directives are sometimes idiosyncratic. They are intended as a reflection of personal values, not a rote rejection of some kinds of life support. They require inquiry on the part of the physician to make certain that the physician fully understands the patient's wishes and is prepared to act in accordance with those wishes. Had Dr. D. but asked what Mr. R. meant by "under any circumstances," or even why he had chosen to express his wishes in that way, he would have spared Mr. R. the prospect of having his actual wishes ignored.

30

"No Feeding Tubes for Me!"

Pauline Randall, a sixty-five-year-old married woman with three adult children, has been suffering from amyotrophic lateral sclerosis (ALS) for several years. Her neurological condition has deteriorated so that she can no longer control any voluntary muscles. Confined to bed in a nursing home in a small midwestern American city and breathing with the aid of a respirator, she communicates through the electronic monitor that responds to eyelid blinks. She can "write" words and brief sentences in this way.

Mrs. Randall understands that her condition cannot be treated and that it will inevitably lead to her death. But she has been an active participant in her health care and has been determined to continue functioning as long as possible.

Her physician, Dr. Samuels, believes that she is not receiving adequate nutrition and that the time has come to insert a nasogastric feeding tube. When he proposes this procedure to her, she blinks quickly, "No more!" He asks, "Do you understand that you will die slowly of starvation if we do not insert this feeding tube?" "Yes," she blinks, "No more."

When Mrs. Randall's family, which has been close and supportive throughout her illness, learns of her opposition, they have divided opinions. Her husband believes that her wishes should be respected, but two of their three children are convinced that her life should be prolonged. The nursing staff believes that she should not be made to suffer any longer.

There is no question that Mrs. Randall is legally competent, that is, that she understands the procedure being proposed and the consequences of refusal. Should her refusal of the feeding tube be honored, even though it will lead to her death?

COMMENTARY
Richard H. Nicholson

In 1860, the English poet, Arthur Clough, wrote "The Latest Decalogue," only one couplet of which is usually remembered nowadays:

Thou shalt not kill; but needst not strive
Officiously to keep alive.

Today those lines are often quoted in the United Kingdom as summing up a proper attitude to terminal care. Repeated use out of context, however—starting with Bernard Shaw in "The Doctor's Dilemma"—has hidden the lines' origin in parody. Clough's poem went on:

Do not adultery commit;
Advantage rarely comes of it;
Thou shalt not steal; an idle feat,
When it's so lucrative to cheat.

Such an error is not untypical of the deceptions and misunderstandings that surround the care of patients with terminal, or inevitably fatal, illnesses. Mrs. Randall understands that her neurological deterioration will lead inevitably to death; yet one wonders whether Dr. Samuels has accepted that she is a dying patient. After all, at a slightly earlier stage of her illness, he acted in a way that would almost never happen in the United Kingdom. He started to aid her breathing with a respirator.

Since she can no longer control any voluntary muscles, such respiratory assistance, to be effective, would almost certainly be intermittent positive pressure respiration (IPPR), probably administered via tracheostomy. The normal way in which ALS patients die, when not attached to a ventilator, is by suddenly, and usually unexpectedly, stopping breathing; at autopsy it is uncommon to find any reason why death happened at that particular point. Artificial respiration is likely to prevent this mode of death, and was therefore a major intervention in Mrs. Randall's dying.

Cynics might suggest that the only reason why a patient like Mrs. Randall would not be artificially ventilated in the United Kingdom is that the National Health Service cannot afford enough ventilators. In fact for many years U.K. doctors have assessed the value of such interventions in terms of the probable quality of life as well as the probable quantity. In the 1936 House of Lords debate on the Voluntary Euthanasia (Legalisation) Bill, Lord Dawson, the royal physician recently revealed to have eased King George V's passing with morphine and cocaine, said:

If one goes back fifty years . . . it was an accepted tradition that it was the duty of the medical man to continue the struggle for life right up to the end. With time that has changed. There has gradually crept into medical opinion, as there has crept into lay opinion, the feeling that one should make the act of dying more gentle and more peaceful even if it does involve curtailment of the length of life.

When you pass . . . to lives which are burdened by incurable disease, and where the gap between that stage of illness and death becomes wider, it may be fully admitted that the difficulty is greater, yet when the patient is carrying a great load of suffering, our first thoughts should be the assuagement of pain even if it does involve the shortening of life.

Pain and comfort will in fact be important considerations in Mrs. Randall's case. Although she cannot move at all, her sensation is probably intact. Without extremely skilled and, above all, experienced nursing care she will frequently be very uncomfortable. Such experience will not be available in a small city where there is probably no more than a single case of motor neuron disease each year. Thus it will be important for her to have very regular small doses of morphine to take away the *feeling* of pain and discomfort; morphine will also take away the *feeling* of thirst or hunger.

Concern for the quality of Mrs. Randall's dying and the provision of appropriate care mean that she is most unlikely to have any sensation of hunger or thirst. Starvation therefore holds no fears for her and, with her intellect intact, she can decide to refuse the nasogastric tube. In U.K. hospices, where such appropriate care is available, it is neither the physician in charge nor the patient who raises the possibility of a nasogastric feeding tube: it is usually the intern or resident. Once the possibility has been raised it will be discussed widely among the doctors and nurses, within the family, between the doctors and the patient, and between the doctors and the family. The conclusion is nearly always that a feeding tube should not be used. This accords with the principle that a doctor is under no moral obligation to do to a patient that which is of no benefit to the patient. Many people in the U.K. would regard as a refined form of cruelty any technical intervention to prolong the life of a patient whose mind and sensation are working, but who is incapable of any voluntary action and whose ability to communicate is minimal.

In the rare event that it is not possible to reach accord among the patient, doctors, and family, the outcome may be different. In Mrs. Randall's case, she and her husband agree, and no doctor would go against their combined wishes. If only Mrs. Randall refused the feeding tube, while her husband and family wanted it inserted, the likely outcome would be whatever the doctor thought best: and that would most likely be to withhold the tube. If Mrs. Randall and her husband and family all still wanted a feeding tube inserted, then it would be inserted, regardless of the doctor's opinion.

Such a case has never been to court in the U.K. If a court were ever called on to decide, it would do so under English common law according to whatever practice a responsible body of medical opinion felt to be appropriate. In other words, if Mrs. Randall refused the tube, the court would uphold that decision, since the majority of experienced doctors in this field would not wish to feed her.

In summary, this case could never have taken the course it did if it had occurred in the U.K. Ventilator support would not have been offered, and a senior physician would not have proposed inserting a nasogastric tube. Both, in the circumstances, would have been regarded as extraordinary, rather than ordinary, means of care, therefore carrying no obligation that they be used. All efforts would be concentrated instead on ensuring that routine care kept Mrs. Randall as comfortable as possible, so that the burden of her inevitable dying was kept to a minimum for her and her family. Such care would include very careful positioning, drug treatments such as hyoscine to reduce salivation when swallowing became difficult, mouth care to prevent thrush, and attention to her bowels to avoid fecal impaction.

Why such cases can and do occur in the United States is sometimes difficult for America's transatlantic cousins to understand. Can it really be explained just in terms of a desire to avoid malpractice litigation? Or does it reflect the essential Puritanism of American society, with its tendency both to demand masochism, and to reject doctrines, such as that of ordinary and extraordinary means, which sound too Catholic in origin?

COMMENTARY

Hans-Georg Koch and Tatjana Ulshoefer

In the Federal Republic of Germany (FRG), the case of Pauline Randall would raise numerous legal and ethical problems, in part because the discussion about euthanasia is burdened by historical experience. The so-called "extermination of unworthy life" during the Third Reich still affects the current debate.

In the FRG one distinguishes among three kinds of euthanasia. What is called "passive euthanasia" means the withdrawal or nonapplication of life-supporting measures. The term "indirect euthanasia" describes measures with the primary purpose of minimizing the suffering of a patient, even if this implies hastening the time of death. "Active euthanasia" means all measures that actively and deliberately induce death, such as the administration of drugs with the intention of terminating life, regardless of motive.

There is a consensus that this last kind of "euthanasia" should be punishable by law. This applies even if it is carried out in accordance with the sincere and expressed wishes of the patient. (The applicable law, section 216 of the criminal code, states that killing on demand constitutes a punishable offense.)

Another preliminary remark seems in order. The discussion about euthanasia in the FRG is largely overshadowed by the debate about suicide. Most of the euthanasia cases that have reached the courts involve patients who had previously attempted to commit suicide. The Supreme Court, in several widely criticized decisions, has stated that suicide is an ethically reprehensible action. These decisions influence the evaluation of the obligations of a physician who attends a would-be suicide. In accordance with these decisions handed down by the court, the physician is liable to be prosecuted for homicide by negligence if he encounters an unconscious would-be suicide victim in a life-threatening situation and fails to administer all required and reasonable aid.

On the other hand, assisting a person determined to commit suicide is not punishable per se, nor is it regarded as suicide if a patient, being aware of his or her situation, refuses life-preserving treatment and accepts his or her inevitable death. This can, in a particular case, lead to conflicting evaluations.

A case comparable to that of Pauline Randall's has as yet, so far as we can determine, not come before an FRG court. Nevertheless, it is generally accepted that a patient has the right to refuse even part of an envisioned course of treatment—such as a specific surgical procedure. Furthermore, in medical practice the use of respirators as well as the insertion of nasogastric feeding tubes are both considered ordinary treatment. Such a wish expressed by a patient has to be respected by the physician, even if it might threaten the life of the patient and is therefore seen by the physician as irrational.

This obligation to respect the wishes of the patient results from the constitutionally guaranteed right of self-determination as well as the right to protect oneself against physical violation. This applies even in cases where a (temporary) physical violation might be medically indicated in order to save the patient from a life-threatening illness. A surgical procedure undertaken without the consent of the patient constitutes an illegal and punishable act.

This obligation to respect the wishes of the patient, however, does not obviate the duty of the physician to counsel the patient and to recommend measures which may be medically indicated. Likewise, it does not release the physician from the duty to render medical and nursing care to the patient, as well as measures that alleviate suffering, as long as the patient so desires.

Although the problem of euthanasia has been discussed in the FRG for a considerable time, there are still no clear legal provisions governing a physician's actions when a patient's life approaches its end. In view of this legal void, various medical organizations have drawn up guidelines for physicians facing a patient's approaching death.

In 1986, an interdisciplinary working group (composed of professors of criminal law and medicine as well as their assistants) produced an "Alternative Draft Bill Concerning Euthanasia" (published by G. Thieme Verlag, Stuttgart and New York). Furthermore, the subject was discussed last year by the criminal law committee of the fifty-sixth convention of the German Lawyers Association.

Given this situation, procedures in the FRG in a case similar to that of Pauline Randall's would presently be as follows:

The case of Pauline Randall would be regarded as falling into the category of "passive euthanasia," meaning the withdrawal of life-prolonging measures. The patient is fully able to express her informed wishes. In such cases, the patient's wishes are decisive, because a physician's duty is to protect life, not to force patients to continue to live against their wishes.

The positions taken by the patient's next of kin, and even more so those of the nursing staff, are irrelevant, as long as it can be assumed that the patient has made an informed decision. Differing opinions of, for instance, the patient's spouse or children do not have to be taken into consideration.

The attending physician would have to respect Mrs. Randall's wishes even if he has arrived at a different conclusion, which he regards as "medically reasonable." He is obliged, however, to counsel the patient and to recommend the procedures he considers reasonable.

Although the physician has to respect Mrs. Randall's right to reject feeding by nasal tube, nevertheless he might continue the other elements of medical care, including all nursing care.

In a somewhat different case Peter Noll, a Swiss professor of criminal law widely known in Germany, acted similarly to Mrs. Randall. When confronted with a diagnosis of cancer of the bladder, he decided against the mutilating surgical procedure recommended by his physicians, although he had a good chance to be cured. In a diary, Professor Noll recorded his thoughts and feelings for posterity. He wrote: "The will to live should not be so strong that one passively endures all pains of life-extending measures" (Peter Noll, *Diktate über Sterben und Tod*, Zurich: Peudo Verlag, 1984).

COMMENTARY
Ren-Zong Qiu

A case like Pauline Randall's is not rare in China, even though it is a country socially and culturally quite different from the United States. In December 1986, a session of the Beijing Colloquia on Medical Ethics (a group comprised of interested professionals in ethics, medicine, and health care administration that meets bimonthly to address topics in biomedical ethics) discussed three cases of pain-ridden dying cancer patients who refused to accept treatment, in addition to three other cases of patients who were irreversibly comatose.

One of these dying cancer patients committed suicide as a result of the physician's refusal to withdraw treatment. The second attempted suicide after a similar denial but failed, whereupon a physician approved his request and he died peacefully. The third is still alive; he thought about suicide after his physician refused to withdraw treatment, but he has not attempted it.

Cases of this sort occur mainly in the middle-sized or big cities and other developed areas where a number of modern hospitals are located. The situation does not occur in the 10 percent of villages where people still live in abject poverty without access to health care and even without enough food and clothing, or in other underdeveloped areas.

Public officers and medical professionals are divided on the question of whether the treatment refusal of a patient like Mrs. Randall should be accepted. A survey conducted by investigators from the Central China University of Science and Technology, the Beijing Union Medical College, the Capital Medical College, and the College of Traditional Medicine in the spring of 1986 found that among 170 respondents including laymen and professionals, 39.4 percent approved of active euthanasia for a pain-ridden dying cancer patient; 31.8 percent approved of treating her with all-out efforts; 16.5 percent advocated ordinary care and food; 10 percent wanted to withdraw all treatments and food and let her die; and 2.3 percent were undecided. So far technology for electronic communication, such as was available to Mrs. Randall, is not available in China, and generally respirators and feeding tubes are classified as extraordinary care.

Although the percentage advocating passive or active euthanasia was rather high (49.4 percent), I doubt that the advocates would definitely follow through in practice. One of my friends was terminally ill with intractable pain and refused further treatment. Both the attending physician and her two children agreed that the treatment would only prolong her suffering and death. But nobody took the move. Why? The cultural climate bound them hand and foot.

The Confucian tradition is deep-rooted in China. There are twenty-four popular models of behavior of the dutiful son from various periods in Chinese history. Some of them made every effort to save their parents' lives, and they still serve as examples of filial piety. According to the Confucian tradition, if the child agreed to the parent's refusal of treatment, he or she would be charged with violating the principle of filial piety. Even if the child did not agree, he or she has to take into account the opinions of relatives, neighbors, and colleagues who may consider such an action a violation of this principle. Gossip is a fearful thing.

Most Chinese doctors and nurses were trained in modern Western medicine (in contrast to those who practice traditional medicine); they have incorporated some Hippocratic principles into their Confucian background. The former's principle of "Do no harm" and the latter's principle of "Ren" (humaneness, loving-people, or beneficence) are fused.

Moreover, their personal experience during the Cultural Revolution made them extremely cautious about this kind of case; some physicians were condemned as murderers solely because they failed to save the lives of patients suffering from fatal diseases. No legal considerations have influenced decision making so far, because courts and lawyers have been prohibited by the government from becoming involved in such cases since the 1950s on the grounds that legal professionals do not have adequate medical knowledge to give judgment. This situation is beginning to change, however, and courts are starting to consider such issues once more.

The salary of medical professionals is fixed and independent of how many patients they treat. And they do not concern themselves with the shortage of medical resources as much as the hospital managers or health policy decision makers. However, economic factors greatly influence the family's decision. If the patient were employed by the government or the military, or worked for a university or state-owned enterprise and thus enjoyed public health services (free medical care) and had a fixed salary, the family would tend to reject the patient's refusal of treatment. The families of patients employed in private or nonstate collective enterprises who are not eligible for public health care are likely to accept the patient's suggestion.

An irreversibly comatose patient who worked in a factory where I did manual labor during the Cultural Revolution has been given all-out life-saving measures in the hospital at the insistence of his children. The hospital proposed withdrawing treatment after several months, but the children rejected the idea.

In my opinion the way out of the dilemma raised in a case like Mrs. Randall's requires a conceptual shift. Medicine should be further humanized, and man's life made more humane. If a terminally ill patient refuses treatment in order to die humanely and with dignity, nobody, including his or her children or physicians, has the right to reject the patient's wishes. Instead they ought to respect the decision. An ethics committee should review the decision to ascertain if the patient is in a terminal condition and if it is his or her real wish.

Mrs. Randall is a competent patient. She understands the procedure being proposed and the consequences of refusal. She prefers a humane death to an inhumane life. Neither her children nor physicians have the right to deprive her of that final decision.

31

When the Doctor Gives a Deadly Dose

At age seventy, Mrs. R. had become severely disabled by cardiac failure due to a damaged mitral valve. With her full and appropriate consent, she underwent a risky valve replacement, which initially went fairly well. However, within twelve hours after surgery, her cardiac output was clearly inadequate. Despite intensive care in the ICU, an adequate blood flow could not be sustained and an experimental cardiac assist device was implanted in her chest. Again, initially she seemed to improve as she was finally "waking up," though she remained moderately unresponsive. A few hours later, however, even with the assist device, her cardiac output again began to fail. No treatment arrested this downward spiral; everyone involved agreed that she would not survive. In addition to the cardiac assist device, Mrs. R. was on a respirator and had seven different tubes going into her body for fluids, medications, and monitoring.

Her surgeon, Dr. L., had remained in the hospital throughout the twenty-four hours since surgery. He talked with the family frequently and encouraged them to discuss their concerns, to visit the patient, and to call in other family members and their pastor.

Since Mrs. R. was vaguely aware and seemed quite uncomfortable, with her family's knowledge she was given morphine. Dr. L. turned off the cardiac assist device and stopped the medications regulating her blood pressure. Since she still seemed uncomfortable, jerking at intervals and furrowing her brow, Dr. L., gave her another dose of morphine. When that had no discernable effect, he asked a nurse to draw up 10 cc of potassium chloride. Then, within sight of most of the ICU staff, he injected it into Mrs. R.'s intravenous line.

Within minutes, she lay still and the cardiac monitor showed no heartbeat. Dr. L. turned off the respirator and went to tell the family that Mrs. R. was dead. The ICU nurses and house staff were very concerned. Had Dr. L. behaved appropriately? What should happen now?

COMMENTARY
Howard Caplan

Dr. L.'s actions in this case are tantamount to euthanasia and therefore illegal. Nevertheless, my opinion is that Dr. L. did nothing morally wrong. He had attempted all reasonable interventions to save Mrs. R.'s life, but not with the purpose that she should experience misery in an intensive care unit for the remaining days of her life. It is most probable that he performed surgery on Mrs. R. with the hope and goal that it provide a resumption of the life she enjoyed prior to cardiac failure. Upon determining that the outcome of the operation was poor, and that further interventions were turning futile and useless, Dr. L. did the humane thing. He provided a quick, painless death, a good death, which is what "euthanasia" really means.

This conflict between law and morality indicates that there ought to be a law permitting mercy killing in appropriate cases, and this case would certainly fall under that category. It is true that the Oath of Hippocrates demands that no doctor ever administer a lethal drug. However, the advances of modern technology require a modification of this principle; reliance on medical technology has brought much pointless suffering to people whose lives can be sustained only with much concomitant suffering. The general principle to guide decision makers ought to be that if there is no hope that medical intervention will restore the patient to comfort, then euthanasia should be available as a choice.

Who should make this choice? We should strongly encourage people to spend some time considering what they would want done should they ever be confronted by circumstances prognostically similar to Mrs. R.'s. Certainly, middle age is not too early to develop a personal philosophy about life and death, and to assess how much life-extending technological intervention is desirable in situations of terminal illness.

The psychological defense mechanism of denial prevents many people from thinking about such matters. Yet human beings are the only creatures on Earth who know they are destined to die. If we refuse to contemplate our eventual death, when illness or old age herald the impending end, we may find ourselves in an intensive care unit, sustained by a variety of life-support systems that do nothing to enhance the quality of our lives.

Dr. L. should be left alone. If any witness to the "crime" is inclined to notify the district attorney, the public will be inundated yet again by journalists, waxing pontifical regarding the ethics of mercy killing, the time-honored sanctity of life principle, and the arrogance of doctors who "play God." If there are people who work in intensive care units who have not yet accepted the inevitability of death, and especially the desirability of death as a means to end pointless suffering, they should find new work in some other area of medicine. My conjecture is that a national referendum on euthanasia would result in the passage of a humane law, offering hopelessly ill patients and their families the right to choose a good death, rather than having no alternative but to experience a bad death.

COMMENTARY
Nancy Dickey

Attending to a dying patient and interacting with the family are always emotionally difficult. Compassion and mental vigilance exhaust physicians both mentally and physically. However, succumbing to the pressures of the moment by "helping" a patient over the final hurdle is neither ethically justifiable nor legally acceptable. The current opinions of the Council on Ethical and Judicial Affairs of the American Medical Association clearly state that a physician may alleviate pain and cease or omit treatment but *should not intentionally cause death*.

Dr. L.'s behavior may be viewed as homicide. Whatever his justification, his behavior is unacceptable by legal, social, and ethical standards. Ethics may at times require one to attain a higher standard than that required by law, but ethical standards should not be lower than legal ones.

Despite recent changes in social perception, the law continues to view Dr. L.'s behavior as homicide. Though the penalties exacted for such behavior have been minimal, the action of taking someone's life, even in the name of mercy, has not been legally sanctioned. Physicians do not have the legal right to actively end someone's life.

Moreover, citizens who know that a crime has been committed have an obligation to report that information. Thus, the health care professionals in attendance with Dr. L. have an obligation to report his action—both to hospital personnel for evaluation and action by the medical community, and to the police for civil action. Dr. L. would then be subject to the legal process of evaluation and to peer review of his behavior.

Some people would argue that there is no difference between allowing an illness to take its course and not instituting all means of treatment versus actively intervening to speed the time of death. I believe that we must maintain our vigilance and carefully safeguard the very fine line that does separate those two notions. We must not allow ourselves to become deities who decide that a particular quality of life is not worth maintaining, that the disease process is too slow or tedious, and that therefore we shall omnisciently choose the moment of death. When treatment no longer benefits the patient, there is no ethical obligation to continue it. When there is little possibility for extending life under humane and comfortable conditions, a physician may permit a terminally ill patient to die. He may allow a relentless course of an illness to proceed to death, but taking a giant step beyond that and *choosing* the moment of death by active intervention is unacceptable.

The physician is regarded by society and individual patients as a fiduciary, a trusted advisor whose duty it is to safeguard the well-being of the patient. Withdrawing technological support and allowing a disease process to proceed to death must be done with great care. To allow a physician to become an executioner, justified by whatever eloquent references to quality of life and patients' rights, would place at risk the role of the healer and the trust of the society in the guardians of health. At no point has medicine, the profession, or its organizations, spoken in favor of euthanasia or intentionally causing death in the form of mercy killing by any name, nor should we now.

Many mechanisms have come into use in the last decade to aid physicians in making these very difficult decisions. Ethics committees and rigorous Do-Not-Resuscitate protocols have been developed in an effort to safeguard the decision-making process from capricious or premature decisions. However, the process is that only—a process. If a physician chooses not to follow it, it cannot benefit either the patient or the physician. More widespread knowledge about such processes and increasing opportunities to utilize these mechanisms should enhance their effectiveness for the profession and the public.

One response to Dr. L.'s behavior would be to report it as a crime. However, I believe that our response should be to educate doctors regarding the ethical nuances of limited treatment versus active euthanasia. This could be done through the peer review mechanism, the hospital executive committee, or the ethics committee.

Despite all of the movement toward death with dignity and rights of patients to terminate treatment, life should be cherished—despite disabilities and handicaps. The uncertainties of medicine should be considered and unless it is clearly established that the patient is terminally ill or permanently comatose, a physician should not be deterred from appropriately treating the patient.

In "making . . . decisions for the treatment of . . . persons who are severely deteriorated victims of injury [or] illness, the primary consideration should be what is best for the individual patient. . . . Quality of life is a factor to be considered."

Statements, currently expressed or previously formulated by the patient, regarding his or her treatment preferences should prevail in treatment decisions. Finally, the compassionate physician, while carrying out the treatment (or nontreatment) plan, should respect the comfort and dignity of the patient. Physicians should be advocates and advisors to their patients, not executioners.

COMMENTARY
Joanne Lynn

This is a very troubling case. Dr. L. has clearly erred. Mrs. R. could have been comforted in ways that are conventional and widely accepted, such as giving more morphine. To use a dose of potassium that will paralyze the heart seems more like giving a poison than giving a pain reliever. It thus seems reasonable to construe his action as being within the statutory definition of homicide. Yet prosecuting Dr. L. for homicide would probably lead to no good for anyone and might make it more difficult to provide justifiable and conventionally acceptable symptom relief in other cases. The wrong in itself does not warrant the penalty that would attach, yet it needs to be condemned so that it will not be repeated.

What should happen? First, Dr. L. should be offered the opportunity for careful consideration, reflection, and counseling. He has been working for too long and was probably too involved in the case, perhaps even too sympathetic to Mrs R.'s plight. He may well be quite resistant to recognizing that others may view his behavior in a negative light and should be granted some time, perhaps a few days, in which to examine his own action and to decide how to make amends.

Second, the family should be supported, as they always should be, through this time of crisis. There should be no deception in the first few days after death, but the exact circumstances should probably be spelled out in a conference with the family a few weeks later. The nurses and others who were witnesses should be asked to write down their observations immediately and the medical record should be carefully guarded against loss or alteration.

The institution's responsible parties should also be involved. These include the chief administrator, attorney, and ethics committee or consultants. All parties should have recurrent discussions over several days.

If all involved, including the family, are satisfied that nothing warrants referral to a criminal prosecutor and if the experience has led to apologies and revised policies that make it clear that this action has not been condoned, then I believe the issue need never be referred to the prosecutor, or even to those who regulate medical licensure in the state. The potassium injection is, to my mind, "over the line" that demarcates acceptable professional behavior; but it is so close to that line that I am loathe to encourage testing its locus and support.

But if anyone involved feels otherwise, or if those responsible for ensuring quality care in the institution feel that there are substantial possibilities of recurrence, the case should be referred to the criminal prosecutor and to the licensure authorities. Most likely, this referral would lead to a dismissal of charges or to acquittal at trial, as the cause of death will be so difficult to prove. However, the experience of a criminal charge and investigation will certainly serve to chasten those who might think of injecting potassium in their patients. Even a conviction might be good for the profession, though devastating for Dr. L.

Granted, there is little analytic difference between giving potassium or morphine in this setting. But there is a strong perceived difference, based largely upon history and the convenience of mixed motives in using morphine. That perceived difference is very important in defending a reasonable range of options for practitioners who are attempting to relieve the symptoms of dying patients. The backlash from prosecuting Dr. L. could well increase physicians' reluctance to provide adequate symptom relief, for fear that deaths accelerated in this way, which already fit within the bare language of homicide statutes, may be construed as homicide.

If this case goes to public investigation, there is probably strong reason for responsible practitioners to step forward to defend other justified and ordinarily accepted trade-offs that can be achieved between the length of a life and the attributes of that life. They would need to proffer examples of good behavior, to help to differentiate it from Dr. L.'s behavior. They would also need to instruct the public that, although wrong, Dr. L.'s behavior should not be penalized severely under criminal law. This sort of case is certain to arise from time to time and is essential in allowing society and the medical and nursing professions to define the bounds of good practice. While Dr. L. will have to bear the weight of the censure, his burden should be lightened by those of us whose range of acceptable behaviors is made more certain and more protected by his being censured.

Selected Bibliography

Part Three: Death and Dying

Battin, Margaret P., and Mayo, David J., eds. *Suicide: The Philosophical Issues.* New York: St. Martin's Press, 1980.
Beauchamp, Tom L. and Perlin, Seymour, eds. *Ethical Issues in Death and Dying.* Englewood Cliffs, NJ: Prentice-Hall, 1977.
Crigger, Bette-Jane, and Nelson, Hilde L., eds. "Dying Well? A Colloquy on Euthanasia and Assisted Suicide," Special Issue, *Hastings Center Report* 22, no. 2 (1992).
The Hastings Center. *Guidelines on the Termination of Life-Sustaining Treatment and Care of the Dying.* Bloomington, IN: University of Indiana Press, 1988.
Kuhse, Helga, and Singer, Peter. *Should the Baby Live? The Problems of Handicapped Newborns.* New York: Oxford University Press, 1985.
Lynn, Joanne, ed. *By No Extraordinary Means: The Choice to Forgo Life-Sustaining Food and Water.* Bloomington, IN: University of Indiana Press, 1986.
Murray, Thomas H., and Caplan, Arthur L., eds. *Which Babies Shall Live? Humanistic Dimensions of the Care of Imperiled Newborns.* Clifton, NJ: Humana Press, 1985.
President's Commission for the Study of Ethical Problems in Medicine and Biomedical and Behavioral Research. *Deciding to Forego Life-Sustaining Treatment.* Washington, DC: U.S. Government Printing Office, 1983.
Rachels, James S. *The End of Life: Euthanasia and Morality.* New York: Oxford University Press, 1986.
Ramsey, Paul. *Ethics at the Edge of Life.* New Haven: Yale University Press, 1978.
Shelp, Earl. *Born to Die: Deciding the Fate of Critically Ill Newborns.* New York: Free Press, 1986.

Research with Living Subjects

INTRODUCTION

While we often tend to think of medical ethics as having to do with the care given by individual doctors (or other caregivers) to individual patients, bioethics has also been shaped in crucial ways by concerns to protect human subjects in biomedical research. Indeed, the Nuremburg Code, promulgated in response to the atrocities of Nazi research during the Second World War, is an important foundation of contemporary medical ethics in the contexts of both research and therapy. As the cases here indicate, our understanding of and concern for informed consent, for example, were forged in the research setting.

Yet biomedical and behavioral research also raise questions differently from individual therapeutic relationships. Research, whether with human or animal subjects, is not conducted primarily to benefit the individual subject, but to benefit others—for the sake of the general public and other researchers as well as current or future patients with the same disease. Thus it becomes especially important to assure that subjects are fully informed of the possible benefits and risks of research and freely consent to participate. So too, subjects must be chosen equitably so that the benefits and burdens of research do not fall disproportionately to particular individuals or groups.

The cases in the first section here—"Consent to Research"—explore what constitutes truly informed consent. Thus one case examines whether someone can be held to a "Ulysses contract": for example, whether someone who becomes incompetent as a result of mental illness can withdraw consent to experimental treatment that he or she gave while competent. Another looks at how differences in worldview and values influence research conducted with subjects from other cultures—especially when researchers from Western countries work with subjects in the developing world.

The second section—"Selection of Subjects and Protection of Their Interests"—focuses on what kinds of considerations should guide investigators in determining who may be asked to participate in research. How should we balance the need to assure that a clinical trial is scientifically valid and that its data can be reliably generalized to other patients against possible harms to immediate subjects? Is it ever permissible to allow healthy subjects to volunteer to be injured in research that will not benefit them directly, but may offer insights that will ultimately help others? One case questions whether scientific data can truly be morally neutral: ought we to use data that derive from unethical research like the Nazi experiments on hypothermia?

Finally, as animal experimentation has become more controversial, questions of the ethics of using nonhuman species to human ends have become more urgent. Can we, for example, as one case examines, use an endangered species such as chimpanzees as heart donors for experimental transplantation procedures? What ethical deliberations ought to arise when we contemplate breeding "oncomice" or other animals susceptible to particular diseases for research purposes, or indeed, when we think of creating new species altogether through techniques of genetic engineering?

32

Can a Subject Consent to a "Ulysses Contract"?

J.S., a twenty-four-year-old male schizophrenic, has been taking antipsychotic medication regularly since the age of fourteen. Four years ago he was admitted to a private mental hospital, where he was treated with moderately high doses of Prolixin, a powerful neuroleptic. He progressed to the point of being treated in the day treatment program while he lived with his parents. Recently, J.S. started to complain of difficulty in swallowing and increased involuntary movement of his legs, arms, and tongue. When symptoms became acute, he was diagnosed to have tardive dyskinesia — an iatrogenic, usually irreversible, and progressive syndrome caused by neuroleptic medication. There is no known successful treatment.

The doctor recommended that J.S. should be placed on a less powerful antipsychotic medication, Mellaril, which he hoped would prevent the tardive dyskinesia from getting worse. After a month on this new medication, however, J.S.'s psychosis deteriorated so severely that he had to be hospitalized again. Five days later, the patient was squatting in the corner of his room smearing feces, spitting on himself, refusing to eat, and burning himself with matches. He refused all medical interventions. When his health and safety became dangerously affected, the hospital invoked the emergency exception to the informed consent law, which permitted physicians to temporarily administer antipsychotic medication against the patient's will. Within a week, J.S. emerged from his profound psychosis and again became affable. In a few weeks, he was able to comprehend his situation: the medicine that prevented him from "going under" was causing him to suffer from tardive dyskinesia, and this condition was likely to worsen so long as he remained on this medication.

At about this time, J.S.'s therapist heard of an experimental program for the treatment of tardive dyskinesia at a nearby research facility. J.S. was accepted into the program, and signed consent forms for treatment with experimental drugs. In the experimental unit, J.S. was first taken off all medication. Within a week he again regressed into an acutely psychotic condition and he refused the experimental medication. Some researchers suggested that J.S.'s parents be asked to invoke a state law that provided for limited guardianship of a patient in need of special services, but the research unit's lawyer counseled against this approach. The researchers then suggested going ahead with the treatment anyway. Since the patient had consented during his competent hours, they argued that it didn't matter if he changed his mind later; the

"Ulysses contract" was binding. (Ulysses had asked his men to bind him to the mast of his ship before sailing past the Sirens, and to refuse his requests to sail nearer while he was under the irresistible influence of the Sirens' lovely song.) Again legal counsel did not agree and the research team finally decided to exclude J.S. from the project. He went back to the hospital where Prolixin was administered. When he returned to "normal" and learned what had happened, he begged for another chance to try the experimental medication.

Who ought to be able to consent to experimental treatment for J.S.? Should the subject's wishes during his competent period be recognized as valid?

COMMENTARY
Morton E. Winston and Sally M. Winston

Two distinct but related ethical issues are raised by this case. The first concerns the decision to continue using a medication that has known harmful iatrogenic effects. Since there is no effective treatment for tardive dyskinesia (TD), decisions to prescribe neuroleptic medications must be made on a case-by-case basis.

Among the possible benefits are the potential for deinstitutionalization and self-sufficiency; the alleviation of suffering; cessation of suicidal, self-destructive, or antisocial behavior; and amenability to other forms of therapy. The risks and costs are the potential iatrogenic symptoms: disfigurement, discomfort, social ostracism, and eventual threat to life. In each patient, physicians must weigh the probable level of functioning with and without medication, speed of progression of symptoms, degree of dose-relatedness, reversibility of the syndrome, and the degree to which the symptoms of TD are masked by the medication that causes it.

Generally, patients and/or their legal guardians are informed of these risks before they consent to treatment. However, because of significant individual differences in responding to these medications, and the progressive nature of the iatrogenic syndrome, clinical judgments need to be continuously reevaluated. In the case of J.S., the physician apparently decided that the danger produced by J.S.'s own psychotic behavior was a graver and more immediate risk than that produced by the iatrogenic syndrome. Since the more powerful neuroleptic will tend to mask the symptoms of TD while causing the underlying syndrome to worsen, the decision does not solve the problem.

The most interesting issue raised by this case, however, concerns the patient-subject's consent to and subsequent refusal of the experimental treatment. We think it is reasonable to interpret J.S.'s initial consent as constituting a Ulysses contract in which he, in effect, instructs others to disregard his deranged protests and to carry out what he had indicated in his competent hours to be his authentic desires.

The function of informed consent is to insure that the individual's own choices and preferences, where known, be given priority in decisions concerning treatment. In cases like this, where a patient is intermittently competent, the most responsible policy is to regard statements made during the most lucid and competent periods as best expressing the patient's true intentions. Given that J.S. predictably regresses into florid psychosis when unmedicated, his refusal of the experimental treatment is probably itself a symptom of his illness, a part of the general negativism of schizophrenia, and should not be interpreted as a withdrawal of consent.

Like Ulysses, J.S. appears to realize that he will need someone instructed in advance to ignore his deranged opposition and steer him under protest into treatment. Unlike Ulysses, however, J.S. did not explicitly indicate in advance that his protests were to be disregarded. However, forgoing the experimental treatment is not in the best interests of J.S. or the research team. Therefore, a "reasonable person" standard would suggest that, if able to do so, J.S. would have acted prudently had he followed Ulysses' course.

Once J.S. refused the experimental treatment, the research team had several options. If the research team had sought to have him declared legally incompetent and placed under the limited guardianship of his parents, they would have had to show that he was unable to make a competent and responsible decision concerning his participation in the experiment, and that the experimental treatment would be likely to benefit him directly in a way unobtainable by any other means. It seems unlikely that a court would have granted guardianship, since the patient was clearly competent when he entered the experimental program, and there was no evidence that the experimental treatment would in fact benefit him, or benefit him more than his normal medication. This is probably why legal counsel advised against this course. On the other hand, to ignore the patient's refusal would appear to abrogate his right to withdraw consent; hence counsel advised against forcing participation.

Since the treatment was experimental, the hospital emergency rule could not be invoked. To give J.S. the experimental treatment along with his normal medication would violate elementary principles of research design which typically aim to control for possible drug interaction effects. Thus, no doubt regretfully, the members of the research team felt that they had no alternative but to exclude J.S.

Cases of this kind could best be handled if there were a regular procedure for drawing up Ulysses contracts, allowing patients to specify in advance the precise conditions under which their requests or protests are to be disregarded, and to designate someone to act as their proxy under those conditions. Ideally, such agreements should not involve complicated legal procedures, but they should provide safeguards to allow competent persons to change their minds. One possibility would be to have the IRB appoint a person to monitor both the subject's initial consent and subsequent behavior in order to determine whether the terms of the Ulysses contract are being fulfilled. Without such agreements, it will be difficult to successfully treat patients such as J.S. who are caught between the Scylla of psychosis and the Charybdis of tardive dyskinesia.

COMMENTARY
Paul S. Appelbaum

The history of regulation of medical research involving human subjects demonstrates a primary concern with two issues: the right of subjects to act autonomously in deciding on participation, and the imperative to protect subjects from harm. Can both these concerns be justified in a manner that would permit J.S. to participate in a research project that holds the potential for substantial benefit to him?

Considering first the autonomy issue, our task is to determine which of J.S.'s decisions—the nonpsychotic decision to participate in the study or the psychotic decision to refuse—represents the most authentic manifestation of his will. I use authentic here to mean the decision that is most congruent with his life history and his sense of himself as a person (see Bruce Miller, "Autonomy and Refusing Lifesaving Treatment," Hastings Center Report, August 1981).

Given the distorting effects of psychotic illness on persons' usual modes of thought, behavior, and communication, J.S.'s decision to participate in the experimental program, which was made while he was nonpsychotic and in a state that the law would define as "competent," is much more likely to represent his authentic desires than his subsequent refusal in a state of psychosis and legal incompetence. This conclusion is bolstered by the fact that although J.S. experienced severe consequences as a result of his initial decision to participate, namely regression to a psychotic state, he chooses to take part in the study when he is competent again. Such first-hand experience with the risks of participation approximates the level of knowledge we would like to see in all subjects who consent to research. Although there may be technical legal problems in honoring J.S.'s previous competent consent at a time of subsequent, even incompetent refusal, allowing him to participate would seem to be the proper ethical course.

Note that no one else needs to decide what constitutes J.S.'s best interests or, at the time of refusal, how he would have decided if he were competent. Like any other competent individual, J.S. has told us his wishes and we must honor them.

Proceeding along these lines, however, raises an additional concern. Ordinarily, one of the most important mechanisms for preventing harm to subjects is to permit them to withdraw from a research project at any point during the study. In the name of protecting J.S.'s autonomy, however, we have deprived him in part of this right. Clearly, some additional means of protection are called for. In such circumstances, an individual independent of the research team—perhaps associated with the IRB that reviewed the project—should be empowered to monitor the situation and withdraw J.S. from the study should significant, unforeseen risks arise.

I conceive the powers of this monitor to be strictly limited. The role does not call for substitute decision making, or for a reassessment of J.S.'s participation unless there is imminent danger from risks of which the subject was unaware at the time of the original consent. As a competent decision maker, J.S. has as much right as any other person to consent to known risks, particularly when the possibility of personal benefit exists. (Many cases of TD do improve or remit with the cessation of neuroleptics, and it is unclear if the syndrome is inevitably progressive even when neuroleptics are continued.)

The implications of this discussion are not limited to situations such as J.S.'s in which the possibility of a competent consent exists. Given the importance of further research on conditions found only in people who can never be expected to give a competent consent—such as patients with advanced senile dementia or severe chronic psychoses—it is crucial to explore means of allowing these individuals to participate in research, while simultaneously ensuring their protection. I am not addressing the question of obtaining initial consent. But once participation has been approved, the presence of an independent individual, charged with monitoring unexpected risks, may provide an important measure of protection to the subjects involved.

COMMENTARY
Nancy K. Rhoden

The distinguishing features of the proposed Ulysses contract are that a person, while competent, embarks on a course of action but suspects that strange, mind-altering forces may come into play and thus explicitly instructs those nearby to ignore future decisions that reflect such unnatural influences. J.S., we must assume, did not initially give a consent even remotely resembling a Ulysses-type contract: regulations governing federally supported research require that subjects be told they can withdraw at any time; in any case, people entering an experimental treatment program rarely agree not to withdraw. Thus legal counsel were correct in refusing the researchers' request to render J.S.'s consent retroactively binding. It would be dishonest, and indefensibly paternalistic, to justify overriding a refusal (even an incompetent one) by reference to a prior consent when the consent lacked the features of a true Ulysses contract.

But even though J.S.'s prior consent could not appropriately be transformed into a Ulysses contract, such a contract could be a prime candidate for getting J.S. back into the experimental program and for ensuring that further incompetent attempts to withdraw will be ignored. A binding consent, particularly for experimental treatment, is highly unusual. But the peculiarities of J.S.'s situation, and those of others like him, present the strongest possible justification for such an approach. The case suggests that J.S. is one of those schizophrenic patients who responds quite well to neuroleptic drugs such that, when taking them, he is in fact reasonably competent, in contrast to his condition when unmedicated. Because of this we can feel fairly confident that his consent while medicated represents his true wishes, like Ulysses' request prior to succumbing to the Sirens' strange spell. Thus the principle of respect for persons would support ignoring J.S.'s refusal and honoring the decision that most accurately reflects his "real" wishes. The principle of beneficence would probably yield the same result, since the experimental treatment is most likely in J.S.'s best interests (unless its risks are unusually high).

But we should not rush headlong to embrace Ulysses contracts for the treatment, experimental or otherwise, of the mentally ill. Our society has a long and shameful history of ignoring mentally ill patients' refusals of treatment and complaints of side effects. Particularly in our understaffed and underfunded state mental hospitals, doctors have treated patients with unnecessarily high doses of neuroleptics without monitoring the patients' responses or attempting to reduce the dosage, and have then ignored patients' complaints of neurological abnormalities until irreversible damage was done. Should we now so readily sanction a binding consent that allows doctors who are experimenting upon victims of this iatrogenic disorder to unhesitatingly ignore patients' attempts to withdraw from the project? We must remember that some attempts to withdraw may be due to unpleasant side effects of the experimental drugs. (Suppose Ulysses had asked that his bonds be loosened because they were choking him.) In addition, many mental patients may be rendered unusually docile, dependent, and easy to control by neuroleptic drugs. Thus an initial consent to treatment may not always represent their true wishes.

Clearly we cannot have a Ulysses contract that makes the consent absolutely binding without regard to the reasons behind a subsequent refusal. It is easy enough to say that a subsequent refusal that is competent—e.g., the patient lucidly states that the new drug is causing severe dizziness and he would rather live with the tardive dyskinesia (or schizophrenia)—will override a prior Ulysses-type consent, while a subsequent incompetent refusal will not. But competency is notoriously difficult to define and determine. Some mentally ill persons, plagued by side effects, may subsequently refuse in such an unusual, oblique, or paranoid manner that their refusal appears thoroughly irrational. Moreover, physicians faced with a patient's attempt to withdraw from an experimental treatment program may be tempted to underestimate the competency of the person who questions their medical judgment (as they may have overestimated the patient's competency when he or she originally consented).

A completely psychotic refusal should not override a valid consent, but we must provide safeguards that will recognize legitimate revocations of consent. Perhaps physicians could give mentally ill patients the option of appointing, during their lucid intervals, a relative, friend, attorney, or other individual (not a member of the treatment or research team) who could act as a substitute decision maker in the event the patient again lapses into incompetency. The various persons involved might still disagree about the patient's competency, but such a modification would allow an independent person, who presumably has the patient's best interests at heart, to consider a subsequent refusal of treatment in light of the patient's mental state at the time of consent, his or her present mental state, any side effects from the experimental treatment, other options, and so forth. Alternatively, patients could choose to make a modified Ulysses contract in which consent would be binding for a specified time period and then reviewed, or in which a subsequent incompetent attempt to withdraw could be overridden, but only after review by an independent psychiatrist or hospital ethics committee. Such modifications could allow valuable treatment programs, experimental or otherwise, to proceed despite psychotic attempts at withdrawal, while building in safeguards to ensure that a patient's legitimate desires are not ignored.

33

Informed Consent in the Developing World

The government of a North African Islamic republic has called upon an American physician, Dr. Arthur Bosley, to determine whether hydatid disease is a serious health problem. This infectious disease is caused by the larval form of the tapeworm *Echinococcus*, whose eggs may develop into numerous large, fluid-filled cysts in the lungs, liver, and other organs. These cysts, which can attain a diameter of 6 inches or more, may distort or displace vital organs or may rupture, causing an immediate and sometimes fatal toxic reaction. Under natural circumstances the tapeworm lives part of its life cycle in sheep and part in dogs. Because sheep play a prominent role in Islamic religious life, a large proportion of the population comes into contact with the parasite.

While there is no effective treatment for most forms of the disease (other than surgery in advanced cases), other sheep-rearing countries have prevented infection by eliminating the parasite. These control measures require expensive regional or national programs for the discovery and proper disposal of infected sheep and for the killing of stray or feral dogs, which might spread the infection. To determine whether it should deploy the resources necessary for such a program, the government wants Dr. Bosley to conduct an accurate survey of the distribution of the disease in humans.

Dr. Bosley believes that the best way to undertake this survey is to test a few drops of blood taken by finger prick and to perform a skin test of the type used worldwide to diagnose allergy. Together with his North African colleagues, all of whom were trained in Europe or America, Dr. Bosley decides to conduct the survey among adult patients attending public clinics, where as many as 100 or 200 patients can be seen each day. A preliminary survey convinces Dr. Bosley that these subjects have an understanding of disease and its causation that is very different from his own. Many of them believe that a disease is caused by the activities of malevolent spirits or persons, and that therapy depends upon removing or placating these beings. However, they also recognize the power of Western physicians to influence symptoms of disease. Dr. Bosley finds that his subjects are particularly pleased with his use of needles as this practice conforms to their own notions of the efficacy of puncturing as a therapy. And it is therapy—not participation in research—that they are seeking at the clinic.

Recognizing that informed consent is a basic tenet of research ethics, Dr. Bosley faces a dilemma. In this particular society and with these particular subjects, can he fully inform them and obtain their consent? Are different standards of informed consent appropriate in different settings?

COMMENTARY
Ebun O. Ekunwe

There are two vital questions raised in this case: Is the proposed study the most effective way of assessing the size of the problem? And, are the tests similar to tests that a doctor may ordinarily perform in diagnosing and managing a patient who comes to the clinic?

Currently, the two tests that Dr. Bosley proposes appear to be the safest and surest means of diagnosing the individual cases of hydatid disease. These data will enable him to determine the distribution of the disease in the study population. Therefore, Dr. Bosley needs to carry out his study as proposed. In answer to the second question, it is quite likely that many patients have had patch tests for various allergies and even more have had blood drawn for "tests."

Accordingly, Dr. Bosley should obtain what is best described as "uninformed consent." In most developing countries, the germ theory of disease causation is yet to be accepted, particularly among the not-so-educated members of the population. Dr. Bosley and his team could spend a considerable amount of time and energy explaining the cause of hydatid disease and still not succeed in getting the people to understand. Since he cannot convince them of the true etiology and pathology of the disease, he should not waste his time.

In most developing countries, a blood test is considered a good thing—if your blood is good, then you are all right. If Dr. Bosley tells the patients attending the clinic that he wishes to do a blood test on them, they would readily consent. In this case, the patient consents without having all the available information at his or her disposal. The researcher is informed on the patient's behalf as he (the researcher) knows that: (1) the procedure is essential to the health care policy decision and (2) the risks involved are tiny and no more than the risk of having regular clinic tests.

Suppose Dr. Bosley and his team were to write out all information on a piece of paper and request that each patient should sign (as in developed countries). He would encounter two major problems. First of all, his population may not be able to read. Even those who can read may not understand all the medical terms that such information is bound to contain. Fear and rejection usually attend a lack of understanding. The second problem is the signature. People are afraid to sign or thumbprint any document. They feel, rightly, that the writer of the document has a hold, usually sinister, on them once they have signed.

If, on the other hand, he spends time verbally informing them, they are going to be suspicious of his intentions. They would consider him the obstacle between them and the services offered by the clinic. In addition, they would feel that he has something to hide—"Many words hide a multitude of sin." Those who have not actually heard him will know him by reputation, through the grapevine. They will in turn stay away from the clinic. In this sense, trying to obtain informed consent may be reverse ethics, as it will keep patients away. Then Dr. Bosley's sample will not be truly representative of the population and the distribution that he arrives at may be vastly different from the true distribution. Besides, he will lose a lot of skin test results, because the patients whose skin has been tested will not all come back to have the result read.

However, Dr. Bosley owes it to his patients and himself to explain that the finger prick will not make them better. If he fails to confess that he does not possess magical powers to use his needle to make them feel better, his program will soon be in disrepute. Before long, patients are going to notice that there is no difference between the health of those who have had the finger prick and those who have not. Finally, even in developing countries, if the proposed tests are different from routine tests, and carry risks of complications and/or pain, then informed consent must be obtained either verbally or in writing.

COMMENTARY
Ross Kessel

This case raises important questions concerning the special problems of obtaining informed consent in a transcultural setting and in particular of the possibility of forcing Western values upon non-Western societies. Many of the same questions may be faced in transcultural settings within the United States.

In considering whether to conduct this research study, Dr. Bosley must weigh the costs and benefits. In considering the best interests of those he is attempting to benefit he must ask how and by whom the seriousness of health problems is ranked; how medical resources are allocated; and whether marked inequalities in access to health care influence the moral choices to be made. Moreover, in arriving at estimates of the risks and benefits of his research he must determine who shall make such estimates. This in turn will lead him to examine whose standards and values need to be considered, and whether local or Western standards of institutional review should prevail, particularly in obtaining informed consent.

Whose standards should operate here? Should Dr. Bosley enforce essentially Western notions of consent upon local physicians with different, and perhaps even hostile, values? Or should he accept some local standard of consent, even if it fails to meet all the guidelines of his American Institutional Review Board (IRB)? He will not receive specific help from the International Guidelines proposed by the World Health Organization.* These accept the principle from the Declaration of Helsinki, revised in 1975, that "each potential subject must be adequately informed of the aims, methods, anticipated benefits and potential hazards of the study and any discomfort it may entail . . . and . . . the doctor should then obtain the subject's freely-given informed consent, preferably in writing" (Recommendation 9, page 38). However, the Guidelines recognize that " . . . those who are *totally* unfamiliar with modern medical concepts" (page 24, emphasis added) and "vulnerable social groups" (page 26) present special problems; and, indeed, state that the involvement of human subjects is only contingent upon freely elicited informed consent *"when feasible"* (page 7, emphasis added).

Turning to the current federal regulations, issued in January 1981, concerning the protection of human research subjects (45 CFR 46) Dr. Bosley will find them similarly flexible. The regulations leave room for American investigators to explore with their overseas counterparts appropriate forms of obtaining consent, without negating the responsibility of IRBs and the Department of Health and Human Services to oversee such research protocols.

For example, a signed consent form need not be obtained if the research presents no more than minimal risk of harm to subjects and does not involve a procedure for which written consent is normally required outside the research context. Moreover, an IRB may approve a consent procedure that omits or alters some elements of informed consent—*or waive the requirement altogether—* if the IRB finds and documents that the subjects are at no more than minimal risk or that the research could not practicably be carried out without the waiver or alteration.

Regardless of these formal requirements, Dr. Bosley will find that the elements of free and informed consent are the same in this study as they would be within the United States. Dr. Bosley's subjects must be both competent and free to give consent, and they must both be given and comprehend enough information to make consent meaningful. However, special moral and sociological problems arise within a transcultural setting in deciding what information to impart, how to impart it, and whether it has been understood.

Dr. Bosley must decide who shall give consent, and under what conditions. He will surely decide that his subjects are fully competent and ought to consent for themselves, and will reject the notion of group or proxy consent whereby a local leader gives consent for all.

Even if the issue of competency is put aside, obtaining individual consent that is free and uncoerced may be no small task in a public clinic. When hundreds of patients must be seen each day there may not be much time or inclination for careful explanations and questions. Moreover, patients in

---

*Anonymous, "Proposed International Guidelines for Biomedical Research Involving Human Subjects," WHO/CIOMS, Geneva, 1982.

the public clinic will likely believe that they are not in a position to refuse consent.

Perhaps the most perplexing questions facing Dr. Bosley are how to adequately inform his subjects of the nature and reason for his study and how to determine whether they have adequately comprehended this information and can therefore provide informed consent. Moral problems arise in deciding what information to impart; sociological problems arise in the method of communication and in determining whether it has been comprehended.

To inform his patients of the purposes and benefits of his study Dr. Bosley will have to enter the belief system of his subjects. In the case of hydatid disease he will find that while they may accept the notion that dogs (animals generally held to be "unclean") may be accepted as a cause, they will have great difficulty accepting his view that so holy an animal as a sheep could be responsible for human disease. Moreover, many of his subjects are likely to be convinced that the final cause of disease is the result of the evil eye rather than the accidental passage of a parasite from animal to man. Dr. Bosley may also have difficulty informing his subjects of the risks of his procedure. He may find, as Teitelbaum* has done, that whatever he may say, diagnostic skin testing and finger puncturing will be "known" by his subjects to be therapeutic. Within their view of illness and its management, the "risks" of skin testing may well be perceived as "benefits," which provide treatment for the unrelated illnesses that brought them to the clinic in the first place. Thus, in trying to inform his subjects about the purpose of his study and the methods to be employed, Dr. Bosley may find himself "lying" in order to stay within, and avoid damaging, their belief systems.

How will Dr. Bosley determine that his subjects have understood the information he presents? Even if he finds competent translators, the cultural gap is likely to prove wide. His best alternative is probably to provide an opportunity for his subjects to ask questions, even though his subjects may have difficulty framing them. Only by this means will Dr. Bosley assure himself that his subjects are adequately (though surely not fully) informed.

In conclusion, Dr. Bosley must proceed upon the belief that his research subjects are fully competent to give free and informed consent. He must develop procedures in the setting of his study that will minimize, if not eliminate, coercion and undue influence both from his own words and actions and from the clinic setting itself. He will need to develop a setting in which his subjects are encouraged to explore with him their understanding of the nature of his enterprise and especially its risks and benefits. He may well decide that his description of the nature and causation of hydatid disease be within the framework of these subjects' views of disease and of their understanding of the benefits to be derived from the study.

*J.M. Teitelbaum, "The Social Perception of Illness in Some Tunisian Communities," *Psychological Anthropology*, ed. T. Williams (The Hague: ICAES, Mouton, 1975); and J.M. Teitelbaum, "Humoral Therapy in Tunisia," *Anthropology and Mental Health*, ed. J. Westermeyer (The Hague: ICAES, Mouton, 1976).

34

When Research Is Best Therapy

Mr. S., a forty-eight-year-old male, was referred to the oncology clinic with a histologically proven diagnosis of renal cell carcinoma, that is, cancer of the kidney. Lung metastases present at the time of original diagnosis have grown. Although there is a small percentage of spontaneous remission with this disease, no curative radiation therapy or chemotherapy is available. The response rate to standard progestational (hormonal) agents or chemotherapy is about 5 percent and those responses usually involve only modest shrinkage. Mr. S. informed his physician that unless some form of treatment would improve his quality of life or extend his period of survival he would prefer to postpone treatment, particularly if a proposed therapy would risk reducing the quality of his existence.

The physician knew that a drug company was financing a randomized trial that would compare gamma-interferon to Depo-provera, a standard progestational agent. As with almost all studies of anticancer drugs, both physicians and patients would be aware of the treatment. Two-thirds of the patients were to receive interferon; those who received Depo-provera and did not respond to it would not be "crossed over" to interferon.

Although no interferon of any kind was then available for nonresearch uses, studies of alpha-interferon in renal cell carcinoma had indicated a 5 to 30 percent response rate. A Phase I* trial of gamma-interferon designed to determine toxicity and recommended dosage level had resulted in six responses from among thirty-six patients with renal cell carcinoma at various dosage levels. No regular Phase II study had been done. On the basis of this evidence, the physician believes that gamma-interferon would be the most promising treatment she could offer Mr. S.

Should the physician ask Mr. S. to participate in this study? If she does, should she make certain he understands that: (1) In her best clinical judgment, only gamma-interferon offers any real hope for his disease; (2) he has the right to withdraw from the study at any time and therefore a right to withdraw if he is randomized to Depo-provera? Does Mr. S.'s agreement to participate in the study entail an obligation to accept either therapy? Finally, should the drug company have conducted a regular Phase II study of gamma-interferon before financing this randomized study?

COMMENTARY
Don Marquis and Ron Stephens

Mr. S.'s physician faces a serious dilemma. She believes that gamma-interferon is the best drug available for his renal cell carcinoma. The only way for him to receive it is by participating in the clinical trial. Since physicians have an obligation to give their patient what in their judgment is the best treatment

---

*A Phase I trial attempts to establish the safety of an agent rather than to access its effectiveness. A Phase II trial is designed to demonstrate effectiveness.

that can be obtained, it might be argued that the physician has an obligation to enroll Mr. S. in the study.

Yet Mr. S. is disinclined to accept ineffective treatment and the physician evidently believes that Depo-provera is very likely to be ineffective. What, then, should she tell Mr. S.? Should she enroll him in the study? One possibility is to suggest that participation is tantamount to a contract between Mr. S. and the drug company; Mr. S. would participate in the study even if he receives Depo-provera in exchange for a chance to receive gamma-interferon. However, this characterization obscures the patient's right to withdraw from the study at any time.

Another possibility is to obtain Mr. S.'s written informed consent to participate in the study, but remain silent concerning both the supposed contract and his right to withdraw in the event of randomization to Depo-provera. Yet since patients frequently do not read consent forms carefully and often do not understand them when they do, it is questionable whether such "consent" would be informed. If the physician is properly concerned with Mr. S.'s autonomy, she should explain that he can withdraw from the study at any time for any reason without his care being compromised, and make certain he understands that this provision holds even if he is randomized to receive Depo-provera.

There are, however, substantial arguments against withdrawing the patient if he does not receive the desired therapy. If every physician adopted this alternative, the study presumably could not be completed. Further, this seems tantamount to *using* a drug company protocol to obtain experimental therapy for a patient while at the same time frustrating the purposes of the protocol.

While it might damage a physician's career in academic medicine, this last course of action is morally preferable. It is the only course of action that does not violate the physician's duty to her patient. The moral bind experienced by physicians who consider enrolling patients in the study suggests that the study itself is ethically flawed. Is this so?

This is a Phase III study of anticancer drugs designed to show that a proposed treatment regimen is better than or at least as good as, but less toxic than, standard therapy. A physician should ask her patient to participate in such a randomized study only if good evidence that one treatment is inferior to the other is not available. Only randomized clinical trials that satisfy a condition of therapeutic equivalence should be conducted.

The physician in this case *believed* that the gamma-interferon versus Depo-provera trial did not meet this standard, not because she was convinced that gamma-inferteron was a proven therapeutic agent for metastatic renal cell carcinoma, but because she had no confidence in the "standard" therapy for the disease, Depo-provera.

There is considerable justification for her conclusion. For some oncologists, Depo-provera has been the drug of choice for metastatic renal cell carcinoma only because there is no other potentially effective treatment. Many would offer it to a patient only if he or she really wanted chemotherapy and then only because Depo-provera does not have serious side effects. In addition, poorly designed studies of the efficacy of Depo-provera have yielded mixed results. Hence the physician's belief that gamma-interferon offered Mr. S. the only real hope of benefit for his disease was probably quite sound.

The trial was badly designed. A Phase III study on gamma-interferon should not have been conducted because there was no established efficacious treatment. The drug company instead should have run a regular Phase II study of gamma-interferon involving fifteen to twenty patients with renal cell carcinoma who would receive gamma-interferon at a dosage schedule suggested by the Phase I trial.

COMMENTARY
Ethel S. Siris and M. Margaret Kemeny

One of the realities of medical practice is that there are some diseases for which no good treatments exist. The difficult question of whether to enroll a patient such as Mr. S. in a clinical trial, with all of its attendant risks and uncertainties, must be faced by both the patient and the physician. Defining the roles and ethical and legal obligations of the three participants involved in the decision to enter a cancer patient into a clinical trial—the personal physician, the patient, and the clinical investigator—provides insight into the issues that arise in this setting.

The personal physician's role includes an obligation to inform the patient of the existence of the clinical trial and to give an objective opinion as to whether enrolling in the study would be in the patient's best interest. There are many considerations in deciding whether to recommend participation in a randomized trial in oncology, including possible inconvenience and considerable expense to a seriously ill patient, the loss of the primary doctor's control of treatment, and the possible risks and discomforts of untested therapies.

Unfortunately, Mr. S.'s doctor is not being objective about the study. Though there are only minimal data on the safety and effectiveness of gamma-interferon in treating metastatic renal cell carcinoma, she has a strong conviction that it is the treatment of choice. She may take this position in part because the results with standard treatment—Depo-provera—are so dismal. However, she also appears to feel that gamma-interferon is intrinsically a better choice, a treatment that she believes should work and be safe. Given the preliminary nature of the studies, some of which examined a different agent (alpha-interferon), her certainty seems premature. The clinical trial is being conducted to provide a more objective basis for evaluating the data.

The physician's beliefs pose a serious problem for her and her patient: She wants Mr. S. to enter the study, but in light of his stated wishes concerning treatment and her strong conviction about the best therapy, she wants him to participate only if he is randomized to receive gamma-interferon. In our view this position is flawed. The physician may certainly convey her impression that gamma-interferon is promising, but she should be careful to avoid creating a situation in which her patient will suffer emotional anguish if he is randomized to the "wrong" treatment arm. Her role is not to make a judgment about which arm of a particular study she hopes her patient will receive, but to decide whether to recommend this or any appropriate study.

The patient's role in deciding whether to participate in the clinical trial also entails certain obligations. The process of obtaining informed consent should make it clear to Mr. S. that he has the right to withdraw from the study at any time. This right includes the option to leave the trial solely because he is disappointed about the treatment to which he has been randomized. We would hope, however, that a patient would not enter a study with the unstated intention of leaving if he doesn't receive the treatment he wants.

It is the investigator's responsibility to be certain that the trial is designed so that it is scientifically and ethically valid, one in which all treatment arms offer equivalent risk/benefits ratios. If the patient understands this and has not been unfairly influenced by unsubstantiated opinions regarding different treatment modalities in the study, he or she should be able to accept his or her assignment in good faith. Though we strongly agree that the patient has inviolate rights, we would also argue that he or she has some obligation to remain in the study out of fairness.

The patient entering a clinical trial in oncology is typically anxious and frightened. The informed consent process, though imperfect, should convey enough information about the study and alternative management strategies to allow the patient to make a rational choice in what is invariably an emotionally turbulent setting. The researcher has the obligation to inform these individuals not only objectively, but also compassionately. All of this takes time, both the patient's and the researcher's. In fairness, Mr. S. should agree to enter the study only if he reasonably believes that it is in his best interest to participate and is committed to fulfilling the protocol requirements in good faith.

Finally, should the drug company have performed a Phase II rather than a Phase III study? Both typically involve controlled trials, with Phase II studies looking for a promise of efficacy of the study therapy in a small number of subjects and Phase III trials seeking definitive evidence of efficacy when the experimental agent is compared with current therapies in a larger number of subjects. When a treatment arm proves significantly more effective than the control arm, the study can be stopped and the new treatment used on a wider range of patients. All new drugs eventually go through the Phase II-III process, since all drugs must be compared to existing treatment regimens. There is no way to assess the efficacy of one arm over another before the clinical trial has been implemented.

The medical community's scientific obligation is to continue searching for better treatments for solid tumors and to test these treatments with an established empirical scientific method. Individual patients and their personal physicians must also recognize their responsibility to society as a whole. Without individuals who freely participate in such studies, many advances in cancer treat ment modalities in such varied areas as lymphomas, testicular tumors, ovarian cancers, and some lung cancers could not have been made. Mr. S. and his physician should carefully consider these issues in the context of his personal needs and wishes as they work together to do what will be best for him.

35

The Last Patient in a Drug Trial

A thirty-year-old man was admitted to the hospital for chemotherapy. Eighteen months earlier he had had an above-the-knee amputation for a malignant tumor of the right foot and was considered free of disease. A month before admission a chest X ray showed multiple areas of metastatic tumor throughout both lungs. For several weeks he was treated with a combination of conventional chemotherapeutic drugs that are sometimes effective against this type of tumor. This patient had no response, however.

Normally, he would now be a candidate for treatment with an experimental drug. In this instance, the drug currently being tested has shown no antitumor effect in any of the eighteen patients with this form of cancer who have received it. Toxicity has been typical for an experimental anticancer agent. All the eighteen patients experienced significant nausea and vomiting for about forty-eight hours after taking the drug. Several patients developed sores and ulcerations in the mouth for several days, and almost all had temporary severe decreases in their blood counts. Two patients developed pneumonia as a result, and were treated with antibiotics.

If no responses were seen, the trial of this drug was originally designed to end for this type of cancer after nineteen patients. The physicians in charge of the trial could then say with 95 percent confidence that the drug would be effective in less than 15 percent of patients with this kind of tumor, and thus that this drug had little usefulness against this form of cancer. This patient is the "last" patient in the trial — unless he responds, the trial will be closed. The patient wants to be treated. The physicians in charge of the trial are anxious to finish the study so a definitive judgment can be made on the usefulness of the drug.

Is the physician obligated to treat the patient with another drug that "might" work rather than to complete the trial? Does the fact that the research team "knows" the drug is ineffective affect the patient's informed consent? Do the physician's obligations to perform scientifically good research conflict with his obligations to this patient?

COMMENTARY
Peter P. Sordillo

The physician who enters a patient in a Phase II trial of an anticancer agent has two goals: to evaluate the usefulness of the Phase II drug against a certain form of cancer and to offer the patient another chance after he has failed to respond to conventional chemotherapy. Occasionally, a patient in whom standard chemotherapy has not worked will respond to a new drug, and sometimes these responses are marked. Likewise, there is no way to assess the value of a new agent other than to test it on patients with cancer, since the effectiveness of a drug against animal tumors frequently does not correlate with its effectiveness against tumors in humans.

The case dramatizes the potential conflict between these two goals. Certainly, the physician does not want to expose his patient to a drug that is likely to make him sick but is unlikely to help him. On the other hand, the physician feels obligated to see that the scientific trials that he conducts are rigorous and valid so that it can be determined which of the hundreds of new drugs being tested every year are useful.

This conflict does not arise only when the "last" patient in a trial is to be treated, however, and cannot be resolved merely by ending the trial at an earlier point. Even after nineteen patients have failed to respond, by the criteria outlined in the case history, there is still a 5 percent chance the drug may be an active agent. Others have argued that it is a much greater error to conclude that a potentially active agent has no value than it would be to conclude that an inactive drug is active. The latter will be quickly discovered, but if a trial finds an active drug to be inactive, that drug may be lost forever. So even after nineteen patients have failed to respond to a drug, the physician may feel he has not "proven" the drug inactive, and may be reluctant to end the trial. Further, even a hint of antitumor activity in such a trial may mean the drug has usefulness for a group that has not been tested (for example, patients not previously treated with standard chemotherapy) or in combination with other drugs. Conversely, even midway through a trial of a drug that has not produced responses (and most new anticancer drugs produce few or no responses), the physician may believe that this drug is *less* likely to benefit his patient than another drug that has not been tested.

Thus, the obligations of the physician to the patient and to do good research, may be in conflict not only when the "last" patient in a trial is being treated, but throughout the trial. Can this conflict be lessened? I would argue that whether a physician advises his patient to participate in the trial of a new drug must depend both upon the status of the trial and the condition of the patient at that particular moment. For example, a physician may feel that a patient who is not healthy enough to live through more than one trial of a drug that proves inactive should not waste his "last chance" on a drug less likely to help him; thus he may recommend that the patient receive something else. On the other hand, there may be less objection to a patient who is expected to have a long life span being one of the last subjects in such a trial. Currently, these distinctions are not made. The toxicity encountered during the trial and the potential harm to the patient must also be weighed. The severe discomfort and the risk of serious infection that often accompany these drugs seem easier to accept early in a trial when there is still a significant hope of benefit than when the hope of benefit is small.

One might claim that imposing such conditions detracts from the scientific validity of the drug trial since we are "selecting" those patients who participate. While this argument may be valid for controlled trials, it does not apply to the noncontrolled Phase II trials of experimental agents as currently conducted. The major purpose of these trials is to detect any sign of activity by a new drug, and the exclusion of sicker patients (who are less likely to respond to agents that are useful) could actually make it less likely that the drug will falsely be called inactive.

Providing information on the status of the drug trial is clearly an essential part of giving informed consent. In current practice, what the last patient in a trial is told about the potential value of a drug is usually the same as what the first patient learns. But the information necessary to provide true informed consent must include not only a description of the drug's toxicity, but also some idea of the success or failure the investigators have encountered during the trial. This need not be a precise statistical statement, but something on the order of: "This drug has been very useful against animal tumors, although so far it hasn't worked on any of the patients on whom we have tried it. We'd like to try it on one or two more people with this form of cancer before giving up on it. If this drug doesn't work, we have other, newer drugs with which we can try to help you." A statement of this sort would provide the patient with some of the information he needs for deciding whether to take the new drug, without foreclosing the possibility that informed patients would agree to participate in these studies.

COMMENTARY
Kenneth F. Schaffner

Medical research represents a quest for useful *warranted* assertions about human beings and their illnesses. Over the centuries many therapeutic regimens of questionable benefit and often considerable harm have been inflicted on patients, from ancient enemeta and bloodletting to more recent gastric "freezing" for duodenal ulcers. Various statistical methods have been developed to test scientifically whether the observed effects of a new drug (or other treatment) are attributable to the drug and not due to chance, biological (including genetic and environmental) variability, clinicians' bias, a placebo effect, or spontaneous remission.

It will not be possible in this short commentary to discuss all the different designs for clinical trials, such as randomized, fixed sample, sequential, double-blind, matched pairs, and the like.* (The trial discussed here is what is termed

*The reader is referred to E.A. Gehan and E.J. Freireich, "Non-Randomized Controls in Cancer Clinical Trials," *New England Journal of Medicine* 290 (1974), 198–203; and more generally to H. Wulff, *Rational Diagnosis and Treatment* (Oxford: Blackwell, 1976), esp. Chapters 9, 10 and Appendix; and to A. Feinstein, *Clinical Biostatistics* (St. Louis: Mosby, 1977). See also D.L. Sackett, "The Competing Objectives of Randomized Trials," *New England Journal of Medicine* 303 (1980), 1059–60.

a nonrandomized Phase II trial.) Suffice it to say that all such trials have as their objectives *validity* or statistical soundness, *generalizability* or wide applicability, and *efficiency* or cost-effectiveness. In my comments I shall focus primarily on the issue of validity and its relationship to the ethics of patient care.

In part because of biological variability, there are few completely deterministic processes or therapies that are 100 percent efficacious in medicine. In order to detect, in as rational a way as possible, those clinical procedures that might be useful, statistical reasoning must be invoked. A clinician who reasons statistically asks whether an observed pattern of patient responses can provide a valid inference for a clinically important effect at some level of probability. (Similar reasoning comes into play in the *design* of a trial.) Sound statistical methodology in a clinical trial is a sine qua non for grounded knowledge of the utility or disutility of a drug. A clinical trial of a drug that is methodologically unsound and/or statistically unconvincing will not persuade other physicians to use (or to discontinue) a particular drug.

Clinical trials, especially the large randomized ones, are essentially a post–World War II innovation. From their inception, investigators have had to wrestle with difficult ethical issues of patient assignment, risks and benefits and more recently with the complexities of informed consent. Clinical trials also illustrate the ethical conflict of the physician as researcher and the physician as therapist.

Statistical validity and the ethical dilemmas inherent in medical research coalesce in this case study. The research physicians wish to be able to conclude with "95 percent confidence that the drug would be effective in less than 15 percent of patients with this kind of tumor, and thus that this drug has little usefulness against this form of cancer." They need one more negative response to achieve these percentages, presumably the patient in question.

Little information is provided about additional features of the research design or why the 15 percent figure was chosen. Apparently this is the control percentage for currently available therapy for this type of tumor in patients at similar stages of disease. The size of the trial needed to achieve the 95 percent confidence level (or analogously a significance level or P value $\le$ .05) can be obtained from what is known as a binomial distribution. To use a loaded coin-toss analogy, the investigators have asked themselves: how many times do I have to toss a coin, which I believe in the long run will turn up heads (therapeutic successes) less than 15 percent of the time, to be sure that I will get this result (< 15 percent) nineteen times out of twenty (19/20 = 95 percent)? More specifically, if we assume a constant run of tails (therapeutic failures), how long must the trial be? The simple binomial formula shows that for eighteen failures the desired probability is .054, whereas for nineteen failures, it becomes .045, thus crossing the "magic" threshold of "significance" or "confidence."

Significance levels of 5 percent or less and confidence regions of 95 percent or more have been adopted, often without question, by investigators and by journal editors who may not publish a trial unless the threshold is crossed.

The 5 percent level is conventional but not completely arbitrary since in a normal distribution approximately 95 percent of the probability falls between +2 standard deviations from the mean. Still, some researchers, such as A. Feinstein, are critical of its dogmatic character.

These considerations underlie the case in question but do not provide any clear answer. Only additional information and ethical principles will provide the necessary guidance. The main ethical principle operative in this case—one accepted by essentially all investigators—is that no patient should be assigned to a trial if he or she and the responsible attending physician justifiably believe that harm will result. If there is another experimental drug available with more likely beneficial results, the patient should be advised of the option or options. If such a drug is not available, there is still a *higher* than 5 percent chance (actually 15 percent) that the drug currently under investigation will work in 10 percent of the cases. This chance is calculated on the basis of probability but should be adjusted to take account of other biochemical, physiological, pharmacological, and clinical information relevant to *this* patient. The attending physician should provide the patient with a summary of this complex and updated knowledge in terms the patient can understand. This summary should include a clear statement of the anticipated side effects of the drug and a report on the efficacy of the drug to date. Should the patient elect the current drug and should it not work, the investigators will have achieved their 95 percent level; but clearly a patient cannot be expected to enter such a trial to achieve "statistical significance."

36

Can a Research Subject Be Too Eager to Consent?

Lila Goldberg, age twenty-one, was admitted as a voluntary patient to the adult psychiatric service of a large university teaching hospital because she had lost thirty pounds in six months and extensive out-patient medical evaluation had failed to reveal an organic basis for the weight loss. After the diagnosis of anorexia nervosa was confirmed, the patient was placed on a high-calorie diet and a behavior modification program supplemented by individual psychotherapy.

One week after admission, Steven O'Connor, a psychiatrist affiliated with another ward, solicited Ms. Goldberg's participation in a research project that would measure the concentration of biogenic amines in the blood and spinal fluid of patients suffering from anorexia nervosa. This investigation was not intended to be of direct clinical benefit to the patient. However, the study could conceivably provide information about the presence of any underlying neurophysiological abnormalities in this disorder. Ms. Goldberg readily agreed to be a subject and signed a thorough informed consent form for the protocol, which already had institutional review board (IRB) approval. As a participant she would have blood drawn by vein several times and would undergo three lumbar (spinal) punctures—procedures that carry a high risk of discomfort and a low risk of infection.

Lila's psychiatric nurse, Sharon Miller, questioned her patient's inclusion in this study. Having observed that all anorectic patients eagerly agree to participate in studies despite discomfort and potential harm, Nurse Miller reasoned that psychiatric illness made an anorectic patient overly cooperative and thereby masochistic. The patient's willing participation in the protocol could be construed as another anorectic symptom. Dr. O'Connor countered that Ms. Goldberg was fully competent to volunteer. Should she be allowed into the study?

COMMENTARY
Spencer Eth and Cheryl Eth

Lila Goldberg, described as an adult who is not retarded, psychotic, or mentally incompetent, has voluntarily entered a hospital for treatment of her mental illness. There is apparently no hesitation accepting her consent for hospitalization, diagnostic procedures, and treatment. Unexpectedly, however, objections are raised to her participation in a research protocol. The argument is based on the peculiar nature of her illness—that anorexia nervosa causes a specific impairment of critical judgment, which greatly increases the likelihood of a variety of self-destructive behaviors.

Anorexia nervosa is a mental illness that primarily affects adolescent girls. Typically, those affected retain their intellectual abilities and can often continue to function until the illness has progressed to the point of serious medical complications. In fact, the contrast between an emaciated appearance and persistent dieting and hyperactivity may be the only clue to this potentially fatal illness.

A prominent personality feature of anorectic women is submissiveness. Many are described as "perfect children." The manifest need to be cooperative, even obedient, propels anorectics into perpetual self-sacrifice. Often the patient's life before the onset of anorexia has been a series of attempts to live up to the expectations of family and friends, along with fears that she will fail to be the "best little girl." Starvation may be the sole area in which she expresses her independence and mastery. The patient is locked into a behavior pattern (starvation) much as the alcoholic is compelled to abuse liquor despite the dreadful consequences.

In situations where the anorectic must satisfy her unconscious need for self-punishment, her capacity to act as a moral agent is diminished. Offering the anorectic an opportunity to participate in an experiment associated with discomfort is comparable to offering a heroin addict the chance to be in a morphine metabolism study. Two dangers of research are (1) probable risks or injuries to subjects that exceed anticipated benefits; (2) the possibility of injury to the person's autonomy and moral integrity. Dr. O'Connor's study clearly carries no substantive physical risk. But without additional protection anorectic patients are vulnerable to moral injury whenever they are solicited for research.

An additional safeguard is needed to supplement rather than replace the anorectic patient's own informed consent. This mechanism might operate as follows: if the anorectic declines to enter the study, her decision alone suffices. If she wishes to participate, then a concurring opinion is required prior to her acceptance.

But who shall serve in this role of patient advocate/guardian? We would eliminate some obvious choices. Local IRBs should not become involved in the mechanics of securing consent. The psychiatrist, whose duty is to provide treatment to Lila Goldberg, faces a double-agent problem of divided loyalties if he is also acting in his colleague's behalf. The patient's parents, if they are available, are usually concerned, but the psychological conflicts at work in anorexia deeply enmesh the family in the patient's illness. One alternative would be a patient representative or subject advocate appointed by the state or by the hospital. However, a much simpler solution is to turn to the professional psychiatric nurse. She possesses the minimum of a bachelor's degree in nursing and two years of psychiatric nursing experience, which should ensure knowledge of the research process, proficiency in interviewing, and the ability to assess the patient's capacity to function in the psychological, social, behavioral, and medical spheres.

The designated nurse should have no vested interest in the research project nor should she provide primary care to the patient. She could be a consultant who would interview the patient until key data were collected. If the patient wished to enter the study and the nurse determined that participation was self-destructive, the patient would be excluded. This independent veto power is analogous to the nurse's role in disapproving a psychiatric patient's pass to leave the hospital if the pass request is deemed clinically inappropriate.

This consent process does not guarantee a wise decision, but it does minimize the risk of collusion with an anorectic's self-destructive impulse. There are drawbacks—added expense and inconvenience, diminution of independent decision making, and the creation of an impediment to research—but the important advantage is that it protects the moral integrity of the patient.

COMMENTARY
Harold Edgar

In all likelihood, Ms. Goldberg should be allowed to participate in the research. Before so voting, I want to discuss the matter briefly with my IRB.

First, Ms. Goldberg has been admitted to the hospital for treatment. Presumably Dr. O'Connor, from a different ward, has consulted her physician to assure that this physician knows no reason—physical or psychological—why

Ms. G. should not consent. If not, Dr. O'. acts wrongly. Does the IRB have a rule covering this situation? Is one needed? Is there any doubt about the impropriety of administering unnecessary spinal taps to patients for whom one is not responsible and about whom one knows almost nothing?

Second, commentators too often ignore nurses and other hospital personnel in discussions of medical ethics. They see patients more often, and in more varied circumstances, than physicians usually do. Nurse Miller, a psychiatric nurse, may be especially capable of discerning a particular patient's inability to understand and act with conventional rationality about a research protocol. Such a patient should not be asked to risk serious pain and discomfort in research not directly benefiting her. I believe lumbar punctures pose such a risk. Am I wrong?

Nurse M.'s objections, however, are not based on observations of Ms. G. She has developed her own theory of anorexia: *all* anorectics are willing to suffer in others' behalf, and this trait is part of their disease. She reasons further that consent produced by "disease" is not free and meaningful.

Her evidence is scant. From what we are told, it is simply that everyone says "yes" to Dr. O'. Are not other explanations of the patients' behavior much more likely? Is Dr. O'. informing patients of the possible discomforts in a fair way? Researchers want potential subjects to say "yes" when asked to join an experiment. Researcher enthusiasm may be desirable, and is inevitable anyway. The policy problem is to temper enthusiasm in order to minimize unnecessary risk taking and to assure subjects a fair choice.

This responsibility now falls partly on IRBs. Few IRBs check systematically whether the research they approve is in fact understood by the patients who sign up. Should they? Broad questions about IRBs and whether there may be better ways of accomplishing their mission are beyond the scope of this commentary. As a practical matter, however, making sure that researchers do not inappropriately encourage volunteering is complex for reasons other than the difficulties inherent in policing a hospital. Briefly, a physician's confidence may be helpful to patients in many settings. Requiring a skeptical presentation can compromise a physician-patient relationship. Moreover, what is a physician to say when the patient asks for an opinion on whether to volunteer? These are problems of research on nonvalidated therapies however. In experiments such as this one patients should be told bluntly that there is no chance, or no reasonable likelihood, that undergoing the procedure will help them. Researchers sometimes shy away from such candor. Consent forms often include boiler plate statements such as "we hope this research may be of benefit to you" in circumstances where there is no such chance. More important, researchers may wrongly convey such impressions in seeking consent.

All the patients Dr. O'. has approached have volunteered. Should this trigger another look at the protocol? Most IRBs do not keep track of such percentages with a view to rechecking the consent process if the level of volunteering seems out of line with our intuitions about readiness to take risks. We should be cautious, however, in assuming that everyone is against risk taking. Persons suffering from a baffling and life-threatening problem might well risk discomfort to help others similarly afflicted. Anorectic patients may have a special desire to learn that their problems have a direct biochemical cause.

The case assures us that the consent procedure is full and fair. Thus, it remains only to discuss with the IRB Nurse M.'s observation. Is it true in the experience of the medical members that anorectics uniformly sign up for research regardless of what it entails? The researchers I have questioned casually say that anorectics are pretty much like everyone else. Some say "yes" and some say "no" to research participation. If that is the case, there is no reason not to proceed with the research.

We presume adults' statements are legitimate signs of their preferences over a vast domain of activity, and we respect such preferences although we realize that people may not truly know what they want. Similarly, we act on the words they say recognizing that people often do not say what they mean or mean what they say.

To be sure, no rule is absolute. We disallow some preferences, and we correct for mistake and fraud in many contexts. But, there is no fraud or mistake here. Moreover, Ms. G. does not fit a narrow category of persons whose ability to process information and relate it to themselves is so sharply limited that to credit their "statements" would undercut respect for the principle of autonomous choice. No claim is plausible that Ms. G.'s agreement is uniquely determined by a condition foreign to her character.

The mentally distressed have as vital a stake as the rest of us, if not more so, in assuring the conservative administration of doctrines that deny significance to individuals' statements of what they want. Surely we are not going to monitor all Ms. G.'s choices, and disregard whichever ones we think occasion more suffering than likely benefit. To assume that her choices in this context require a unique capacity beyond that required for everyday affairs is to elevate medicine and research to an undeserved status. To make informed consent the tool for finding such a capacity will convert it into an elaborate fiction.

37

Can a Healthy Subject Volunteer to Be Injured in Research?

Anthony Breuer

A sixty-three-year-old woman thought to be suffering from Amyotrophic Lateral Sclerosis (ALS), or Lou Gehrig's Disease, came to a major medical center for a second opinion. Here the diagnosis was confirmed. She agreed to participate in a basic research project directed at exploring cellular mechanisms that might cause ALS, a fatal disorder of the nervous system. The project had passed rigorous peer review, was funded by the National Institutes of Health, and had been approved by the Institutional Review Board of the medical center. During the informed consent interview the patient was accompanied by her sixty-five-year-old husband, a retired carpenter who was in good health.

Part of the research protocol required excision of the motor branch of the median nerve in her left (nondominant) severely afflicted hand. The patient and her husband understood that the removal of this small ALS nerve would permanently limit her ability to move her thumb with the same facility as before the biopsy, but would not affect her ability to flex or bend the distal part (phalanx) of the thumb. The patient agreed to the biopsy specifically because she wished to contribute her nerve to this research effort. She fully understood that this was not a treatment protocol and that her participation would be of no immediate benefit to her.

At the same time the patient's husband volunteered to undergo biopsy of a motor branch of his own normal median nerve to serve as an experimental control. He knew he would lose most of the function of the thumb in his left (nondominant) hand. But, he assured the physician, he was not doing carpentry and neither needed nor intended to work during his retirement. He wished to contribute to the research effort and to the understanding of his wife's disease.

The offering of a normal nerve as a control for an investigation into a fatal disease process raises a serious question for the physician/researcher. The husband, who is not the patient, is volunteering to be a research subject. Should the clinical researcher accept the offer and operate on his thumb?

COMMENTARY
Robert J. Levine

In this case there is an easy way out. A normal median nerve can be secured from an amputated arm (for example, from a patient with an osteosarcoma) or, in accord with the provisions of the Uniform Anatomical Gift Act, from a brain-dead person. In general, when we can, we should redesign research to replace a risk of injury (in this case, a 100 percent risk) with mere inconvenience.

But let us suppose that the research objectives can be achieved only by taking the motor branch of the median nerve from the hand of a healthy person. Why not? Principle 5 of the Nuremberg Code should cause us to hesitate: "No experiment should be conducted where there is an a priori reason to believe that death or disabling injury will occur except, perhaps, in those experiments where the experimental physicians also serve as subjects." Should we consider whether a neurologist could get by without motor function in his or her nondominant thumb? If so, then perhaps we can meet Nuremberg's rigorous standard.

This, however, is not the final answer. Consider Nuremberg's use of the term "disabling." Since this man does not intend to do carpentry in his retirement, he would not be disabled in the sense used by the Workers' Compensation Board. On the other hand, try tying your shoes or opening a pistachio nut without using both thumbs. Not impossible, but quite difficult. At a minimum, the prospective subject should be informed of all anticipated consequences of his offer.

Suppose the fully informed retiree still freely offered to donate his nerve. Then we must wonder if his offer is truly "free." Does he think that his offer will be rewarded by the doctors' paying special attention to his wife's needs? Does he see this as a means of expiation of some real or imagined sin against his wife? These are the sorts of concerns that informed the Declaration of Helsinki's Principle III.2: "The subjects should be volunteers—either healthy persons or patients for whom the experimental design is not related to the patient's illness." Admittedly, this is a principle that we violate daily without remorse.

We live in a society that disapproves strongly of pointless acts of self-mutilation: consider our revulsion from the self-laceration of the more extreme punk-rockers. By contrast, we generally approve heroic acts done for altruistic reasons. While a soldier is not required to hurl his body on a hand grenade to save his comrades, those who have done so have received posthumous Congressional Medals of Honor. In this context, the sacrifice of the ability to open pistachios easily may be regarded as reasonable if, in turn, one might save thousands from the scourges of Amyotrophic Lateral Sclerosis. In the absence of the urgency created by a live hand grenade, however, one should consider very carefully the conditions under which such a sacrifice could be considered permissible.

In order to justify acceptance of an offer of the sort made by this man, in addition to the general norms that guide the conduct of all research involving human subjects, the following conditions should be met: (1) The problem to be solved must be very important; the dreadful disease ALS qualifies on this count. (2) There must be strong theoretical reasons to predict that the research will make a major contribution to the solution of the problem. (3) There should be no alternative approaches to the solution of the problem which would result in lesser disability to any individual. (4) The subject should meet very high standards of comprehension and voluntariness. (5) The investigators should make a commitment to rehabilitate the subject to the extent they can with the aid of other professionals such as physical therapists; there should be no charge to the subject for the necessary therapy.

Having allowed the proverbial camel's nose under Nuremberg's tent, can we be sure that the rest of its carcass will not follow? No! Therefore, as an IRB member I would vote to disapprove this project until it was discussed and approved by an authoritative national ethical deliberative body such as the recently abolished President's Commission for the Study of Ethical Problems in Medicine and Biomedical and Behavioral Research or the Ethics Advisory Board.

COMMENTARY
George A. Kanoti

Is it ethical to agree to a person's free choice to undergo a nonreversible injury and thus compromise the principle of "Do No Harm"? Clearly the husband had no ethical obligation to participate in this research, but does he have the right to volunteer?

No overt coercion appears to be present, but there are subtle coercive elements. The husband's feeling for his wife and his frustration at the lack of knowledge about her lethal disease could lead him to consider sacrificing his own healthy nerve to advance knowledge. Since it has been only a few weeks since ALS was confirmed, the researchers should be cautious about the adequacy of the consent. The prestige of the researcher and the institution also can contribute to the decision to volunteer.

The physician is pulled by contrary obligations. On one hand, it is important to answer a medical question in a scientifically valid manner by comparing the activity in a diseased motor nerve with that of its exact normal counterpart. The availability of a perfect control would improve understanding of ALS. But the researcher also has an obligation not to produce harm. The husband is not ill, nor does he have a disability. He would suffer loss of flexibility in his thumb if the median nerve were surgically removed. This would limit his ability to grasp and hold objects in that hand. The physician also realizes that this proposal is freely volunteered. It is an opportunity that rarely presents itself. One benefit might be to the volunteer's self-esteem; that is, his sacrifice will further knowledge of this terrible disease.

Ethically, the volunteer's proposal falls within the category of an act of supererogation or altruism (above and beyond the call of duty or obligation). In applying the principle of supererogation to a specific case, one must be sensitive to the unique factors of the case. In this instance we have a retiree, a former carpenter, who obviously has used his hands in his trade. We also know that the loss of motion in the thumb is not total, but is limiting. We are not sure exactly how limiting the loss of the nerve would be on the manipulation of tools. We also have to make certain that the request is motivated by a genuine interest in advancing knowledge and not by some psychological reaction to the illness in his wife and the frustration of a lack of knowledge about the causes and cure of ALS.

The best solution would be to acknowledge the offer, request further information about the need for full use of the thumb, and advise a period of several months for both physician and husband to reevaluate the request. And, the researcher should make every effort to obtain a nerve biopsy from a brain-dead donor, perhaps as part of a transplant donation effort, during this period. If the effort to obtain an alternative nerve biopsy fails and all parties remain convinced that the choice is free and knowledgeable, the procedure can be performed.

COMMENTARY
Douglas P. Lackey

One could easily imagine an IRB rejecting this protocol. The benefits of the research are conjectural and distant; the harm is certain and immediate. The subject's consent cannot quash the general prejudice against deliberate mutilation, especially when the voluntariness of the consent is tainted by the stress of dealing with a spouse's severe illness.

No right of the carpenter would be violated by this refusal. In my experience on an IRB, I have encountered cases in which cancer patients have demanded access to experimental protocols and cases in which families of Alzheimer's patients have demanded enrollment of senile relatives in experimental regimens. In all these instances, IRBs have properly maintained that no one has a right to be an experimental subject.

Nevertheless, assuming that the research has scientific merit and that the nerve used as a control can only be obtained from a living subject, I think that the experiment should proceed.

In cost-benefit analyses of research protocols, the IRB should weigh expected costs against expected benefits, where an "expected cost" is the probability of a loss multiplied by its severity. No special moral weight should be given to a loss the probability of which happens to be 100 percent. (Likewise no loss should be dismissed as negligible merely because its probability is low.) There is a common psychological tendency to prefer a greater expected loss of low probability to a lesser expected loss of very high probability. This tendency is irrational and should be resisted in the formation of policy.

Far from impugning the validity of the carpenter's consent, I would give it relatively high weight. Many prospective experimental subjects, reading the list of possible side effects, reason that since the side effects have low probability, they will not occur. On this assumption they volunteer for the experiment. This amounts to rating the expected disvalue of their improbable side effects as zero, a certifiable mistake in moral mathematics. (Across thousands of experiments, some subjects who say "it won't happen to me" must be mistaken.) The carpenter cannot be making this mistake, since he knows for sure what is in the bargain. His consent to mutilation is at least as informed and rational as the consent subjects commonly give to experiments that have improbable but catastrophic side effects.

There is a tendency among researchers and many IRB members to regard people with medical problems as morally ideal subjects for research on those problems, even when the prospect that the research will produce therapy for these subjects is nil. ("They have an investment in the disease," I have heard it said.) On the other hand, the participation of normal subjects, who have no investment in the disease, is viewed as altruism verging on the irrational. There is relatively little resistance to using severely ill Alzheimer's patients as subjects in Alzheimer's research, despite the logical tangles of proxy consent.

But the carpenter's sacrifice will be seen as abnormal and will be referred to journals as a problem in medical ethics.

I think that philosophers should be the last to assume that all action not directly linked to self-interest must be dismissed as irrational. The carpenter's desire to find some way to share his wife's fate is rooted in feelings, but these feelings are at the center of human life. For the bureaucracy to block this attempt on moral grounds would be a most inhumane application of humanistic ethics.

38

Nazi Data: Dissociation from Evil

Dr. A. is a researcher currently studying hypothermia. Most of his data come from experiments with fully informed volunteers whose responses are carefully monitored as their body temperature is lowered in a cold water tank or shiver chamber. Dr. A., of course, also relies on results gathered by previous hypothermia investigators.

Among this material, however, are certain data that trouble him. These are the observations of Nazi researchers at Dachau, who casually sacrificed an unknown number of lives in hypothermia experiments. After careful review, Dr. A. believes the Nazi data are reliable. Dr. A. considers this data to be particularly important, since he is both unwilling and unable to take his research subjects as far as the Nazis took theirs; at the same time, he is appalled at the prospect that a published report of his own investigations should be linked to crimes against humanity.

Dr. A. examines several options. He could simply reconcile himself to using the Nazi data; or reject the data on moral grounds and only cite other legitimate research; or use the data but cite it only with an explicit condemnation of Nazi methods and some account of his own ethical reservations concerning its use. Dr. A. is uncertain, however, if this last option would be a sensitive gesture or would merely add an element of hypocrisy to his use of the material.

How should the Nazi data be regarded? Is the data tainted by Nazi crimes or is it morally neutral information? Should researchers treat this information any differently than data gathered in more conventional ways?

COMMENTARY
Mark Sheldon and William P. Whitely

The Nazi data challenge Dr A. to turn inward and focus on his role and responsibility as a medical researcher.

In the interest of possible future good, perhaps even saving lives, is it acceptable to make use of data collected through mutilation, torture, and death?

Is it better not to use the material at all? Is this a sacrifice a moral civilization must make in the memory of those who were lost to the silence of history? The fundamental obligation of medicine is to protect and preserve life. Thus, if Dr. A. believes that use of the data will contribute to the preservation of human life, he should cite it in his own research.

As a reseacher, Dr. A. is motivated by a desire to contribute to scientific understanding and to improving and preserving life. Nevertheless, he realizes that the data are not morally neutral. Nazi medicine lost sight of its duty to preserve life. Dr. A. is aware of the barbarity that produced the data and he must wonder if the men, women, and children who were tortured and murdered will be further violated by use and citation of the data. This question is difficult because it is impossible to know what the victims themselves would have wanted done with the data. It is also impossible to discern what effect using the data will have on society, on the collective memory of the Holocaust, or on the future of medical research. Because of these uncertainties, Dr. A. must acknowledge that by using the data, he may contribute to the desecration of the victims and their memory.

Kristine Moe maintains that use of data from Nazi research is justifiable under certain conditions. The data must be reliable, unavailable from any other source, capable of contributing to the greater good, and publication must be accompanied by a clear condemnation of the means by which the data were collected ("Should the Nazi Research Data Be Cited?" *Hastings Center Report*, December 1984). Moe's conditions give Dr. A. some guidance on what he should do. The first two conditions are clear. They are scientific issues stipulating that Dr. A. should not use the data if it is unreliable or if similar information is available from ethical studies. Dr. A. appears to have resolved these questions responsibly.

The third condition is confusing. It suggests that Dr. A. should try to calculate both the harmful and beneficial effects of using the data and arrive at an estimate of the "greater good." It is not clear how Dr. A. would conduct these calculations or whether anyone would agree with his conclusion. The "greater good" is an abstract notion and it is difficult to know when it has been adequately met.

The central issue and the concern that originally called Dr. A. to this profession, however, is the desire to contribute to humane understanding to preserve life. If the data can preserve life, Dr. A. not only can, but should use it.

The fourth condition requires a clear condemnation of the means by which the original data on hypothermia were collected. This condition is also difficult because it is not obvious how the condemnation should be accomplished. What specific characterization should be given to the Nazi experiments? "Inhuman" is an understatement that does not reflect adequate condemnation. "Bestial" and "vile" would be more satisfactory. Or should Dr. A. focus on the victims rather than the perpetrators? Should he describe the terrible suffering of the victims so that the reader understands the human cost of the data? If the data are a regular and important part of his work, should he try to educate his colleagues and the public by speaking and writing about the medical crimes?

By using the data, Dr. A. may be desecrating the memory of the victims. Thus he is faced with a profound challenge creatively and continuously to sustain a sense of condemnation that keeps alive the memories of the victims and fights against a future that replicates the past.

COMMENTARY
Brian Folker and Arthur W. Hafner

In some ways, the issue faced by Dr. A. is one of meaning. The Nazi data are unique in that they are imbued with meanings seldom encountered in the realm of rational, scientific enquiry. This dimension of the data has gone virtually unacknowledged in current debates over their proper status. Most who oppose use of the data identify condemnation of the Nazi researchers as their principal objective. It seems reasonable, however, that consideration of the meaning of the data in a contemporary context should be an equally important factor for those faced with a choice such as Dr. A.'s. Researchers need to fully understand what their use of the data implies, and this requires an answer to two separate but related questions: What meanings are inherent in the Nazi data? What would be the full value of any gesture one might choose to make regarding these data?

Perhaps the most intriguing question on which the issue of proper use turns is whether or not scientific data can acquire a moral taint. Common sense seems to indicate that a parcel of information about the physical world is morally neutral. Since our society so highly esteems an understanding of the physical universe, some might even argue that any such information is inherently valuable. Why should this be any different for some apparently reliable data (for instance, what researchers at Dachau learned about the resistance of the human body to cold) simply because the circumstances under which they were gathered horrify us?

However, regarding the data as morally neutral ignores an important aspect of human discourse. Disseminated through contemporary journals, such data become tokens in the daily exchange of ideas and information between scientists. Any communicative token—be they words, symbols, or a set of research data—achieve a good part of their meaning through association. A cross is only the transection of two pieces of wood, unless one happens to be a Christian; a swastika is a similar figure, unless one happens to identify with the National Socialists—or their victims. It is of course correct to observe that, unlike a cross or swastika, the data in question have a concrete, primary meaning that is not necessarily associated with crimes against humanity. In the practical world of exchanged meanings, however, the historical associations are both undeniable and overwhelming.

Is it possible for scientists to ignore these meanings or at least place them in brackets and set them aside? It would be easier to say yes if the world of scientific discourse were closed. Many researchers are motivated by a powerful desire to discover truth or save lives. They may, after careful consideration, decide that the demands of their calling outweigh the data's associative meanings, no matter how horrific. Such researchers must first consider, however, the exchange that transpired between science and the public. We are unavoidably identified with the words, ideas, and symbols in which we trade, and responsible for all the meanings they convey. Researchers must be concerned with the perception that they are sometimes insensitive to the ethical dimensions of their work. If a scientist cavalierly gives inhumanely extorted data a place in that work, public confidence is rightfully shaken.

Our ability to punish Nazi scientists by refusing to cite their data has vanished after the lapse of almost half a century. Nevertheless, this outwardly directed meaning represents only a portion of the total significance such a gesture may contain. Such expressions serve also to make important statements about the people who perform them. Indeed, it is the self-defining nature of our use of the Nazi data that is most important.

Dr. A. should reject the Nazi data. We would not wish our names, our work, or our laboratory to be associated with such heinous meanings. This course of action grows out of convictions that contemporary scientific inquiry can and should proceed in a thoughtful, morally reflective atmosphere. However, each reseacher must make such a decision for him- or herself, cognizant of the fact that the moral meaning of the data is an inescapable presence that must be weighed against a legitimate need for the information. Whatever decision a researcher arrives at should not stem primarily from a desire to condemn the Nazis or even to commemorate their victims but rather out of a concern for himself as a moral being.

COMMENTARY
Willard Gaylin

Despite the oft-repeated Luddite statement that in science "anything that can be done, will be done," much that could be done in human research and that would have been beneficial to do, was not done because it was inhumane. We do not separate twins at birth to study the influences of heredity and culture on identical genetic creatures. We do not inflict injuries on volunteers to test therapeutic procedures. We do not allow people to "volunteer" for radiation experiments or burning mutilation—even though the data accumulated could be of enormous help in saving lives; more people suffer from severe burns than from freezing in cold water. We do not, to be specific, replicate the Nazi experiments. On a utilitarian caculus it might be worth it. "We" do not do it. The Nazis did.

The Holocaust is beyond comprehension. The destruction of six million Jews for no other reason than that they were Jews would have been sufficient to mark this as a monstrosity of the first order. The torture and pain, humiliation and degradation visited upon them adds its dimension of surrealistic bewilderment. That this was done not by barbarians in some precivilized time, but by what had once been considered the most civilized country in Europe—by the descendents of Goethe and Kant, the *Landsleute* of Beethoven and Bach—drives us into a blind alley of disorientation. That it was done with the scientific elegance and obsessive meticulousness characteristic of German technology is an absurd and painful paradox.

To examine the detailed activities of the camps is to risk being turned to stone. But even when one protects oneself from the Medusa's head, and examines it only through reflected images of the *Zuschauenden*—the onlookers—our sensibilities are assaulted by disbelief and despair. Explain the silence of the German and Austrian people who knew and in their silence collaborated; the uncharitable indifference of those Christian institutions of charity, the Protestant and Roman Catholic churches; the absence of humane grace on the part of our most humanistic leaders of the western world, Winston Churchill and Franklin Delano Roosevelt. The indifference of the world at large is what makes of the event an unfathomable morass.

After forty years of attempting to "understand" the Holocaust I have reluctantly admitted defeat. If one cannot understand then what can one do? One can remember. One can make sure that others remember. And one can refuse to be added to the list of onlookers, which brings us to the current case. There is an easy technical way out. "Dr. A. believes the Nazi data are reliable." Why should one believe anything from the Nazis is reliable? But it is not necessary to find technical reasons for avoiding the substantive problem. There is no ambiguity here. Let us accept the ingenuous faith of the researcher. We cannot cite these atrocities. To use this data is to become an onlooker, and beyond that, an accomplice. To publish this data in a scientific journal is to legitimize it.

We cannot remain silent while others rationalize the use of such data. By remaining silent we join all those other silent onlookers. The great poet of the Holocaust, Nellie Sachs, fixed their guilt:*

You onlookers

Whose eyes watched the killing

As one feels a stare at one's back

You feel on your bodies

The glances of the dead.

. . .

You onlookers,

You who raised no hand in murder

But who did not shake the dust

From your longing

You who halted there, where dust is changed

To light

*Nellie Sachs, "You Onlooker." In *O the Chimneys* (New York: Farrar Strauss, 1967), p. 19. Poem trans. by Ruth & Matthew Mead.

To use this "data" is to give it, beyond credence, honor. The Nazi medical experiments were but threads in the tapestry of evil that was the Holocaust, but no thread must be dignified by its utility. We must not add our numbers to the multitudes of onlookers who slept peacefully through the nights of anguished cries while dreaming their sweet dreams of a better tomorrow.

39

The Heart of the Matter

A heart transplantation team at a major urban teaching hospital invariably has more candidates for heart transplantation than hearts available to transplant. The program is known to benefit both low-risk and high-risk patients. Nevertheless, 30 percent of the candidates die before a heart becomes available. Members of the transplant team, who are both medical practitioners and scientific researchers, consider alternative sources of organs and decide upon the hearts of chimpanzees.

The researchers realize that they are entering upon relatively uncharted waters, despite the close evolutionary link between human beings and chimpanzees. However, they have previously performed a series of preparatory experiments transplanting hearts between cynomolgus monkeys and baboons. Though all the hearts were ultimately rejected due to the incompatibility of the two species' tissue types, there was temporary survival—an average of eleven weeks—sufficient to "buy time" for potential transplant recipients.

If the analogy between monkey/baboon and chimpanzee/human being holds, the chimpanzee heart could serve as a temporary "bridge" to a human heart, if and when one becomes available. For various reasons, medical and otherwise, the transplant team considers the chimpanzee heart preferable, as a bridge, to an artificial, mechanical heart. Moreover, it is possible that the chimpanzee heart could become a permanent replacement, if problems of immunological rejection could be overcome. Still further, this experiment might lead to scientific knowledge allowing the use of other types of animal hearts, for example, those of pigs or cows. This would solve—practically, if not ethically—the chronic problem of the insufficient supply of transplantable hearts.

Confounding this possible human benefit and heady medical technology are certain inexorable facts. Chimpanzees are an endangered species. There are about 100,000 chimpanzees left in the world and about 2,500 in captivity in the United States. International trade in chimpanzees is banned, breeding in captivity is difficult, and capture of wild chimpanzees is "inefficient" in terms of preserving individual lives. For every wild chimpanzee captured and delivered to its destination, as many as ten other chimpanzees die.

Moreover, captive chimpanzees are much in demand for other forms of scientific and medical research. Finally, the scientific merits of using chimpanzees in research and particularly in this medical therapy carry a correlative ethical albatross. Can we, for such a purpose, ethically justify the use of such a complex and elaborate form of animal life, in several behavioral activities so close to our human selves?

Should the transplantation team go ahead with its experiment? Should the project be approved by the institution's Institutional Review Board (IRB) and Institutional Animal Care and Use Committee (IACUC)?

COMMENTARY
Strachan Donnelley

If the transplant team is embarking upon uncharted waters, the ethicists are in the same boat. There seem to be no adequate or widely accepted ethical principles with which to decide this case. We should perhaps immediately ascribe to Socratic wisdom and state frankly that we know that we do not know. Yet I think we can make some headway and point to the problems that we need to resolve.

There are numerous ethical issues surrounding this xenograft—the transspecies transplant of a chimpanzee heart into a human being. The IRB must struggle with the problem of what would constitute adequate informed consent for this unprecedented "innovative therapy" or experiment. Both the IRB and the IACUC must satisfy themselves that the medical professionals/researchers are fulfilling the ethics of good science—that the preparatory experiments were sound and that there is a reasonable expectation of good results—both for the human research subjects/patients and for the advancement of significant scientific knowledge. However, the latter question is intricately tied up with perhaps the most difficult and interesting ethical issue—this particular use of chimpanzees in scientific research and medicine.

A singular virtue of this case in animal ethics is that it bypasses the usual ethical concern with animal pain and suffering and focuses directly on the issue of the ethically legitimate and illegitimate uses of animals for human purposes. This issue hinges crucially on the relative moral status of human beings and the various species of animal life. If one tends toward extreme positions, there is no ethical dilemma. If animals have no moral status and are not objects of moral concern, we can freely use them for our own purposes (e.g., as supplying hearts as "bridges" to human hearts). If we accord chimpanzees a moral status near, if not equal, to our own, we should prohibit their use in most, if not all, painful or ethically harmful research and certainly in this particular experiment.

However, if we tend to neither extreme, but consider chimpanzees as important objects of concern, though of less ethical significance than human beings, then things become decidedly less simple. We are confronted with ultimate questions about our status in the overall scheme of the world and about our proper relation to nature and the realm of animal life. Concerning all this, there is no philosophic or ethical consensus, though I would argue for a fundamental ecological perspective and a conception of man as within nature.

From such a perspective, animal individuals and communities of individuals are understood to be essentially interconnected. Individual animal lives are lived out on various species-specific levels of activity, some more complex, elaborate, and, thus, ethically significant than others. Organic, worldly "activity" is taken to be the "ultimate good," and thus the fundamental focus of ethical concern. Our final ethical duty is therefore the protection of the ongoing realm of life as a whole, with its various interlocked levels of animate being. Our penultimate ethical duty is concern for finite and mortal individual lives (the concrete instances of life), relative to their unequal status of ethical significance.

According to this philosophically speculative and tentative position, it would be unethical to use chimpanzees for merely therapeutic purposes—that is, to use individual chimpanzees for the sake of individual human beings. Given the open-ended demand for "bridge hearts," this already endangered species of richly significant life would soon be extinct. Human life would remain finite, mortal, and vulnerable to all the vicissitudes of worldly, metabolic existence, while the particular and complex goodness of chimpanzee being would have vanished from the world. The ethical costs of such human self-concern, both for human beings and for the animal kingdom as a whole, seem unjustifiable.

However, if this procedure were deemed a potentially significant scientific experiment that in no way threatened the presence of "chimpanzee being" in animate nature, then it might be ethically justifiable. If there was the real potentiality of the use of animal hearts of nonendangered species (e.g., pigs or cows), if we deemed this an ethically appropriate use of individual animal lives, and if the chimpanzee experiments were crucial to the possible realization of this novel therapy, we could ethically justify the use of a limited number of chimpanzees—if this were an adequate allocation of a very scarce animal research resource and if we satisfied the ethical demands of experimentation on human research subjects.

These are all very big "ifs." Ethical caution should here carry the first word, in the face of parochial human self-interests and medical technological hubris. However, a possible ethical justification could be based on the intrinsic goodness of organic, worldly activity and the varying ethical significance of different levels of animate being. This, of course, would be to subscribe to a substantive speculative vision of the world. Yet this seems the fate of all ethical positions—that they are ultimately based in some particular metaphysics.

COMMENTARY
Willard Gaylin

Following the wisdom of the Queen of Hearts ("Sentence first—verdict afterwards") I will start with my conclusions. Although trees may have standing, animals have no "rights." In the world of morality—as in the world of politics—the animate (and the inanimate) exist, are valued, respected, esteemed, judged, considered, dealt with or destroyed, all in service of the purposes and interests of humankind.

This position has in the past been attacked as being unfairly anthropocentric. I acknowledge my bias, although I would point out to critics that the position was most firmly established in the religious tradition of the Old Testament and confirmed in that same tradition by such modern philosophers as Kant. With the inherent self-confidence of his Lutheran morality, Kant said, "The first time he [man] ever said to the sheep, "Nature has given you the skin you wear for my use, not for yours," . . . he became aware of the way in which his nature privileged and raised him above all animals." We stand above the general animal host.

I oppose the attribution of rights to animals because I fear it diminishes the special status of Homo sapiens. The respect for human beings demands a dignity granted our species beyond any qualitative comparison with others. We are *sui generis*. We also pay a price. This unique nature imposes a special moral obligation on our species, which is why only we human beings are able, and willing, to agonize about other species.

There is no way to defend or argue the special dignity of humankind within the brief context of a case history. But even within the severity of my position the case of the chimpanzee hearts raises moral dilemmas. It *is* directly within the purposes of humankind to treat animals with compassion, empathy, sensitivity, and understanding; to have reverence for those common qualities we share with the higher primates; and to be aware that with the mutability of our nature the way we honor and revere other creatures and other things will define the degree to which we have been true to our humanity. If human nature is so perverted as to be indifferent to suffering and blind to beauty, what is left of that nature is no longer "human"—therefore not worthy of its special role in the moral universe.

This does not mean that living things may not command respect. But all animals are not created equal. This is recognized implicitly in the Animal Welfare Act. In this act "animal" is defined as "warm-blooded animal." As Sara Swenson has noted, the word "animal" itself is here defined in anthropocentric terms of the animal's usefulness/relationship to human beings, rather than by criteria such as intelligence or biological complexity.

Some animals have less value than inanimate structure; some animals have negative value. I do not grieve for the destruction of T. pallidum, that beautiful and delicate spiral organism that is the cause of human syphilis. To destroy this entire species would be a blessing, whereas if someone were to blow up the Grand Tetons or willfully destroy Botticelli's "Primavera," a greater moral crime would have been committed through the destruction of these inanimate "things."

Nonetheless, this case is a difficult one. Heart transplantation is not necessarily my highest priority of research in this period of limited resources. But in this specific case it deals with the survival of children which, indeed, is high on my priorities. However, it places at risk that creature most nearly human, and therefore most worthy of respect, the chimpanzee.

To debate the principles, beyond the case history, let us now not concern ourselves with the value of heart transplants, or other specifics of the current state of scientific knowledge. Let us assume a valuable and available technology, and go straight to the heart of the moral dilemma.

Chimpanzees have enormous charm, sensitivity, great intelligence and a strong kinship with humanity. Should this be sacrificed for human ends — and with what limits? The implicit issue evolves into the following dilemmas: Given a promising or proven procedure would you sacrifice a chimpanzee for a trivial human need? I suspect most of us would not. Would you sacrifice a chimpanzee for a child's life? I suspect most of us would. Would you sacrifice the entire species of chimpanzees for the entire species of Homo sapiens? I suspect most of us would. And now finally the hard question. Would you risk sacrificing the species of chimpanzees to relieve the pain and suffering and premature death of many children? Here, I, at least, emphatically would. Others would not.

Our current understanding of anthropology is replete with the suggestion of humanoid species — higher than the chimpanzees — which have died out for unknown causes of climate or competition. Such is the "cruelty" or actually the moral indifference of nature. It is only with the introduction of human sensibility, human empathy, and human contacts for identification that we — alone among creatures — consider the "rights" of other species. It is the nobility of the human being that some of our misguided members might sacrifice their own children for the preservation of a kindred, living creature. I am pleased for the presence of such advocates (they honor our species) even while I reject their sentimentalities. I am, however — even with my coarser sensibilities as expressed by my willingness to sacrifice the chimpanzee — still, I hope, within the limits of decency that define that glorious discontinuity — Homo sapiens.

40

New Creations?

In the past three decades, researchers have been able to make many mammalian cells grow as cell lines in culture. These cell lines have been essential to the growth of modern cell biology, and have had many therapeutic spin-offs, such as the production of diagnostic monoclonal antibodies. The use of cell lines is even supported by many animal rights campaigners, as they have spared some animals from being used in research.

In the last few years, a special kind of cell line derived from early embryonic cells has also been developed. These cells, called embryonic stem cells (ES cells), are derived from preimplantation blastocysts and can be subjected to genetic manipulation. A major practical application of ES cells is to allow the selecting out of desired genetic variations. Cells carrying the altered gene(s) can then be injected into a blastocyst of the same species to genetically engineer an animal with a desired trait, such as early tumor formation. (A slightly different technique was used to create the famous patented Harvard "Oncomouse.") The animals made will be intraspecies chimeras, but their progeny will not be because only a single egg or sperm cell is used. Some of these reproductive cells will be genetically derived from ES cells of the chimeric animal. In this way a new genetic strain of animals is made.

ES cells could also be injected into a blastocyst of another species to create a transpecies chimera. New species can also be created by simply mixing very early (preblastocyst) embryonic cells from two different species. The most publicized example of such a cross-species chimera was the "geep," formed by mixing the embryonic cells of a goat and a sheep. While most of the research has been done in mice and farm animals, researchers have developed similar cell lines from human embryonic tumor cells.

Given the effects of this research on the animals involved, and the potential implications of future research, is it ethical for research using ES cells or chimeras to proceed?

COMMENTARY
Darryl Macer

In medicine, scientific research, and agriculture, the use of ES cell lines presents definite advantages in breeding, limited clonal reproduction, and the development of new animal strains. Research on ES cells is a very rapidly developing new technology, and since it involves changing life-forms themselves, respect and caution are required of any researcher. Considering the wide genetic variation occurring naturally, new animal strains should not be thought of as unique, artificial forms of life. Nor has past experience with recombinant DNA indicated any *inherent* danger in mixing genes from different species. A first question to address, then, is whether the benefits to our knowledge and technological advances are worth the harms to the animals.

Many human genetic diseases are untreatable, and even if the gene(s) involved are known it can take many years to understand the cause. Some animals have been made using ES cells to be laboratory models of human disease, and will substantially advance the research leading to cures. Animals have also been made to be sensitive for drug testing, and if cloned animals are used this can greatly reduce the number of animals—as well as the time—required for such tests, prior to clinical trials. ES cells are also being used for basic research into gene expression and development, which, while having fewer immediate benefits, will have broader long-term benefits in agriculture and medicine.

An important objection to this research is that we should not deliberately create diseased animals. If we begin from the premise that it is wrong to make diseased animals, unless there is some perceived benefit to other animals or humans, the central research question is how much scientific benefit can be reasonably expected to come from the creation of these animals. Here we have to weigh not only benefits and harms, but also uncertain benefits with certain harms, namely, the suffering of diseased animals. Although the prospective benefits suggest that we should assess the ethics of proposed research on a case-by-case basis, this assessment should be guided by a limit that created animals should not suffer beyond the falling thresholds acceptable for vivisection.

Some current research using ES cell lines raises questions about whether animals are being used without any clear sense of what benefits are expected. For example, some research has used ES cell lines to test the effects of blind mutations to multiple genes, with the principal goal seeming to be to maximize the number of mutated genes per animal. Researchers then analyze the animals that survive this process in a manner analogous to that in which mutated yeast and bacterial cells are used to study gene mutations. While this approach may increase the pace of research, it may be unethical in that it imposes more pain on animals than is caused by vivisection upon known animal varieties. Moreover, if we do not know what genes we are mutating or the effects of a given mutation, how will it be possible to determine whether the research in question is potentially beneficial or ethical? In general, there needs to be a more thorough examination of the ethical limits of breeding mutated, transgenic, and chimeric animals for both research and agriculture.

Research involving potential human ES cells is more dubious. Skills in human embryo manipulation are improving, and several babies have been born following preimplantation genetic biopsy; at the pace at which embryo manipulation advances, it may not be long before there are practical uses for ES cell lines. In addition to research on the roles of genes in development, some research might be extrapolated for use in corrective germline therapy. This would be ethical, however, only when we have first achieved precision with research on animals.

Moreover, such research should be deferred until society has come to a consensus on the time and developmental limits of human embryo experimentation. If we are prepared to justify some human embryo experiments for their scientific or medical benefit, then research on embryos involving ES cell lines could also be reviewed by regulatory authorities. The criteria here might be the extent to which research is directed toward developing therapy to treat the symptoms or the causes of some genetic diseases.

Scientists have come to accept regulation upon their work. The control of the use of some developments in genetic manipulation, such as the temporary ban during the 1970s and current controls on human gene therapy and human embryo examination, show that limits can be placed. These examples illustrate that, if the legal-ethical debate catches up with the science, common fears of a slippery slope need not be so great.

COMMENTARY
Roger A. Balk

This case is problematic in the way it links together events and processes that are distantly if at all related. Growing cell lines in culture and developing embryonic stem cells are related only to the extent that both make use of cell cultures. A major question that may be raised by the creation of transgenic animals is the kind of potential moral threat this activity represents.

The case suggests that the creation of a transspecies chimera is a major problem in and of itself. At the risk of trivializing the discussion, we could observe that this is nothing more than the creation of another jackass, and while mule drivers may be a special breed, neither they nor their charges are commonly regarded as a new species. Of course, to many, and not just animal rightists, the questions of a species barrier is a significant point for moral and ethical concern, and to this matter we will return in due course.

The fact is that embryonic stem (ES) cell research is a very exciting technological development for those engaged in transgenic animal research. It introduces DNA by viral transduction or transfection into embryonic stem cell lines. The process involves isolating inner mass cells from a blastocyst and maintaining them in culture as pluripotent ES cells. ES cells are selected in which the incoming DNA recombines with homologous chromosomal sequences to create a mutation in the target gene. These cells are transferred into a recipient blastocyst and germ-line chimeras are generated. The chimeras are founders of lines that carry the selected mutation. The process as a whole is called homologous gene targeting.

There is tremendous potential use for homologous gene targeting in developing therapies for human genetic disorders. Targeting mouse homologs of these genes would produce animal models of specific human diseases. It may also be possible to propagate other stem cells in vitro just as it is possible to propagate ES cells—such as the recent isolation of mouse bone-marrow stem cells that retain their ability to regenerate the entire blood cell population. When it becomes possible to identify and propagate the corresponding human bone-marrow stem cells, the cells of someone suffering from a severe hemoglobinopathy could be targeted with sequences of normal globin genes to correct the genetic defect. Moreover, the fact that this process can occur in vitro suggests that a potential replacement for animal models may exist in this technology.

A process with this kind of potential cannot be regarded as benign, and the question of what ethical and social controls should be placed on its development and use is a very real one.

While the creation of cross-species chimeras may get news headlines, it is not really very newsworthy. It does not in itself represent a change in species. A goat with a few sheep genes is still a goat. The major challenge presented by such mutants would appear only if it were decided to wipe out all the sheep and goats in the world except for the offspring of this combination. The future of this population based upon a single animal source could be threatened, since it lacked the genetic variation that is the basis for survival in terms of Darwinian evolution. To replace the cumulative wisdom of natural selection for human purposes by interfering in massive ways with the future of germ lines is worrisome, to say the least. As it might be applied to commercial agriculture, the technology will require careful scrutiny and undoubted regulation. To my mind, the issue of intervention, not that of the sanctity of species (a dubious biological notion at best), is the real cause for concern. The appropriate response is to limit specific human designs strictly, rather than outlaw a very promising technology.

The speed at which developments are taking place in this one area of biotechnology poses a genuine problem even for those who are active participants in these changes. For those of us who must come by our understanding of these events at second hand, it is downright daunting. The series of experiments that enable these new techniques to be developed are abstruse to the nonspecialist; often a whole new field is there before anyone is actually aware of its presence. Even more depressing is the poor record of the regulatory process in the United States in coping with these issues. When we add to this the fact that no ethical or social impact review is a part of the patenting process, it is easy to form the view that the whole undertaking has gotten out of hand.

This case presents no ethical challenges to the technique of ES cell research. The problem will arise when a specific proposal is made to target cells that control, say, some aspect of human behavior. The question is how we as a society are going to get wind of these developments, and what means we are going to devise for controlling the problems that grow out of them.

COMMENTARY
Benjamin Freedman and Marie-Claude Goulet

> *Revenons á nos moutons.*
>
> —Maître Pantelin

Is this form of research ethical? The question has been asked a thousand times before, on topics from AIDS to zoonosis. It will, in the future, be asked ten thousand times more. We know the canonical form the answer must take: "It is ethical, provided...." And we know how to fill the hole left by the ellipsis: The trusty, rusty old bioethical tool kit is unpacked. Risks, benefits, liberties, all are arrayed on the bench, and forced into the approximately fitting slot of autonomy, beneficence, and so on. The approach has served us well before, on many questions, and no doubt will in the future as well. But the activity in question—transspecies manipulation—is different.

We are not, in the most relevant sense, talking of transspecies *research*. Research is a preliminary to a change in practice, and the ethics of research is the ethics of a means. But transspecies manipulation is, recursively, the change itself; research into doing it does it. (And new organisms do tend to take on a life of their own.)

It makes no sense, then, to talk of this as research; but even if it did, it would make no sense to use the old research ethics vocabulary in this context. The conscious, calculated modification of organisms to achieve a genetic complement unknown(and commonly unachievable) in nature, represents a new departure in human capacity, and a new stage in the history of this world over which we have claimed regnance. Before trying to parse the ethics of this practice, we need to choose an appropriate attitude for reflection. The attitude that must be rejected is one of business as usual. The appropriate emotion is awe.

John Mendeloff has noted features of reasoning common to bioethical commissions.* Areas of common agreement are sought—in particular, legitimating analogies: old, accepted practices that appear to be relevantly similar to the novel issue in question. A limited agenda is set, confining the question within narrow limits. The adoption of a legitimating analogy implies that no novel ethical concern is raised; the narrow agenda excludes all slippery slope arguments. Yet transspecies manipulation is of its essence a new departure, and our current fumbling attempts are ushering in a new era of biological (and biologistic) history. The standard maneuvers of commissions—"muddling through," in Mendeloff's phrase—so useful in seeking a consensus view, are peculiarly inapt for transspecies manipulation.

We can trace the malignant influence of these habits of thought within the numerous documents that have been issued through the standard consultative process, even when the genetic manipulation of human somatic cells is under practical consideration. (Unnoticed by most commissions, even current proposals for human somatic cell genetic intervention bear a transspecies component, in their functional incorporation of noncoding regulatory sequences drawn from mice or viruses.) The (Australian) National Health and Medical Research Council report on somatic cell gene manipulation sees it as ethically comparable to "many drugs" (p. 15), or "conventional treatments" or "drugs and vaccines" (p. 16), or "cancer chemotherapy" (p. 18)—very much business as usual. The statement on gene therapy issued by the European Medical Research Councils in February 1988 states, "Insertion of genetic material into somatic cells and their subsequent transplantation is not fundamentally different from any form of organ transplantation or blood transfusion."(!)

Undeniably, somatic genetic manipulation shares some features in common with other forms of treatment. The creation of chimeric forms of life has its own legitimating analogies, for example, selective breeding, cross-pollination, and the deliberate induction of mutagenesis. But both forms of genetic manipulation are in other respects strikingly new departures: planned maneuvers, in principle irreversible, that effect alterations of individual or species at the

*John Mendeloff, "Politics and Bioethical Commissions: 'Muddling Through' and the 'Slippery Slope,' " *Journal of Health Politics, Policy and Law* 10, no. 1 (1985): 81–92.

biological lowest common denominator, the molecular genetic level. That level of change is plenipotent. While dramatic changes in organisms or progeny can be induced chemically, surgically, by controlling the environment, or controlling breeding, the potential of these agents of change remains a subset of the prospects opened up through genetic manipulation, which in principle permits all possible biological changes to be actualized.

Of course, it will be responded, current molecular biologic and embryologic manipulative techniques are primitive, clumsy. Their current and imminent use will be restricted to the benign (correction of lethal single-gene defects in newborns, induction of more efficient strains of cattle and grain, for example), and to the occasional side-show ("geeps").

The objection utterly misses our point, which is not concerned with the *use* of transspecies manipulation but with its *meaning and import*. Future generations will look back at our geeps and see in them the muted harbinger of all that was to come. Future cartoonists will draw geeps as emblematic of prehistory, as Gary Larson, in *The Far Side*. draws wheels hewn of stone. The current induction of transspecies change is a cusp, and one that seems to us closer to an unimaginable future than to a comfortably familiar past.

As is often the case, though, it is easier to be critical than constructive. Transspecies manipulation is not business as usual; but what approach would be better? We will need to canvass our traditions, religious and cultural as well as ethical, for clues; and we may find, as we had discovered in reading traditional Jewish sources, that genetics and speciation are central to some concepts of creation.* We will need to entertain and explore new principles of reasoning, too. An ethics of changing—changing of species as well as of individuals—is one possible arena for consideration, with departures from a natural baseline themselves requiring justification, independent of such familiar grounds of ethical critique as risk. (Further problems are in turn suggested, as choosing a benchmark for change from a world in random as well as purposeful flux.) Inquiry should be above all wide ranging; in the dictionary of ethics, the entry under "wicked" should read "seriously lacking in imagination."

We are not suggesting that transspecies manipulation be banned, nor are we prepared to say how it should be controlled. We are simply wondering how we should think about it. All that we are certain of is how this inquiry should start: with somber awe.

Selected Bibliography

Part Four: Research with Living Subjects

Annas, George J., Glantz, Leonard H., and Katz, Barbara F., *Informed Consent to Human Experi-
mentation: The Subject's Dilemma*. Cambridge, MA: Ballinger, 1977.
Barber, Bernard. *Informed Consent in Medical Therapy and Research*. New Brunswick, NJ: Rutgers
University Press, 1980.

---

*Benjamin Freedman, "Leviticus and DNA: A Very Old Look at a Very New Problem," *Journal of Religious Ethics* 8, no. 1 (1980).

Beecher, H.K., "Ethics and Clinical Research," *New England Journal of Medicine* 274 (1966): 1354–60.

Christakis, Nicholas A. "The Ethical Design of an AIDS Vaccine Trial in Africa," *Hastings Center Report* 18, no. 3 (1988):31–37.

Dickens, Bernard M., Gostin, Larry, and Levine, Robert J., eds. "Research on Human Populations: National and International Guidelines," *Law, Medicine & Health Care* 19, nos. 3–4 (1991).

Fox, Michael Allen. *The Case for Animal Experimentation*. Berkeley: University of California Press, 1986.

Fried, Charles. *Medical Experimentation: Personal Integrity and Social Policy*. New York: American Elsevier, 1974.

Jones, James H. *Bad Blood: The Tuskegee Syphilis Experiment, 2nd edition*. New York: Free Press, 1992.

Katz, Jay, Capron, Alexander M., and Glass, Eleanor S., eds. *Experimentation with Human Beings: The Authority of the Investigator, Subject, Professions, and State in the Human Experimentation Process*. New York: Russell Sage Foundation, 1972.

Levine, Robert J. *Ethics and Regulation of Clinical Research*, 2d ed. New Haven: Yale University Press, 1988.

National Commission for the Protection of Human Subjects of Biomedical and Behavioral Research. *The Belmont Report: Ethical Principles and Guidelines for Protection of Human Subjects of Research*. DHEW (OS) 78-0012. Bethesda, MD.: U.S. Government Printing Office, 1978.

President's Commission for the Study of Ethical Problems in Medicine and Biomedical and Behavioral Research. *Protecting Human Subjects: The Adequacy and Uniformity of Federal Rules and Their Implementation*. Washington, DC: U.S. Government Printing Office, 1981.

Regan, Tom. *The Case for Animal Rights*. Berkeley: University of California Press, 1983.

Rowan, Andrew N. *Of Mice, Models, and Men: A Critical Evaluation of Animal Research*. Albany: State University of New York Press, 1984.

Mental Incompetence

INTRODUCTION

Contemporary medical ethics almost routinely stresses the importance of respecting individuals' autonomy in seeking ways to enable them to participate significantly in—if not always to make outright—decisions regarding their care. In one sense, Living Wills and other forms of advance directives extend decision-making capacity even to individuals who are no longer competent. But is respect for autonomy always to be privileged? When might duties of beneficence prevail?

The cases in Part Five examine considerations that come into play in making decisions for the mentally incompetent. Those in the first section—"Involuntary Treatment"—raise questions about the degree of competence a patient must have to make properly "informed" decisions to accept or refuse treatment. Should a neurologically impaired individual be allowed to refuse treatment that would restore him to a significant level of competence, for example? When moral suasion fails, may legal coercion be used to compel someone to undergo therapy that physicians or others hold to be in the patient's best interests? These cases also raise questions of when the interests of others may legitimately have a claim on caregivers. For example, may an emotionally disturbed teenager be forced to take medication to control preterm labor for the benefit of her fetus?

In section two—"Decisions on Behalf of the Incompetent"—cases examine how those who decide for others balance the benefits to be gained by treatment against the harms that treatment may cause. Does prohibiting a mother from having her retarded daughter sterilized truly serve the child's interests? Though she may never be competent to be a parent, are we right to insist that she remain celibate and so deny her the potential goods of affection and sexual expression? So too cases raise the issue of assessing the potentially competing interests of patients, their families, and the broader society. Does society have such an overriding interest in prosecuting criminals that it can force treatment of mentally ill defendants to enable them to stand trial? Can an attorney ethi-

196

cally advise her client to refuse neuroleptic medication at the cost of prolonged incarceration in a psychiatric facility?

As these cases demonstrate, the problems of decision making become even more complex when decisions must be made for incompetent persons. We owe special obligations to vulnerable individuals who cannot choose for themselves, both to respect them as members of the moral community and to protect their interests.

41

"Ain't Nobody Gonna Cut on My Head!"

A fifty-six-year-old farmer, accompanied by his wife, consulted the Neurology Service of Veterans' Hospital because of memory difficulty. For two years the patient had been having increasing trouble with technical aspects of farming. More recently he had been talking about his brother George as if he were alive although he had died two years earlier. He gave his own age as 48 and the year as "1960, pause . . . er, no, l970." Examination revealed that the patient walked with a wide-based gait (a standard sign of brain pathology) and decreased cerebral function but was otherwise normal. The patient had no difficulty with simple coin problems and could repeat six digits.

Pleading pressing business, the patient declined hospitalization to determine the cause of his decreasing cerebral function. His wife tried to persuade him to enter the hospital, but when the resident suggested that she might assume guardianship for her husband through court action, she declined.

Six months later the patient's condition had worsened. Through the urging of the county agent the patient had leased most of his farmland to his neighbors and now did no work. His gait had become so wide-based that acquaintances mistakenly thought him inebriated. He urinated in his pants about once a week, and recently seemed not to care. He sat watching television all day, but never paid any attention to the program content.

Examination at this time showed an apparently alert man without speech difficulty but with considerable mental deterioration. The patient gave his age as thirty-eight, the year as 1949, the president as Eisenhower, and the location as a drug store in his home town. He failed to recognize the name Lyndon Johnson, but upon hearing the name John F. Kennedy he spontaneously volunteered knowledge of his assassination. The patient could not subtract 20 cents from a dollar but could name the number of nickels in a quarter. He could recite the months of the year and could upon request from his wife give fairly long quotations from the Bible.

The resident and the attending physician urged hospitalization. They told the patient they would evaluate him for treatable causes of mental deterioration and memory deficit. In view of his wide-based gait and urinary incontinence in association with dementia, it was likely he had occult hydrocephalus. It was explained that this disorder caused decreased mental abilities by interference with absorption of cerebrospinal fluid. The mental deterioration in these patients is partially (as in his case now) or completely (as in his case six months ago when first seen) reversible. The treatment is to place a plastic tube through the skull to drain the cerebrospinal fluid from the brain to the vascular system; this was explained to the patient with diagrams. The patient immediately rejected the surgery, summarizing his thoughts with these exact words: "Ain't nobody gonna cut on my head." The patient's wife again attempted to persuade the patient to accept hospitalization and, if tests confirmed the clinical impression, surgery. The attending physician argued to the wife that the patient did not have the mental competence to decide his own fate and the wife should become the patient's legal guardian through court action and force hospitalization. The wife politely but vigorously rejected this course of action, pointing out that in her family the husband made all important decisions.

The resident and the attending physician differed in opinions at this point. The resident thought the patient should be followed in the outpatient clinic until he perhaps changed his mind. The resident pointed out that though the patient had decreased mental abilities, he still retained enough intelligence to decide his own fate. The attending physician wished for court action to make the patient the ward of one of his relatives or, if necessary, the temporary ward of the hospital, and to force hospitalization and therapy.

COMMENTARY
James M. Gustafson

The principal substantive moral issue in this case is the status of the right of the patient to determine his own bodily destiny. He refuses to consent to a procedure which is likely to relieve his disability, though apparently he understands in lay terms what is involved in the surgery. At his level of competence he is "informed," but he refuses to give "consent."

The principle of informed consent is based upon one moral assumption and upon one philosophical judgment. The moral assumption is that individuals have a right to refuse treatment even when in the judgment of others that treatment is in the patient's own best interests. A person has a right to determine his or her own destiny. The ground of this assumption is historically located in the libertarian tradition of Western culture; it stems from the same tradition that values civil liberties, that believes that the state exists properly only on the basis of the consent of the governed, and so forth. The philosophical justification for the individual's right to self-determination has been made in various ways: the right is "natural"; capacity for self-determination is what makes humans distinctive as a species and from this is derived both its value and the right; individual rights are conferred by God; excessive incursion on self-determination leads to repression and in turn to social unrest, and for this reason the right is to be protected.

The serious philosophical judgment on which the principle of informed consent is based is that persons actually have a capacity to determine their own destinies. Every case of this sort opens the historic debate about "free will" if the case is carried beyond the immediate clinical circumstances.

This case can be analyzed on the basis of two questions which follow from the two previous paragraphs. (1) Are there *moral* grounds for exerting persuasive, or legal and coercive, measures to override this man's presumed right of self-determination? Do his obligations to his family and to the community (or, to make the point in a weaker way, do the interests of his family and the community) provide a sufficient basis for intervention without his consent? How one would answer this question would depend upon the status of the right of self-determination in relation to the claims of communities (his family, the neighbors, etc.) to limit and even override that right. (2) Are this man's capacities to judge rationally and to act in accordance with a rational judgment impaired by his illness to the extent that he cannot properly exercise his moral right to self-determination? Is he, to use the common term, really "competent"? Does his impairment provide "excusing conditions" so that just as he is not held accountable for his wide gait, so he is not accountable for his rejection of the proposed therapy? Given the assumption of "free will" in the consent procedure, can his will be judged to be "less free" than is necessary and sufficient to make a sound judgment? The attending physician could justify his "wish" for court action on the basis of either or both of the matters raised by these questions.

In this case I would argue in favor of the attending physician's "wish." My principal argument would be on the basis of the patient's limited capacities to exercise his right of self-determination. Note that an empirical judgment about those limits is involved. A hypothesis (and that is all it is) would be required to support the argument, namely, if this man's capacities were not so impaired he would consent to the surgery. Procedurally, I would support the steps taken in the report of the case; that is, first seeking voluntary consent of the patient, then of his family, and only as a last resort seeking a court order. I am prepared also, however, to argue that this man has obligations to his family and to the community that he ought to take into account in making his own judgment. His failure to consent is, it appears, costly to others; others are dependent upon him and, thus, also have a claim on him to consent to a procedure that would permit him to fulfill his duties to them. Procedurally, if such a line of argument failed to persuade him, and then his family, there would be a moral justification for court action. At the base of my conviction here is a significant qualification of the individual libertarian tradition in the direction of a more "social" view of persons and of duties and obligations of persons to other individuals and to communities.

COMMENTARY
Francis C. Pizzulli

At first blush, the attending physician presents a fairly convincing case for initiating state intrusion into the patient's brain. As the title of the case implies, the proffered therapy is fairly characterized as "brain surgery" and thus avoids categorization as "psychosurgery," replete with its politically value-laden premise of experimental treatment for the purpose of controlling socially deviant behavior. If, indeed, the preliminary diagnosis of occult hydrocephalus is sound, the operation would be tailored to rectify an accepted organic brain pathology. Though this entails the concomitant effect of controlling aberrant behavior (e.g., urinary maintenance and dementia), the presence of excess cerebrospinal fluid calls into play a well-defined medical/disease model which makes less persuasive the need to inquire into the motives of the physician as a check against the potential transmogrification of psychiatrists into thought-controllers.

If one were to accept the physician's evaluation of the mental incompetency of the patient, coerced institutionalization and treatment could be defended on a number of grounds. The procedure is relatively nonintrusive; to wit, it is a safe, nonexperimental operation which involves no destruction of brain tissue and is intended to control behavior that ranks rather low on the continuum of volitional and autonomous functions. Not only is this intrusion minimal, but an array of humanitarian and utilitarian impulses militate for intervention. Does not the state have a moral obligation to the patient's former self to restore it? Or an obligation to construct a new self for the person, at which point he would be released to exercise his autonomy to its fullest potential? And would not this restoration to optimal functionality redound to the benefit of his family and community?

Even if we were to assume the patient's competency, the cost of overriding his competent judgment would be measured in terms of a single interference with personal autonomy at a particular time, presumably to be outweighed by the personal and social interest in a long-term increase in autonomy achieved by effective treatment.

Is there a decisive rebuttal to the physician's benevolent despotism? From a traditional legal perspective the case for involuntary commitment (i.e., enforced hospitalization) in this instance is rather weak. There is no mention of antisocial activities by the patient, which would warrant a finding of "dangerousness to others." To say that occasional urinary incontinence and mindless fixation upon the boob tube—behavioral traits found in many "normal" persons—constitute dangerousness to oneself reflects a most extreme paternalistic bias.

Even if the criteria for involuntary commitment are met, the case against intervention by no means falls. We cannot conclude that because an individual may no longer be competent to care for himself generally (e.g., due to memory deterioration), he is thereby incompetent to pass informed judgment upon such an intrusion as the proposed organic therapy. The notion of limited competency, besides having legal recognition, is rooted in the empirical observation that certain mental illnesses do not completely obliterate a person's ability to make decisions. While the patient may no longer recall dates and ages, it is hard to envision how memory deficit can totally discredit the capacity to understand the consequences of an operation, and to immediately summarize the resident's explanation and conclude with a refusal, as the patient has done. Even if we were to adopt the simplistic view that there is no competency where the refusal only occurred because of the mental deterioration, there is no evidence to indicate that the patient is other than strongly individualistic, and would not have decided likewise prior to the onset of deterioration. Moreover, the competent spouse's concurrence in his decision might be construed as evidence of agreement with his lifelong views on brain surgery.

To respond to the invocation of a classic Benthamite calculus that would override limited, albeit informed, judgment to refuse therapy, we might profitably view the case from a rule-utilitarian perspective. While it may be true in this particular case that only a minimally intrusive operation is needed to arrest mental deterioration and partially restore memory function, we should ask what the consequences would be of a practice of substituting the state's judgment for individual informed consent in order to achieve the incremental gain in utility involved in curing those who suffer from marginal mental impairment. Is it too far-fetched to conclude that the result would be a society in which democratic values of personal autonomy, freedom, and privacy would be subjugated to the ideal of state control over various kinds of behavior?

There is one final barrier to coerced surgery, assuming for the sake of argument that there are grounds for civil commitment and that the patient does not have the limited competency to give informed refusal to treatment. Shall the next-of-kin be designated as the proxy, with the power to give or withhold consent? To argue in the negative, because it is suspected the spouse will only rubber-stamp the incompetent's decision, conflicts with the legal presumption of identity of interests among kin. Likewise, to propose a third-party guardian who will rubber-stamp the physician's decision, on the ground that it will enhance the well-being of the patient and his family, arrogates to the physician the right to define that well-being, instead of allowing it to be defined within the privacy of the family.

In sum, only a highly paternalistic society could tolerate the intrusions upon autonomy and privacy that would flow from a practice of coercion in cases such as that at hand.

42

The Woman Who Died in a Box

One frigid January day Rebecca Smith, age sixty-one, was found dead of hypothermia in her makeshift home—a cardboard box covered by a rug—on a New York City street. The Red Cross had reported her unusual living arrangements to the police two weeks earlier. Social workers had visited her, offering food and help in moving to a city shelter. A mobile unit designed to help geriatric patients had approached her. A psychiatrist had visited her and declared her an "endangered adult," part of the procedure that would have allowed the authorities to hospitalize her under seventy-two-hour protective custody. But before the order could be carried out—the first time the city had attempted its implementation—Rebecca Smith died.

Before she joined the ranks of New York's homeless street people, Rebecca Smith had lived a rather different life. One of a family of thirteen children in Virginia, she had graduated from Hampton Institute as valedictorian. But she was hospitalized as a schizophrenic for ten years and underwent electroshock therapy. When she was released from the hospital, her daughter said, she was a changed woman.

In 1959 Mrs. Smith came to New York to live with her sister and then entered a mental hospital in Long Island. She was later released from the institution and decided to strike out on her own. That meant living on public assistance, taking Thorazine, and going to a medical clinic. In 1981 she failed to appear for recertification interviews with social workers and from then on—until her death—she lived on the streets.

Could Rebecca Smith's death have been prevented? How far do society's obligations extend toward those who are in need but who refuse to conform? Does society have different obligations to intervene in protecting those it considers mentally ill?

COMMENTARY
Kim Hopper

On March 19 this year [1982], I joined a hundred others across from the White House in a memorial service for the homeless poor who had died on the streets of six American cities this winter. Forty crosses were driven into the ground of Lafayette Park, joining over 500 already in place, the reported toll of the last five years or so in eleven cities. As it happened, the name on the cross I carried, the name I shouted out in the bright sunshine that day, was Rebecca Smith.

Rebecca Smith's death has drawn much more attention than her life ever did; it has been the subject of two editorials in the *New York Times*, another in the *Washington Post*, and of several commentaries on local TV news. But listen for a moment to the words of Betty Higden in Dickens's *Our Mutual Friend*: "You pray that your Granny may have the strength enough left her at the last . . . to get up from the bed and run and hide herself, and sworn to death in a hole, sooner than fall into the hands of those Cruel Jacks we read of, that dodge and drive, and worry and weary, and scorn and shame, the decent poor" (cited by Steven Marcus, "Their Brothers' Keepers," 1978).

What little we know of Rebecca Smith's life suggests that she may well have read about, and directly encountered, "Cruel Jacks" in the course of her institutionalized life. Mental hospitals were forbidding places in the 1950s and 1960s, and patients often fared as badly there as the "decent poor" had a century earlier in England.

There is a danger in discussing Rebecca Smith's death—that it will be taken for more than it should be, as emblematic of a general refusal of assistance on the part of the homeless. From there, it is a small step to reviving the stale myth that the legions of the homeless poor on our streets are there because they choose to be. The recent history of New York's sheltering efforts suggests otherwise.

Since the *Callahan v. Carey* suit* was filed in October 1979, more than 1700 new emergency shelter beds have been provided by New York City. All were filled this winter. An additional 175 homeless men and women avail themselves each night of the twenty-four-hour drop-in facilities at the Moravian Church and Olivieri Center. Dozens more found respite this past winter, courtesy of the churches and synagogues that opened their doors to the wandering poor. Did these people materialize out of thin air? Or, as appears to be the case, were most of them making their way wretchedly until a more decent option presented itself?

It is difficult to attribute the recent surge in the sheltered population to more rational behavior by the homeless. If anything, observers agree that recent recipients of shelter have more tenuous mental health than traditional clients of the public shelters. The decisive difference appears to be the range of options offered the homeless poor: as that range has increased, so has their demonstrated willingness to come in out of the cold. It takes some flexibility, a modicum of decency, and respect for the heightened sense of self-protection that life on the streets can breed. It takes patience—but that is all.

But exceptions do occur. We don't know exactly what Rebecca Smith was offered, or what she understood the offer to be. A lot of people tried, but there was neither world enough nor time. City attorneys waited until a Friday afternoon to file papers in court, assuring inattention for another two days. Does that imply misgivings about their own resolve? This was, after all, the maiden application of the Protective Services Law. The process has since been streamlined to minimize gratuitous delays. Thus, several people may subsequently have been spared death by exposure. Clearly, once the protection of due process is secured, it is a civil obligation to take emergency action to save from imminent death one who is unaware of the peril.

But in the unforgiving light of hindsight, more than "what should have been done" is illuminated. Private shelters are filled with wary, once-desperate men and women who formerly saw no alternative to the degradation and danger of the public shelters than to live apart from them and to die decently when that failed. Betty Higden would have been one:

> Comprehending that her strength was quitting her, and that the struggle of
> her life was almost ended, she could neither reason out the means of getting

---

*This class action suit successfully argued that conditions in the public shelters for men were so dangerous, dirty, and degrading as to constitute a genuine deterrent to their use by homeless men. It was settled in August 1981 by means of a negotiated consent decree that not only recognized a legal right to shelter but also established certain qualitative standards that public shelters must henceforth meet.

back to her protectors, nor even form the idea. The overmastering dread, and the proud stubborn resolution it engendered in her to die undegraded, were the two distinct impressions left in her failing mind.

Betty Higden's prayer—"to die undegraded"—was heard. She died, alone and unseen, by the roadside one night, the money to pay for her burial sewn into her gown. There is a defiant dignity in such a death, one that refuses to exonerate a society inured to her suffering. It was as if she had demanded, not justice at last, but injustice consistently applied. There were to be no eleventh-hour "heroics," no final capitulation to the indignity of a pauper's death. This recognition, that even the desperately poor may prize self-respect above a forced and servile dependency, should arrest easy ruminations about "what should have been done."

Rebecca Smith's is not a "right to die" case, any more than Betty Higden's was. It is rather an object lesson in how comfortably we tolerate routine misery and how quickly we will pounce to sequester evidence of that fact.

Of course, there is an out. One could argue that others have found their way to refuge before death, that it needn't be shameful, and that were more decent shelter available, Rebecca Smith might not have had to die to force the issue. But to raise the question of intervention only at the hour of her death is seriously to cheapen the worth of her life.

COMMENTARY
Nicholas N. Kittrie

Despite my continuing concern for the excesses of the "therapeutic state"— which has permitted involuntary sterilization, lobotomies, electroshock, and indeterminate incarceration for those suffering from mental illness, while forbidding these procedures to be applied to convicted criminals—I believe that New York has failed in its duty toward Rebecca Smith. This conclusion follows from general principles of enlightened jurisprudence, which are applicable community wide, regardless of the psychiatric status of Rebecca Smith or the mental illness laws of New York.

The balance between personal autonomy and communal responsibility is difficult to strike. Excessive stress on autonomy is likely to reinforce individualism, but also to introduce alienation and community disintegration. Emphasis on communal responsibility, on the other hand, while strengthening collective bonds, could result in paternalism and possibly even in authoritarian suppression. Different societies strike the balance differently. While American jurisprudence, in its commitment to liberty, has not usually articulated "Good Samaritan" laws for the community or individual citizens, both the Italian and French Penal Codes specify penalties for "any person who neglects to afford the necessary assistance" to a "person wounded or otherwise in danger."

One may doubt the desirability or effectiveness of decreeing that an individual citizen become a Good Samaritan under the penalty of criminal law or of interfering with an individual's voluntary exposure to danger—including motorcycle riding, smoking, or sky diving. Yet one can readily concede the importance of communal efforts on behalf of those who appear to be *involuntarily* stranded or in danger.

Rebecca Smith was exposed to evident, continuing, and increasing danger on the public streets of New York. Suppose she had stepped into the middle of oncoming traffic. Would the state agencies have felt the need for a complex and time-consuming procedure to remove her to safety? Would it have mattered whether or not she suffered from one mental illness or another, or from none? In a reasonably humanitarian, welfare-oriented society, at the moment of risk the state must step in, at least temporarily, to rescue those disabled from their own pursuit of "life, liberty and property." This rescue the state owes to its citizens regardless of color, creed, sex, fortune, or mental ability.

What if the citizen for a second time marches into the middle of the traffic, climbs onto the rooftop, or threatens to jump from the bridge? Even for a person who is sane, the state is expected to make a second rescue effort. Moreover, under common law such willful citizens could be charged with disturbing the peace, attempting suicide, or some other obscure legal violation, thus affording the state the justification for temporary restraint.

If minor sanctions are to be attached to deliberate, repeated risk takers, they should apply whether the risk takers are competent or incompetent. But I am strongly opposed to attaching a psychiatric label to people in order to permit greater intervention and control over their lives than over the community at large.

Rebecca Smith died before New York City authorities could implement her hospitalization under its new protective custody law. Yet for at least three decades, under special laws, the mentally ill, alcoholics, and drug addicts have been confined on the basis of psychiatric labels, without conforming to the standards of "due process" and "probable cause" required under the criminal law. At the height of the therapeutic state, in the 1950s and 1960s, efforts were made to greatly and unduly broaden the insanity defense, as well as to altogether prohibit criminal sanctions against public drunkenness. But the late 1970s brought an antitherapeutic movement of similar extremity. While therapists of two decades ago called for voluntary and involuntary "treatment" of all deviants, today's therapeutic nihilists wish to totally abolish the insanity defense and to condemn to benign neglect those who require assistance.

Neither extreme supplies even and civilized justice for America. Rebecca Smith's life should have been saved, even at the cost of a temporary loss of freedom. But the same conclusion should apply to all citizens similarly situated, regardless of their psychiatric diagnosis. The New York seventy-two-hour temporary custody law, designed exclusively for those allegedly mentally disabled, proved not only unjust, but also ineffective.

43

Preterm Labor and Prenatal Harm

Ms. W. is a nineteen-year-old unmarried woman pregnant for the third time, having previously had an abortion when fifteen, and a daughter now ten months old. She was admitted to the hospital in the twenty-sixth or-seventh week of gestation and placed on intravenous medications (magnesium sulfate) to stop her preterm labor. Two days later, Ms. W. asked her physician, Dr. C, to discontinue the medications because she was "tired of being in the hospital and the medications and the fetus were too painful and uncomfortable." Dr. C. explained that the potential risks of premature delivery include: respiratory immaturity, intraventricular hemorrhage, neurologic handicaps, and even fetal death. He advised her to continue the medications for two to three more weeks to give the fetus more time to mature. These critical weeks would enhance the fetus's chances of survival (from 50 percent at twenty-six weeks gestation to 90 percent at thirty weeks gestation) and decrease morbidity, reducing the risk of chronic lung disease (from 50 percent at twenty-six weeks to 20 percent at thirty weeks gestation) and neurological handicaps later on in life.

Ms. W. continued to refuse treatment, and a psychiatry consult was obtained. Ms. W. was found to be extremely immature, emotionally labile and unrealistic, to have a very poor social situation (battered by family members), to have sometimes had suicidal ideas, to have used illegal drugs in the past (but not recently), and to have a long-standing personality disorder (histrionic personality). Meanwhile she continued to refuse the medication to stop labor and threatened to leave the hospital.

Dr. C. contemplates three options: Respect Ms. W.'s wishes and risk delivering a very premature fetus who may expire or may survive and be handicapped secondary to prematurity and its complications; refuse to abide by her wishes, but transfer care to a physician who is willing to do so; refuse to abide by her wishes and try to obtain a court order to force Ms. W. to undergo treatment.

What should Dr. C. do?

COMMENTARY
Bonnie Steinbock

Dr. C.'s first alternative emphasizes respect for patient autonomy, expressing the principle that competent adults have the right to refuse medical treatment. Ms. W. has been diagnosed as having a "personality disorder," but that does not make her incompetent. Nor does it seem that her doctor has serious doubts about Ms. W.'s competency to make decisions. Rather, Dr. C. thinks that she is making a *bad* decision. However, respect for autonomy does not permit using psychiatric diagnoses to force patients to make good decisions.

The third option is based on concern for the fetus. It balances the relatively minor inconvenience to Ms. W. of staying in the hospital and continuing the medications against the extremely serious threat to the fetus of her refusal. A woman who chooses not to terminate a pregnancy has certain moral obligations to the child she has decided to bear. To be sure, she is not required to undergo serious risks to her own life and health, but no such risks are at stake here. These obligations make her refusal unjustified and unfair to the fetus who may die, or perhaps worse, survive and suffer neurological damage in later life.

Both options exert a pull on us, because both represent important moral principles. By contrast, the second possibility—transferring Ms. W to a physician who will abide by her wishes—seems a mere cop-out. It serves to relieve Dr. C. of responsibility for what happens. It does not address the underlying issue: should doctors resort to the courts to protect the unborn?

In a recent column, Alan Dershowitz claims that the law should protect fetuses-who-will-be-born from mothers who "selfishly refuse to follow elementary precautions necessary to give their babies a fighting chance after birth...a mother who has assumed the responsibility of bringing a child into the world should be required to undertake certain minimum steps before birth to assure its health." Dershowitz is aware of the risks of allowing doctors and judges to compel women to accept treatment for the sake of the unborn; the recent tragic story of Angela C. is a case in point. However, he argues that it is the job of the law to draw lines and come up with a middle ground that affords maximum protection both to the mother's autonomy and the fetus's health.

This sensible-sounding solution ignores the reality of the medical setting. The judge is usually faced with an emergency and the need for an immediate decision. Moreover, the doctor is the expert. Dr. C. maintains that the baby's health will be severely compromised if the judge does not act. In this situation, how much weight will be given to the pregnant woman's autonomy?

Making adversaries out of mother and fetus is likely to result in more harm than good. Many women will avoid a physician altogether during pregnancy if failure to follow medical advice can result in forced treatment or involuntary confinement. We need to find other options that will protect babies without turning women into (in George Anna's apt phrase) "fetal containers." Accordingly, I recommend that Dr. C. do more to find out why Ms. W. is so unhappy in the hospital. Perhaps the conditions prompting her refusal can be changed. Perhaps she has other concerns about her baby's future that can be addressed. Instead of threatening Ms. W. with legal action if she does not behave, the doctor should communicate to her his concern for her health and well-being. He should acknowledge her right to make the decision, but also do everything he can to get her to delay making a final decision. Every day that she can be persuaded to wait will benefit the fetus. If Dr. C. is unable to communicate effectively with Ms. W., another doctor, nurse, or social worker should be found who might be able to persuade her to remain in the hospital. He might ask Ms. W. to visit the neonatal intensive care unit so that she can see for herself the effects of a premature delivery. He should remind her, as gently as possible, that if she leaves the hospital, she might end up having to care for a very handicapped baby.

This sort of psychological approach does not take a stand on the relative importance of autonomy and beneficence: that is its strength. Most such cases could be resolved if physicians developed the ability to listen sympathetically and hear what their noncompliant patients are telling them.

COMMENTARY
Don Marquis

Dr. C. is considering taking action that would deprive Ms. W. of her liberty and override her right to control her own body. Any reasons for such an action seem to leave women with fewer rights than men. How could such a Draconian and presumptively inequitable measure possibly be justified?

Presumably *Roe v. Wade* prohibits interference with a spontaneous abortion a woman wants as much as it renders unconstitutional the prohibition of an induced abortion a woman wants as long as the fetus is not yet viable. However, could *Roe* be used to justify interference with Ms. W.'s liberty on the grounds that her fetus is viable?

Suppose we define the age of viability as the gestational age at which some percentage of fetuses, no matter how small, has survived outside the womb and eventually left the NICU. It follows that Ms. W.'s fetus is viable, because fetuses as young as 24 weeks have survived. However, this definition of age viability seems arbitrary. Why not define age of viability in terms of a larger survival percentage? Surely a Draconian measure cannot be justified by appeal to an arbitrary definition.

There is a less arbitrary way of determining viability in this case. Let Ms. W. deliver. If the baby dies in the NICU, then one could argue that it was not viable. If the baby was not viable, then it was not protected by *Roe*. If the child lives, it does not *need* protection from *Roe v. Wade* and the concept of viability will not provide the needed basis for interfering with Ms. W.'s liberty.

Is there any other basis for intervention? Consider the following argument. Should Ms. W.'s fetus be delivered now, there is a substantial risk of permanent lung, brain, or retinal damage. Because the damage may be permanent, the result of the premature delivery may be a *child* or an *adult* who is mentally retarded, is blind, or has cerebral palsy. Such a *child* or *adult* has the right not to be harmed, of course, the right not to be harmed by a preventable premature delivery. This argument appears to justify intervention by Dr. C.

But it might be objected that since Ms. W. cannot legally be compelled to donate bone marrow to another even if needed to sustain life, she also cannot be legally compelled to donate her body even if needed to prevent risk of harm. The trouble with this position is that we believe that children have a right to care from their parents that they do not have from strangers. Consequently, the claim that Ms. W. does not have a legally enforcable duty of care toward a stranger does not entail that she has no such duty of care toward her own *child*: She clearly *does* have such a duty. Hence, it becomes apparent that the basis for intervention by Dr. C. is the doctrine of child abuse or neglect. The human being who may be harmed is a child of Ms. W., not someone else.

This reasoning does not imply that Ms. W.'s right not to be confined involuntarily is overridden by her child's right not to be harmed. However, the following argument is available. Premature delivery entails a significant and unavoidable risk of permanent, substantial injury. Confining Ms. W. against her will entails the *certain* loss of her *liberty*, but no comparable risk of injury. A comparison-of-harms analysis leads to the conclusion that Ms. W.'s right not to be confined involuntarily is overridden by her child's right not to be subjected to the significant risk of permanent, substantial, preventable harm.

This conclusion is based entirely on the *uncontroversial* rights of *postnatal* children and some general moral analysis. Hence, it does not presuppose that fetuses have any rights at all and is compatible with a doctrine of abortion on demand. It follows that the constraints on Ms. W. imposed by this analysis are less severe than they appear. Prior to the gestational age when Ms. W.'s fetus had any chance of independent life, Ms. W could have chosen abortion. In this way, fetal viability is critical to moral analysis of this case.

COMMENTARY
Sahar Kayata

Dr. C.'s decision should balance infant and maternal interests, while keeping in mind his own legal liabilities. The infant's best interest is to remain in utero to allow for further maturation and to minimize any potential harm. About 80 percent of neonatal death *not* due to lethal abnormalities occur in infants born prematurely. Chronic lung disease of prematurity, cerebral palsy, mental retardation, retinopathy of prematurity and life-threatening feeding problems are probable complications in infants born at twenty-six to twenty-seven weeks gestation but are less common in infants born after thirty weeks. Due to their prematurity, at least half of the infants born prior to twenty-six weeks gestation have some type of intracranial hemorrhage. Twenty to forty percent of these infants will end up with a severe handicap such as complete paralysis, blindness, deafness, profound mental retardation, or will require tube feeding. In other cases of intracranial hemorrhage, the child may suffer from lesser degrees of paralysis, seizures, impaired intellectual function, or loss of vision or hearing. Other common complications in twenty-six-week infants include: infection due to the immaturity of their immune system, cardiac problems, limitations of liver function, and lung immaturity that may be life-threatening. Although two or three weeks additional gestation may seem a short time, the benefits the infant acquires are immense and multiple.

For Ms. W., hospitalization by itself is inconvenient and the tocolytic agent (magnesium sulfate) can cause discomfort, flushing, a feeling of weakness, nausea, dizziness, and occasional headaches. Furthermore, she has a personality disorder that may lead her to amplify the side effects of the medications, and may interfere with her ability to assimilate information and to take an active role in decision making, especially when fear, anxiety, and stress are superimposed.

Studies have demonstrated that tocolytics can suppress preterm labor and effectively delay delivery in 60 to 80 percent of the patients. In the majority of cases, this is achieved in a few days, and the pregnant woman can be discharged. There are contraindications (such as severe hypertension, bleeding, infection, fetal distress, fetal anomalies, etc.) that would prohibit using tocolytics and make preterm delivery inevitable, but none of these are present in Ms. W.'s case, making her a very suitable candidate for tocolysis. Dr. C. feels that tocolyties are strongly indicated with no predictable harm to either the mother or the infant. Consequently, Ms. W. has a moral obligation to protect the imperiled infant she carries. Although she has the right to bodily integrity and self-determination, these principles do not grant her the right to refuse treatment that would greatly reduce the risk of harm to her child.

All persons have obligations to refrain from harming children after birth. Similarly, they have obligations to refrain from harming children by prenatal action. Therefore, in theory, the child who is severely handicapped as a result of harmful prenatal conduct could sue the mother and/or the obstetrician. Pediatricians are required by law to report any suspected cases of child neglect and/or abuse since they are "children's advocates." Analogously, it can be argued, obstetricians should act as "infants' advocates," especially in situations where the mother has a psychiatric disorder. Dr. C., however, would then be legally liable to treat Ms. W. against her wishes. Neither patient autonomy nor the doctrine of informed consent requires physicians to accept patient refusal passively and without inquiry, protest, or argument. Persuasion and voluntary compliance are, of course, the preferred techniques, but when they fail, a court order becomes a necessity. In this case, since neonatal harm is expected while the net risk to the mother is low, Dr. C. would be justified in overriding Ms. W.'s refusal.

44

Sterilizing the Retarded Child

A retarded eleven-year-old girl from the city of Sheffield, England, had been booked to enter a hospital on May 4, 1975, for a sterilization operation. The girl, known as "D.," suffers from Sotos Syndrome—also called cerebral giganticism—an unusual group of congenital abnormalities including epilepsy. Characteristics of the disease include large hands, feet, and skull; poor coordination; and endocrine problems of unknown etiology. Intelligence ranges from normal to severe retardation, with most mildly retarded. ("D." had a normal intelligence range, a fair academic standard, and the understanding of a nine- to nine-and-a-half-year-old.)

While authorities in the genetics of Sotos Syndrome are uncertain about its inheritability, they believe that it is not one disease but a heterogeneous group of disorders, and that it may be either a recessive trait or a new dominant mutation. Most cases of Sotos Syndrome have been sporadic, occurring equally in both sexes. Those afflicted do not seem to have a higher incidence of relatives affected than does the normal population, and the risk of genetic transmission is not known. There have been reports, however, of its occurrence among first cousins, identical twins, and between father and son.

"D.'s" father died in 1971, leaving the mother to raise the girl and two other daughters in very difficult circumstances. The mother, a part-time cleaner, is very hard-working, sincere, and devoted. The girl sleeps with her mother in one bed; their two-bedroom house has no toilet; and they live under conditions described as appalling.

In 1973 "D." was transferred to a school specializing in children's behavioral problems, a move reported to be a success. Her progress in education and behavior was evident. But by the time "D." reached puberty at the age of ten, the mother had grown concerned, fearing her daughter might be seduced and have an abnormal baby, for which she would then have to care. She stated: "I don't think my daughter will ever be responsible enough to bring up a family. I don't think she will improve enough to look after children." However, "D." had not yet shown any interest in the opposite sex, and her opportunities for promiscuity were virtually nonexistent since her mother was always at her side.

Dr. Ronald Gordon, a consultant pediatrician at Sheffield Northern General Hospital who had taken an interest in the family, said that there was a risk that any child borne by "D." would be abnormal and that the girl's epilepsy might cause her to harm a child. He thought that she would always remain so substantially handicapped that she would be unable to care for herself or any children she might have. He maintained that his recommendation to operate was based on his clinical judgment; furthermore, he claimed that he and the gynecologist, Dr. Sheila Duncan, should be the sole judges of whether surgery should be performed, provided that there was parental consent. Dr. Gordon also asked the mother, who consented to the sterilization, to discuss the operation with her daughter.

Mrs. Margaret Dubberley, an educational psychologist at the school the girl attended, strongly opposed the operation and brought legal proceedings aimed at having the girl made a ward of the court. The headmaster at the girl's school believed it was unrealistic to be dogmatic about "D.'s" future, a view supported by some medical evidence. Mrs. Dubberley was further supported by the National Council for Civil Liberties and by a movement in the House of Commons opposing the operation.

COMMENTARY
LeRoy Walters

Before we examine the normative issues in "D.'s" case, it will be useful to analyze precisely what kind of sterilization is being proposed on her behalf. Since there is no evidence to indicate that the sterilization of "D." is medically required for the diagnosis or treatment of an existing illness or injury, the proposed sterilization can be categorized as *nontherapeutic*. A more complex question is the voluntariness of the proposed procedure. The surgery envisioned is clearly not compulsory, or involuntary, in the sense of being performed against the expressed wishes of the daughter. However, "D." is legally a minor and is probably not mentally competent to provide voluntary consent to the surgery on her own behalf. Perhaps a third category is required—nonvoluntary sterilization, or sterilization in the absence of the prospective sterilizee's consent or refusal. The proposed sterilization in "D.'s" case would seem to correspond most closely to this third category; that is, if performed, the sterilization would be nonvoluntary and would be authorized by the substituted judgment of the mother and the two physicians.

Under what conditions can nontherapeutic, nonvoluntary sterilization be morally justified? I would like to suggest three formal requirements which should be applied to this and similar cases. First, there should be *just cause*, or a sufficiently weighty reason, for the proposed sterilization. A just cause is required because sterilization in the absence of consent constitutes a significant invasion of the body and a rather massive intrusion into the sphere of reproductive privacy that has recently been recognized by Anglo-American law. The second requirement is that sterilization should be a *last resort*, since it is generally irreversible and since equally effective, reversible contraceptive techniques are available—for example, the pill. The third formal requirement is *due process*, or an adequate procedure for representing the interests and protecting the rights of all parties concerned.

The proposed sterilization of "D." satisfies none of these formal requirements. First, there is no just cause for the sterilization of "D." It is not clear whether sterilization was recommended by the mother and the pediatrician primarily for the benefit of "D." herself, for the benefit of her mother and sisters, or for the benefit of a child which might potentially be conceived and born to "D." (Another logical possibility, not mentioned in this case, would be sterilization for the benefit of society as a whole.) However, no convincing arguments are presented to support any of these possible justifications. The evidence concerning the probability of "D.'s" producing handicapped children is inconclusive at best. In addition, the prognosis for "D.'s" own intellectual development is uncertain. It is at least possible that with the aid of continued special education she will one day be able to make informed decisions concerning her reproductive capacities.

Second, the proposed sterilization of "D." is clearly not a last resort. In the case report there is no evidence to indicate that reversible contraceptive techniques were either considered or tried. Until such alternatives have been demonstrated to be infeasible, consideration of an irreversible surgical procedure is premature.

Third, the proposal to sterilize "D." also fails to satisfy the due process requirement. Quite possibly the physicians and the mother based their decision primarily on the best interest of the child, as they perceived that interest. However, the "clinical judgment" of the physicians extended far beyond the bounds of the medically indicated. Even the mother, whose response in very difficult circumstances is understandable, did not sufficiently consider the rights of her child. In cases where the performance of an irreversible, nontherapeutic procedure on a child is contemplated, due process seems to require either the appointment of a guardian for the child or formal approval by an independent review committee. This at least seems to be the view of the U. S. Department of Health, Education and Welfare (as expressed in the sterilization restrictions published in the *Federal Register*, February 6, 1974) and the British Department of Health and Social Security, as outlined in a discussion paper, "Sterilization of Children under 16 Years of Age" (cited in the *British Medical Journal*, November 8, 1975, p. 356).

It is easy to forget that the momentary act of nonvoluntary sterilization has lifetime consequences for the person undergoing the procedure. A sociological study by G. Sabagh and R. B. Edgerton in *Eugenics Quarterly* (December 1962) reported that, of forty retarded persons who had been sterilized prior to their release from the institution, many understood "the meaning and implications of sterilization" and 68 percent "disapproved of the sterilization procedure which they had undergone."

In sum, the proposed sterilization of "D." in this case fails to fulfill the requirements of just cause, last resort, and due process. The preferable alternative would be to employ nonpermanent contraceptive techniques as necessary, in the hope that one day "D." will attain sufficient intellectual maturity to make her own reproductive decisions.

COMMENTARY
Willard Gaylin

When analyzed in terms of the specific data presented in this case, a court decision to prevent irreversible surgery seems reasonable enough; and that is, in fact, what took place. The child is, after all, still young; the nature of the mental impairment is still unclear; the degree of retardation (and possible maturation that can be expected) has yet to be defined. There will be a time for a reevaluation when the facts of her destiny become clearer.

The actual response the court's decision elicited, however, was not what one would expect for a prudential compromise, but more like that which is accorded a victory of the forces of good over those of evil. The applause in Britain and elsewhere was as unanimous and hearty as though Tinkerbell's life depended on it. One suspects that it was not the eleven-year-old girl and her future that were being judged, but a cliché. For years sterilization of the mentally retarded has been an issue fraught with emotion. The ominous implications of genetic engineering, cast in the shadow of the recent Nazi past, make the problem too easy by evoking an instinctive and intuitive response to the connotation of the words employed rather than their explicit meaning. Here was an issue that managed to unite educational psychologists, the medical establishment, the civil libertarians, and the House of Commons on one side—with only the unfortunate girl's mother in opposition. Any moral issue in biomedicine these days that commands such unanimity warrants a reexamination.

What is needed is some understanding of the value of sterilization in the mentally retarded. An automatic negative response is not warranted; and the reason is precisely the one sometimes relied upon by opponents of sterilization—that we now recognize the mentally retarded as a broad spectrum of individuals who, while limited in their capacity for certain functions of the healthy mature adult, are not limited in all.

One of the great disadvantages of IQ as the measurement of retardation is that it forces us to see the retarded of all ages as children. We describe them as "having the mentality of a six-year-old." No mentally retarded individual has the mentality of a six-, eight-, twelve- or fourteen-year-old. A six-year-old is a learner par excellence, with unbounded intellectual curiosity, and a potential for mastery of new material that a thirty-six-year-old would envy. He is, however, immature, childish, and incapable of making the decisions which his profound intelligence might imply. A thirty-six-year-old with severe retardation to a point where he can neither read, write, count, tell time, nor follow street directions, can still be a mature adult in a host of ways beyond the capacity of the six-year-old. The price we make the retarded pay for their incapacity in one area is the sacrifice of capacity in certain other areas which could be compensatory if allowed to develop.

Because we cast mentally retarded adults as children, we are appalled, for example, at the thought of their having a sexual or even a social life. Deprived of the joy and privilege of parenthood, for which they may have no capacity, they are punished further by being denied the privilege and pleasure of affection, tenderness, romance, and sexual contact for which they may indeed have a capacity.

A mentally retarded individual ought not be given the responsibility of raising a child, and indeed a mentally retarded woman could be terrified of the changes in her body which pregnancy would produce. Sterilization could allow for the kind of innovation in social living lacking at most facilities for the mentally retarded. There is no reason why community living—even a family-type living—that involved affection, tenderness, and sexuality could not be a fundamental part of their lives and partly compensate for their lack of ordinary intellectual pleasures. Instead we punitively add one deprivation onto the other.

Sterilization is, after all, simply a word. There is nothing in the procedure itself that is innately evil. We allow sterilization when its benefits for the individual outweigh its costs. It is a legitimate procedure, offensive to some for religious reasons but not to others. In this matter, society ought to respect the individual conscience and the individual value.

When, as with the retarded, the concepts necessary for intelligent decision making are beyond a person's intellectual grasp, we would be wise to leave the power of the delegated autonomy in the hands of the family. If that is abused, all sorts of legal mechanisms exist for rectification. What state right warrants intrusion into the decision making? If it is established (first by the family, then if there is suspicion of abuse, by courts), that the mental retardation is of a degree that precludes the role of parent, the young woman will be deprived only of the "privilege" of conception and, presumably, abortion. She will gain, however, new freedoms, and her parents will gain peace of mind.

The incursion into the powers of the family by the state, here as in other places, is often cast in the noble language of rights. What is really at issue in many arguments about "fetal rights," "infant rights," and so on is in reality the relocation of delegated autonomy and power from one institution—the family—to another—the state. Too often the kind of government intervention we have been seeing in these difficult cases, where right and wrong are too finely balanced for comfort or confidence in any decision, represents arrogance rather than compassion. It is unseemly and demeans the state, for more often than not the state is acting not *in loco parentis* but simply as Nosey Parker.

If "D.'s" incapacities to be a mother are still evidenced when she is fifteen years of age, she, through the agents of her care, that is, her family, ought to have the right to exercise the privilege of sterilization.

45

Should Competence
Be Coerced?

D.L. was arrested and charged with rape. He is accused of assaulting a neighborhood woman with whom he is only casually acquainted.

According to police records, D.L. manifested psychotic symptoms including auditory hallucinations and paranoid delusions at the time of his arrest. He was quickly transferred to the forensic unit of the state psychiatric hospital and examined by a psychiatrist, who concluded after a thorough examination that he was not competent to stand trial. Following a brief court hearing, D.L. was returned to the forensic unit to receive treatment, including neuroleptic medication, designed to return him to a state of competency. Competency—which includes such factors as being able to understand the criminal charges, understand the elements of a criminal trial, and participate in one's defense—is required for a defendant to be able to stand trial.

Shortly after being placed on medication, D.L.'s symptom remitted. According to the state-appointed forensic psychiatrist who examined him, D.L. is now oriented to time and place, is not hallucinating or delusional, and is able to participate in his own defense in court. The psychiatrist thus has informed D.L.'s court-appointed attorney, the prosecutor, and the court that he is competent to stand trial.

D.L.'s attorney originally planned to enter a plea of "not guilty by reason of insanity" on his behalf. The attorney is convinced that at the time of the rape, which D.L. admits having committed, he was psychotic and unable to distinguish between right and wrong. However, now that D.L. has been medicated, is competent, and appears quite "normal," the attorney is concerned that a jury will have a difficult time believing that D.L. was insane at the time of the rape.

On the advice of his attorney, D.L. refuses continued neuroleptic medication. He believes that it is in his best interest to risk the likely return to psychotic symptoms to avoid having to face a jury as a competent defendant. D.L. understands that this may mean that he will remain for years on the forensic unit of the psychiatric hospital, technically awaiting competency.

The prosecutor is outraged that the defense attorney has advised his client to refuse therapeutic medication in order to avoid trial. She argues that the defense attorney is seeking to deprive his client of needed medication, contrary to his client's best interests, and also is undermining the state's legitimate interest in resolving a pending criminal matter.

Does D.L. have the right to refuse treatment of his psychotic symptoms to avoid trial in criminal court? Is it proper for D.L.'s attorney to advise his client to do so?

COMMENTARY
Frederic G. Reamer

By now it is well accepted that voluntary psychiatric patients have a broad based right to refuse treatment, as long as standard informed consent procedures are followed. Parentalism has its limits. However, there is no consensus with respect to involuntary patients. Case law is evolving and there are a number of conflicting court decisions. It is not clear to what extent involuntary patients, particularly those who are hospitalized following arrest on a criminal charge, forfeit the "right to refuse" held by voluntary patients.

Ordinarily, debate about the right to refuse centers on risks to the patient or to third parties who may be affected by the patient's decision to forego treatment. In this case there is also an additional concern: whether the public's interest in resolving a pending criminal matter should take precedence over the patient's right to self-determination.

Only the most orthodox libertarians would argue that a psychiatric patient has an inviolable right to determine his or her own fate. There are ample precedents where compelling public interest trumps individual rights. For instance, the well-known *Tarasoff* case, and others like it, demonstrates that prima facie rights ordinarily held by recipients of mental health services sometimes give way when they clash with public interest. Similarly, the widely respected *Wigmore* criteria make it clear that there is a limit to psychiatric patients' right to privileged communication in the face of some form of public peril.

The challenge in the present case is locating the fine line that separates justifiable coercion from gratuitious intervention. Viewed narrowly, D.L. may have the right to refuse medication if it cannot be demonstrated clearly that he poses a threat to himself or others. In the end, however, it seems clear that what D.L. and his attorney propose is just one of a large number of imaginative but questionable tactics that a defendant might engage in to avoid criminal trial. In principle, a defendant can refuse to leave his jail cell to be transported to court, shout at the judge continously to disrupt judicial proceedings, refuse to disclose his identity to the judge, or engage in other courtroom antics designed to postpone or prevent a trial. Defendants who engage in such practices typically are threatened with contempt for interfering with the court's mission, and an attorney who encourages such behavior may be censured. It may not be pleasant, but criminal defendants often are required to do things they do not want to do to facilitate their adjudication. Why should a manipulative tactic involving refusal of medication be regarded any differently?

And what about the attorney's behavior? Although some might give him points for creativity and novelty, the attorney's advice seems to land outside the boundaries of professional responsibility. Is it right for an attorney to advise a client to engage in a practice that threatens his health and may lead to long-term languishing in a psychiatric institution? Although restoration and maintenance of the client's mental health by use of medication may come with a significant price, is it not odd for an attorney to encourage a client to engage in what is cerainly a self-destructive health care practice. Certainly we would not tolerate an attorney who advises his or her *competent* client to take drugs that will induce psychotic symptoms to avoid trial. Is not the advice offered by D.L.'s attorney equally unacceptable? Such advice runs counter to the proscription in the attorneys' code of professional responsibility prohibiting practices that damage clients. In effect the attorney's advice may lead D.L. down a path toward emotional and cognitive imprisonment as an alternative to incarceration in a prison cell. Under these circumstances, can D.L.'s consent be considered truly voluntary?

One might expect D.L.'s attorney to claim that deliberately returning his client to a psychotic state is necessary and justifiable to demonstrate to a jury his client's insanity at the time of the rape. This argument fails because if the withdrawal of medication successfully reproduces D.L.'s psychotic symptoms, it is unlikely that he will be competent to stand trial and have to face a jury.

A hard-nosed attorney might argue that I have interpreted too narrowly the lawyer's obligation under existing standards of professional responsibility. But the attorney's stratagem in this case goes too far. He has crossed the outside border of overzealous representation of his client.

COMMENTARY
Michael J. Kelly

D.L. is, according to this scenario, able to participate in his own defense. His psychotic symptoms have "remitted." He is competent to make decisions for himself, to decide what is in his best interests. He knows the consequences of his decision to refuse treatment, namely that he will remain in the forensic unit of the psychiatric hospital.

If we take seriously the autonomy, or the right, of an individual to make choices affecting his or her life and liberty, we can understand how D.L. might choose this alternative to avoid the danger of being incarcerated as a convicted rapist in a prison facility. Surely this is not an irrational decision. It is instead a decision people similarly situated might make in consideration of their own best interests. Only if we assume that the forensic unit of the psychiatric hospital is a far worse setting or outcome than a prison can we maintain that D.L.'s decision is irrational. D.L. has connected a decision to real facts by a process of reasoning or reference.

So D.L. clearly has the right to refuse treatment of his psychotic symptoms to avoid trial in the criminal court. That much is clear.

How proper was the lawyer's advice? Lawyers counsel clients in many different styles, ranging from a high respect for autonomy, in effect telling the client "you decide," to the paternalistic approach of "let me tell you what you should do." Regardless of the style or approach, a responsible attorney would discuss with D.L. the alternatives and attempt to understand, and help D.L.

work through his interests, concerns, and long-range goals before approaching the decision of how to proceed.

The attorney's advice to refuse medication could well be a short-range strategy. Perhaps the attorney believes the chances of conviction for rape would be reduced if D.L. spends some time on the forensic unit of the psychiatric hospital. Or the attorney may have reliable information about prison realities for criminal defendants (for example, that rapists or individuals with D.L.'s characteristices are peculiarly subject to sexual assault unprotected by prison authorities). Even if D.L. asked his lawyer to make the decision for him (a not uncommon phenomenon in professtional practice), the decision to forgo neuroleptic medication may be appropriate and respectful of D.L.'s autonomy as a decision maker, so long as the lawyer knows her client well enough to project that such a decision is an honest reflection of D.L.'s values and perceived interests.

In weighing the pros and cons of proceeding to trial or refusing to take medication, the attorney's description of the risk of conviction is the most critical element. As any physician who has described the risk of death to a patient knows, some risks generate such strong emotional reaction that emphasis on the risk can virtually assure a decision. A lawyer can easily manipulate a client by focusing on terrifying risks. The fear of some people about going to jail is so intense that they would take virtually any action to avoid it. If the attorney overemphasizes the risk of a jail term, she distorts significantly D.L.'s decision.

The susceptibility of clients and patients to manipulation through nuanced counseling is the basis of enormous professional power. This power is often abused. But when it is harnessed to the well being of patient or client, it becomes the source of that magical healing that is the special joy and purpose of being a professional.

The question of coerced medication confronting D.L. and his attorney remains a matter of deep constitutional controversy. In its February decision in *Washington v. Harper*, the Supreme Court permitted states that follow appropriate administrative procedures to medicate forcibly mentally ill prison inmates who are "gravely disabled or represent a significant danger to themselves or others." D.L. is not a prisoner because he has not been convicted, but *Washington v. Harper* may well signal future developments that could apply to competence-to-stand-trial and civil commitment settings. The irony is that D.L., who has refused medical treatment to avoid trial, may be compelled by the state to take medication that would put him back in the courtroom. Yet the dissent of Justices Stephens, Brennan, and Marshall provides a needed reminder of the limits to coercing competence in our society:

> The invasion of a citizen's liberty...is degrading if it overrides a competent person's choice to reject a specific form of medical treatment...When the purpose or effect of forced drugging is to alter the will and the mind of the subject, it constitutes a deprivation of liberty in the most literal and fundamental sense...The liberty of citizens to resist the administration of mind altering drugs arises from our Nation's most basic values.

Selected Bibliography

Part Five: Mental Incompetence

Annas, George J. "Foreclosing the Use of Force: *A.C.* Reversed," *Hastings Center Report* 20, no. 4 (1990): 27–29.

Buchanan, Allen E., and Brock, Dan W. *Deciding for Others: The Ethics of Surrogate Decisionmaking.* New York: Cambridge University Press, 1989.

Chervenak, Frank A., and McCullough, Laurence B. "Justified Limits on Refusing Intervention," *Hastings Center Report* 21, no. 2 (1991): 12–18.

Chodoff, Paul. "The Case for Involuntary Hospitalization of the Mentally Ill," *American Journal of Psychiatry* 133 (May 1976): 496–501.

Culver, Charles M., and Gert, Bernard. *Philosophy in Medicine: Conceptual and Ethical Issues in Medicine and Psychiatry.* New York: Oxford University Press, 1982.

Edwards, Rem B. *Psychiatry and Ethics: Insanity, Rational Autonomy, and Mental Health Care.* Buffalo: Prometheus Books, 1982.

Gutheil, Thomas G., and Applebaum, Paul S. *Clinical Handbook of Psychiatry and the Law.* New York: McGraw-Hill Book Co., 1982.

Macklin, Ruth. *Men, Mind, and Morality.* Englewood Cliffs, NJ: Prentice-Hall, 1982.

Macklin, Ruth, and Gaylin, Willard, eds. *Mental Retardation and Sterilization: A Problem of Competency and Paternalism.* New York: Plenum Press, 1981.

New York State Task Force on Life and the Law. *When Others Must Choose: Deciding for Patients without Capacity.* New York: New York State Task Force on Life and the Law, 1992.

Szasz, Thomas. *The Myth of Mental Illness: Foundations of a Theory of Personal Conduct.* New York: Harper & Row, 1974.

Allocation and Health Care Policy

INTRODUCTION

The cases in Parts One through Five have illustrated ethical concerns in a variety of different patient care and research settings. But they have all focused on questions involving individuals, whether they are patients or research subjects. With this final group of cases we turn to larger issues of health policy.

The first section—"Allocation of Scarce Resources"—examines ethical dilemmas that arise when patients make competing claims upon finite available resources. What criteria should weigh most heavily, for example, when the state must decide whether to transfer an elderly resident from a nursing home to a less skilled, and less costly, residential facility? Should the goal of providing care as efficiently as possible to as many patients as possible prevail over considerations of the distress individual patients may suffer in the process? Or, how are we to choose between two patients who simultaneously require the special services of a single medical team? Physicians also may have competing duties to their patients and to the institutions in which they practice such as hospitals and HMOs. Can duties to patients ever come second; ought physicians to "game the system" to be sure their individual patients get the best possible care? What obligations do caregivers—and society—have to patients who fail to comply with medical recommendations or are "difficult" in other ways?

Cases in the second section—"Organ Procurement and Transplantation"— explore issues surrounding the distribution of organs among potential transplant candidates. Such cases raise in a special way questions about how we draw the boundaries of our moral community. Given that the number of persons in need will nearly always exceed the number of available organs and that transplantation is a sophisticated and costly procedure, must potential recipients belong to the same community as donors, or should this "gift of life" be given strictly on the basis of medical criteria? Should we encourage new strategies for procuring organs—such as establishing a new category of "brain absent" persons to allow us to harvest organs from anencephalic newborns who have no higher brain, or allowing women to conceive and abort their pregnancies solely to provide fetal organs for transplantation?

The final section—"Health Care Policy"—sets questions of individual medical care in the larger contexts of societal goods and the kinds of policy decisions called for in the face of ever-increasing health care costs. Some cases regard the relative moral responsibilities of employers (and society) for employees' health problems. Can a company be held responsible for an employee's alcoholism, for example, or dismiss an employee for not revealing a chronic illness? Other cases raise questions of health care policy more broadly. How are we to balance the very real needs of individual patients with the equally compelling needs of classes of patients? For example, in the context of finite budgets, how can we compare the benefits of providing AZT to persons with AIDS against those of providing adequate prenatal care to all pregnant women? When is home health care a "medical necessity" that ought to be covered by insurers, and when is it the kind of "custodial care" that is properly the responsibility of social service agencies? Finally, as chronic illness comes more and more to be an important factor in health care, how should we use resources to provide palliative care when we can no longer hope to cure?

46

Forced Transfer to Custodial Care

Lawrence Hessman

Mrs. B., seventy-four, diabetic, and partially blind, has lived in a nursing home for the past ten years, and the state Medicaid agency pays her expenses. She feels secure in the home, where she has made many friends.

The state is trying to save money by caring for its elderly medical patients at the lowest possible cost. Many patients are being transferred from nursing homes to less costly facilities that basically offer only custodial care. The goal is to move as many patients as possible out of facilities providing inappropriately intensive medical support to institutions offering maintenance meeting state-approved standards of quality, but without the medical services now deemed unnecessary.

An arbitrary grading system has been established to evaluate nursing home patients to determine their suitability for transfer. Patients are assigned a certain number of points according to their ability to dress, feed, clothe themselves, and the like. If the number of points the patient receives is higher than a designated total, officials feel that the patient can be transferred without any harmful effects.

When she is evaluated, Mrs. B. receives more than the designated number of points, and the decision is made to transfer her. She is not consulted, nor is she given a voice in the decision. She is simply moved—forcibly and against her wishes—to a custodial care institution. The evaluation does not take into account the psychosocial impact of the move or the personal dimensions of Mrs. B.'s adjustment to the home she had been in for the last decade.

Is the state's conduct ethical? Since it is paying the costs of care, and since it has assigned a higher priority to other areas of medical care for funding, does it have the right to disregard individual patients' wishes concerning the location of their care?

COMMENTARY
Charles Fried

This case is sad and appealing, but raises no difficult questions of principle at all. Presumably the nursing home from which Mrs. B. would be moved is deemed inappropriate to her care because it provides a more intensive level of medical supervision than she requires. And, obviously, overall costs of any program cannot be contained if a patient's friendships and preferences require that that patient continue to occupy space in a medically more intensive (and therefore more expensive) environment than is medically indicated.

The situation must arise fairly regularly with patients who would be more comfortable in the more pleasant, caring, and competent surroundings of an acute care hospital than in a nursing home. Surely, however, to be moved by such considerations and, thus, in effect to turn acute care hospitals into nursing homes would make the present disastrous situation regarding hospital costs even worse.

The state agency has to do what it is doing (assuming that it is doing what it is doing intelligently and fairly). If it did not, then some portion of its limited health care budget would be wasted, and persons with more acute needs would be inadequately treated. In other words, if Mrs. B. were to win, we must assume that there would be losers in even more desperate straits than she is.

Of course nothing requires the state to act without consulting Mrs. B. or hearing her side of the case. But this is not the same thing as giving her "a voice in the decision." Competing beneficiaries of limited funds would of course all love to have a "voice in the decision," when that means giving them a veto over unfavorable decisions. Mrs. B. should certainly be able to present her case and to explain why either an exception should be made or why the state agency's guidelines when applied to her case do not require that she be moved. But to allow the matter to depend on her choice is preposterous.

Of course her physician should make every *proper* effort to have her remain in those circumstances which are most favorable to her. He should make sure that the appropriate agency is aware of the extent to which a move might be detrimental. But it is no part of his duties as her physician to falsify the facts (as doctors sometimes do in efforts to procure certain governmental benefits for their patients) nor to use irregular pressures on her behalf. It would be wrong for a lawyer—and it would certainly be wrong for a doctor—to do this. In the end, if the state agency does move her, the responsibility is not her doctor's but that of the agency. It is no more his responsibility than would be the decision of the Social Security Administration to deny a disability benefit when a patient's doctor was unable in all honesty to come forward with a diagnosis justifying such benefits.

COMMENTARY
Robert Michels

Institutions make decisions that affect the lives of individuals and may affect them adversely. When this occurs (as it did with Mrs. B.), we must ask whether it was "ethical," whether it should have happened, and, if not, what should have been different.

This case is simple enough. Mrs. B. is old, sick, disabled, and lives in a nursing home. Yet life is not all bad; she feels secure and has many friends. The state is paying her bill, and the state wants to save money. For administrative reasons it wants to move her, judging that she is "suitable" for transfer to a cheaper setting. Against her will, and without her participation in the decision, she is moved.

The case is sad as well as simple. On the face of it, it should be otherwise. Mrs. B. should be allowed, at age seventy-four, to finish her days where she feels happiest. State-supported nursing homes are hardly palaces, but this one is Mrs. B.'s home, and the state should forcibly remove a citizen from his or her home only under extreme circumstances. True, it is paying the bill, but one of the marks of a civilized society is that even dependent citizens have rights and privileges.

However, that is not the whole problem. Health care is expensive, and the resources allocated to it force us to make choices. Perhaps if Mrs. B. stays in the nursing home, a young man with asymptomatic hypertension will not be detected by a screening program, or a slum child with cerebral palsy will not have two weeks at a summer camp, or the Methadone Maintenance Center will have one fewer social worker. These are the real effects of budget cuts and reallocations.

What are we to do? Mrs. B. earns our sympathy, but the needs are greater than the resources. Somewhere choices must be made. Are cases like Mrs. B.'s the inevitable result? Are there ethical guidelines as to how the choices should be made?

First, the question of resource allocation cannot be ignored. The public must constantly be reminded of Mrs. B.s as it decides how much should be devoted to health care and how it should be distributed. It might be that the state should not be forced to choose between Mrs. B.'s life and other alternatives, but that citizens should support, or demand, that it provide all of them, sacrificing other goals in the process. But the recent trend of political decisions has not been in that direction.

Second, there are guidelines that should apply to state decisions that directly affect the lives of individuals. The state is planning a transfer of patients from one institution to another, but Mrs. B. is an individual who lives in her home, and the state's procedures should recognize that to one who lives there, institutions are homes and each individual is different.

The decision-making process should be able to make individual decisions about individuals, not simply apply "arbitrary" systems of classification. The noxious character of institutions stems from their tendency to classify people arbitrarily rather than to respond to their individual needs and desires. Further, Mrs. B. should be able to participate in the process—in fact, her participation should be required. This is part of recognizing that she is a person, not a line on a state budget. Finally, the state's guidelines should take into account the meaning of the move to Mrs. B., as well as her physical capacity to adjust to it. There are at least two reasons for this: the less important is the clinical fact that her ability to function in the new institution is largely determined by the meaning she attaches to going there. The more important one is that she is a person, and to consider her physical capacity without concern for her psyche is to treat her solely as an organism.

It would seem that the state fell short on several of these, and, therefore, was "unethical." However, we should recognize that the state might have followed ideal procedures and reached the same conclusions, forcibly wrenching Mrs. B. from her home, if its citizens have other priorities that are higher than the care and comfort of the needy.

COMMENTARY
Steven Sieverts

One would wish that this pathetic case were purely conjectural, but, alas, it reports a scenario which has played many times in the past few years. The imperative of health care cost containment has become excessively dominant in some government agencies, seemingly overriding all other considerations. All too often, the Mrs. B.s have indeed suffered as a consequence of how some public administrators have behaved under that kind of pressure. Cost-cutting, when it becomes obsessive, can offend human decency.

From an ethical standpoint, however, I suggest that the issue in this case is misrepresented. The question is not whether the Medicaid agency has the right or obligation to assure that beneficiaries are receiving at public expense only appropriate services to which they are entitled under law. Clearly it has both.

Rather, the issue is the unacceptable manner in which the state officials and the health professionals seem to have behaved in this case and in other cases like it. The Medicaid law and the state regulations simply do not instruct bureaucrats to force our nurses and social workers to carry out sudden and inhumane transfers of elderly poor patients without any prior consultation. They also do not require the negligent public administration and professional management that kept this patient in too intensive a facility for a decade, not only wasting money but probably making her more dependent and less self-reliant than was necessary. They do not force procedures that ignore common decency.

This case presentation asks: since (the state) is paying the costs of care... does it have the right to disregard individual patients' wishes on the location of their care? Let us ask the question another way: do individual citizens have the right to receive, on demand, publicly financed services to which they have no entitlement? The answer, when it is phrased that way, seems clear: obviously not. Any health insurance program—public or private, categorical or universal, limited or comprehensive—must employ procedures to assure that beneficiaries receive only that to which they are entitled.

Those of us who are health care administrators and those of us whose jobs involve the financing of medical care have a constant obligation to assure that our front-line personnel do not implement necessary policies in ways that trample on patients' rights and sensitivities. This requires clearly written policies and rules as well as sensitive management. In this case, the ethical issue may be in part that the public administrators' instructions to the social workers and nurses in the field may have been so poorly phrased (or poorly intended) that insensitive or brutal behavior was subtly encouraged. The crux of the matter, however, is that health care professionals charged with a demanding task—arranging for the timely and humane transfer of a patient to a more appropriate facility (or finding a legitimate and appropriate alternative course of action)—chose to behave in a way that violated not only basic standards of civilized human behavior but also strongly established ethical principles governing how health care professionals are to act with respect to patients.

If the law or the rules tend to promote unethical behavior, it is an ethical obligation of the administrators and professionals to get them changed—and failing that, to interpret them humanely and even to ignore or disobey those aspects that violate basic principles.

The state regulations were indeed badly written, but that is not the main issue. The central point is that the administrators at the top and middle, and the professionals who actually deal with patients, have an overriding obligation to care about the welfare of those patients. When the implementation of rules, even stupid rules, is done in ways that deny basic human rights, such as the right to be consulted and heard about one's own health care, primary blame must be affixed on the people responsible for that implementation, not on an impersonal "state."

47

The Last Bed in the ICU

At the age of seventy, Mrs. A. has been admitted to the hospital for the fifth time in as many years for treatment of respiratory difficulty. The last time she was in the hospital she had nearly died. She has severe emphysema, and when she developed a cold, her deterioration was so rapid that only artificial respiration in the emergency room saved her life. However, it proved very difficult to wean her from the respirator. She spent four weeks in the Intensive Care Unit and required constant care from the medical staff, principally Intern B. After she was discharged, she remained short of breath even while watching television.

Now, five months later, she has contracted another cold, but this time Intern B. has managed to treat her without resorting to the ICU and the respirator. During her illnesses, Mrs. A.'s two sons have been in constant contact with the medical staff. They have been anxious, agitated, and demanding.

It is now 2 A.M. and Intern B. is again called to see Mrs. A., who is becoming increasingly lethargic. It is obvious that she is in respiratory failure and will probably die before morning if she is not given a respirator.

However, hospital policy requires that respirators be used only in the ICU, where the required supporting staff and facilities are available. There is only one bed open in the ICU. The residents like to save one bed for an emergency. As Intern B. approaches, Mrs. A.'s sons are waiting. He knows their questions: What's wrong now? What will you do?

What should the intern do? And on what basis should he make his decision?

COMMENTARY

R. B. Schiffer

Mrs. A.'s sons, speaking for her, may ask for the respirator and ICU intervention. Should this request be granted?

There are a number of reasons why decisions concerning medical interventions for the seriously ill should be made by the patient, or by the patient's representative. But they do not apply in this case. Although Mrs. A.'s family has the right to refuse the ICU transfer and respirator, they do not have the right to demand it. Self-determination with regard to medical care is one thing, but a just allocation of scarce resources is another. The first right belongs to the patient, but the second is a claim which society makes upon the use of its health care resources.

Shall the physician decide? This would be an odd way to decide such questions (although in fact many are decided by physicians). Physicians, like families, have vested interests in some patients compared to others. And little in their educational background qualifies them as experts in the just allocation of scarce lifesaving medical resources.

Still, I believe the physician has an important contribution to make. In this case, there is a single patient and an available, but costly, resource. We must first ask whether the scarce resource at issue *can* justifiably be used by the patient. We can separate this question from that of whether the resource *should* be so used. The physician might be in the best position to answer this first question.

Logically, there are two steps in deciding the allocation of a scarce medical resource for a seriously ill patient. The first is medical or clinical in nature; the second moral. The principle which guides the first step is usefulness; where there is no benefit, there is no obligation to intervene. Indeed, in a setting of scarcity, there may be a moral obligation not to expend resources from which a particular patient has no reasonable expectation of benefiting. The principle which guides the second step is that of justice; the fair allocation of scarce resources when not all who might benefit can be treated.

Suppose the family in the case had heard of the wonders of coronary artery bypass surgery, and demanded it for Mrs. A. This request would be denied for medical, and not moral, reasons. Such a procedure would be irrelevant for her, and would not improve her pulmonary dysfunction.

If it is the physician's responsibility to distinguish a useful from an irrelevant intervention, how should this be done? The case illustrates how difficult this problem can be. Is this woman medically eligible for the respirator/ICU intervention? Can we say that she has a reasonable expectation of clinically benefiting from this intervention? This I find a real dilemma.

Although medical eligibility is usually explained in terms of "usefulness" or "fruitfulness," it is difficult to find a clear statement of what this means clinically. An intuitive view of this concept might include the notion of an increased span of survival, that is, improved mortality. This view, however, raises the quality-of-life issue. The patient group for which these decisions are made is usually very ill. If the ICU machinery should prolong Mrs. A.'s existence, without clinical improvement, would we really describe her as having benefited?

Is clinical morbidity, then, the yardstick by which we should measure usefulness? If the contemplated intervention in this case held reasonable promise of improving level of consciousness, or of restoring respiratory function, should we say that the patient is medically eligible without regard to questions of mortality? This seems odd as well. What if she also had a metastatic malignancy, which augured death in days to weeks? Under these conditions it would not seem that she was clinically eligible for the expenditure of a scarce medical resource.

If there are problems with either significantly improved mortality or morbidity taken separately, perhaps their *conjunction* should guide physicians in determining medical eligibility. That is, for a mortally afflicted patient to be medically eligible for a specific scarce lifesaving medical resource, there should be in the responsible physician's judgment some reasonable expectation of significant clinical improvement in both mortality and morbidity. From the few details we know in Mrs. A.'s case, she does not seem medically eligible for the ICU transfer, and it should not be offered to the family. Although her life span might be prolonged, there is no ground for expecting any significant improvement in her condition.

COMMENTARY
Benjamin Freedman

It is often said that questions of medical ethics fall into two categories: some concern procedures for decision, others the substance of decisions. The distinction, while intuitive, is not easy to sustain. How can we determine which procedures ought to be followed unless we know what values out to be sought? On the other hand, what means are permissible in seeking to implement values?

The issue of procedure pervades the case of Mrs. A. with five decision-making agents entering the stage, each with a special claim:

1. *The hospital* has arrived at a policy judgment that respirators may be used only in the ICU. The reason for arriving at this policy—that the necessary superstructure for effective use of the respirator is available only in the ICU—seems to be an instrumentally rational policy. For such a policy to

be followed, what requirements ought to be satisfied? Clearly, the empirical judgment which dictated the policy should be supported by the best data and technical judgment available. We cannot be certain that this is the case here; "hospital policy" can be made by physicians, health-care personnel, hospital administrators, or other groups.

Even assuming that the best available empirical investigation has been heeded, two further questions for instrumentally rational policy arise. Are the means morally acceptable? Is the end desirable? Both questions are ethical in nature. If the end sought in the ICU regulation is the efficient use of respirators, we quickly smoke out value judgments lurking in factual language. What do we mean by "efficient"? Is efficiency to be sought at all costs? If there are no more respirators available than ICU beds, then it may make sense to limit their use to the ICU, but if additional respirators are available and a patient will die if one is not used, then the refusal to use one under less than ideal conditions seems morally questionable.

2. *The residents* "like" to leave one bed in the ICU open for emergencies. This preference has the flavor of something approaching a gentleman's agreement; for reasons which may be too obvious to require examination, a practice has developed. We often speak of some practice as our "policy." Yet this kind of policy differs crucially from more formal policies in that it need not have been, prior to establishment, publicly debated and announced. The unfortunate result is that what seemed not to require examination often turns out not to stand up under examination. In any event, "practice as policy" does not *bind* those adopting it. In contrast to other kinds of policies, informal agreements may be informally broken. The intern need not feel bound by it. He is an independent moral agent, and should evaluate both the general worth of this policy and the appropriateness of applying it here.

3.*The intern* takes policies of the hospital and the residents and finds himself bound to interpret them. As courts have occasionally acknowledged, interpretation of a policy is an act of policy making in itself. If, for example, the intern decides against admitting Mrs. A. to the ICU, giving as his reasons the policies of the hospital and the residents, he must himself have decided that Mrs. A.'s condition is not an emergency. In spite of the fact that without the respirator she will die, this decision could be acceptable—in the case when, for example, she would die despite its use. But without such a circumstance, the rights and wrongs of the matter should not be decided upon in the heat of action by the intern alone.

Some elements of the decision must be decided by the intern and/or his supervisors: Mrs. A.'s prognosis at the moment, for instance. But other questions would profit by more public examination in which invidious presuppositions, biases, and idiosyncratic views would, it is hoped, disappear. In this case the medical facts alone cannot tell us what is morally required. Even if the respirator will only prolong the patient's uncomfortable life, it is still a moral question whether that prolongation is of sufficient value that the treatment is morally required or permissible.

4. *The relatives* may wish to be involved in, and not merely informed of, the decisions being made in this case. Certainly the relatives' wishes should not necessarily be definitive in deciding what should be done in this case. If the agents responsible for hospital policy (rather than just the intern) decide that treatment that will only prolong life in a diseased state does not qualify one for a respirator (either in or outside the ICU), and if the patient and family are made aware of this before entering the hospital, their views about treatment should not override that policy. Furthermore, the script, curiously, has left out the main protagonist. What are Mrs. A.'s views? If she is totally unable to communicate, the relatives may have a more significant place in the decisions, but if she is able to communicate and there has been no formally announced hospital policy against treatment in her case, then surely she should have some say in the matter.

5. *The patient* has been in this situation before. Has any effort been made to uncover what she feels about the aggressive efforts made in the past to maintain her in her morbid state?

Assuming that we may find out — possibly from the relatives — Mrs. A.'s wishes, I believe those ought to be respected. At worst, this would put her in conflict with the intern's individual judgment that her case does not constitute an emergency. A person's right to treatment should not be invariably subject to a physician's opinions, even when those opinions are based upon a mixture of medical and value judgments. It may be true that only a physician can assess the weight of the medical factors; it does not follow that the physician will do so correctly. If we must err, let us err on the side of individual dignity and autonomy.

The larger moral is that no quick delineation of policy in the heat of a medical crisis is likely to prove adequate for solving moral problems.

48

Two Cardiac Arrests, One Medical Team

George Burnham and Donald Mattison were patients in adjoining rooms in the rehabilitation division of a state medical center. George was a thirty-three-year-old, severely retarded man who had lived in state institutions since the age of three. His family had had no contact with him for over twenty years. George had been trained to feed himself and to keep himself reasonably clean, but at the age of twenty-five he had suffered a cardiac arrest that left him with some paralysis. After rehabilitation he only occasionally lacked bowel control. A second recent cardiac arrest left him semi-paralyzed and totally incontinent. The chances of his regaining even his former level of continence, the staff felt, were hopeless.

Donald Mattison, a forty-eight-year-old businessman, active in community and church affairs, married, and the father of four, had suffered a minor stroke, which left him slightly paralyzed. In his six weeks on the rehabilitation ward he had regained almost total use of his arm and leg. His prognosis for full recovery seemed excellent.

The hospital has at least one cardiac arrest team on duty twenty-four hours a day, and one crash cart in every patient area at all times. The possibility of simultaneous cardiac arrests seemed remote. If it were to happen, there would not be time to transfer an additional crash cart from another patient area, since the rehabilitation ward is served by an extremely slow elevator.

But in this case the improbable happened. George had a cardiac arrest at 3:00 one morning. Within four minutes the cardiac team had arrived in his room and was ready to begin work. At that very moment Donald also had a cardiac arrest. Knowing of the simultaneous cardiac arrests, every team member hesitated. Two also knew both patients' histories; the others, including the team leader, did not. After a moment, the team leader said, "First come, first served. Let's go to work." With no further hesitation, the team began to resuscitate George.

Without the emergency aid, Donald died. George was resuscitated, but suffered yet another cardiac arrest at 8:20 the next morning. This time another team was unable to revive him, and he too died. Did the team leader make the right decision in resuscitating George instead of Donald? Is "first come, first served" the proper principle to apply in such cases?

COMMENTARY
Kevin M. McIntyre and Robert C. Benfari

The most painful of all medical care decisions concerns life-preserving measures which, because of limited resources, require certain individuals to be excluded in favor of others. How does one weigh the relative rights of individuals to such care? Whenever possible, decisions to withhold lifesaving therapy should be made in advance. But in the absence of a clear expression that lifesaving care should be withheld, the person in charge must assume that care was intended. Should incompetency, the patient's family status, capacity to contribute to society, and related considerations be woven into the decision-making process? Let us consider each case on its own merits, then look at the priorities so as to answer the troubling question: "Who shall we permit to die?"

George has just suffered his third cardiac arrest. Since there was sufficient clinical information from two prior arrests to anticipate that cardiac arrest might occur again, in the absence of directions not to resuscitate we must assume that care should be initiated, as it was. George's severe retardation does not per se justify withholding resuscitative efforts, nor does his additional brain damage and total incontinence. The courts have indicated (in the *Dinnerstein* and *Spring* cases) that cardiopulmonary resuscitation (CPR) as well as other forms of lifesaving and life-prolonging therapy can be withheld in appropriate circumstances. But an appraisal by either care-provider or family of the "quality of life" of the lifelong incompetent as a basis for withholding such therapy has been specifically rejected (in the *Saikewicz* and the *Storar* and *Eichner* cases).

Recently, the highest court in the State of New York ruled without equivocation that there exists in some circumstances a positive obligation to provide lifesaving treatment to the terminally ill lifelong incompetent based on the common law requirement that a guardian act only in the best interest of the ward. While some may disagree, that decision supports the conclusion that there existed an obligation to treat George unless a court had already determined that withholding CPR was in George's best interests.

As for Donald, there are no indications that he had refused or would refuse resuscitation. He had a good prognosis for full recovery. He was young, married with four children, and employed.

Assuming that George would have received the full attention of the CPR team had Donald not arrested, how is one to proceed fairly? With a single crash cart and one cardiac arrest team, if we attempt to initiate CPR for both men, it is likely both will die. Donald's prognosis is better than George's. In addition, Donald's wife and children are emotionally and economically dependent on him so that there are broader societal costs were he to die. On balance, the choice clearly favors full commitment of CPR to Donald. Should we then abandon poor George? Or is it possible to allocate care in such a way that he may survive without seriously compromising Donald's chances?

One approach would be to initiate basic life support (artificial ventilation and external chest compression) immediately for Donald, using a single member of the team, and, as quickly as possible, attempt to defibrillate George. If initial attempts at defibrillation were unsuccessful, or if the attempt took more than thirty to sixty seconds, we would abandon efforts with George and concentrate totally on Donald. If George were in asystolic cardiac arrest (no electrical activity, as opposed to chaotic electrical activity in ventricular fibrillation) we would terminate efforts on his behalf because the likelihood of successful resuscitation would be very small and the time required would very likely preclude Donald's resuscitation.

This approach is based on the following considerations: (1) both George and Donald have a right to lifesaving treatment; (2) George's immediate prognosis is poorer than Donald's; (3) the societal costs of Donald's death would be substantially greater than those of George's; (4) George's best chance of returning to his previous state is immediate defibrillation.

Even the brief delay to defibrillate George may decrease the likelihood of successfully resuscitating Donald. But if Donald could be effectively ventilated (providing adequate air exchange in and out of the lungs of a patient whose breathing has ceased) and receive effective external chest compression (for the purpose of circulating blood in a patient whose heart has stopped beating) for a period not to exceed thirty to sixty seconds before all energies were directed toward him, the delay should not entail great additional risk. The small increase in risk to Donald must be balanced against the alternative, which would be to withhold all chances of survival from George. Would that conscientious decision making were as simple as " . . . first come, first served!"

COMMENTARY
Margaret Battin

To consider what would have been the right course of action for the crash cart team leader, let us look at two aspects of the case: first, the distributive principles to which one might appeal in order to honor fundamental moral commitments, and second, the procedural strategies one might use to put them into practice.

Of the many possible principles, at least three are plausible in this case:

Better prognosis. "When both cannot live, treat the one with the better prognosis." This principle, similar to that used in military triage, would clearly have preferred Donald. It reflects a moral commitment to maximizing the preservation of life. It should be applied only where the disparity between prognoses of competitors for treatment is relatively great: it will decide between two individuals when only one is likely to survive if treated, but it will not decide cases where the disparity is uncertain or small (for instance, which patient will receive a kidney, if one's recovery would probably take five weeks and the other's six). This principle can be applied without reference to George's retardation: if the medical history of arrests had been reversed, he would have been preferred.

Social worth. "When both cannot live, prefer the one who has greater value for other persons." This principle, although often attacked as inviting racism, sexism, and bias against the elderly, retarded, and mentally ill, may also be understood without bias: it prefers the person whose continuing life is of greater importance to others. This need not automatically mean Donald. Though George was seriously retarded, he might have contributed significantly to the life of the patients and staff of the ward; conversely, though Donald had prominent public status, he might have been a vicious abuser of relationships with his wife, children, and associates. However, we have no evidence for any such claims, and it is highly likely that Donald had greater value for other persons. Like "better prognosis," this principle is also to be applied only where the disparity between competitors is great; it will not decide, for instance, between saving the parent of two children and the parent of three. Correctly applied, it reflects a fundamental moral commitment to protecting important human relationships.

First come, first served. "When both cannot live, treat the one who is presented for treatment first." This principle, which the leader of the team chose to follow, is blind to the particular characteristics of competing individuals; since George's arrest occurred first he is to be saved, but it could have happened the other way around. Insofar as the principle is neutral to persons, it is similar to random selection, and seems to reflect a moral commitment to the equality of all.

We might praise the team leader's choice as reflecting a primary commitment to the equality of persons. But is this what the team leader's choice really shows? Note that both the other principles—"better prognosis" and "social worth"—would have required the team leader to make a comparative judgment about the conditions and circumstances of Donald and George. But the person-neutral "first come, first served" principle requires no background information about the competitors, presupposes no disparity except time of presentation for treatment, and will decide every hard-choice case except genuinely simultaneous ones. Did the team leader's choice (and do "first come" institutional policies) actually reflect a commitment to human equality, or the fact that this distributive principle is easier to apply? The fact that every member of the team "hesitated" before treating George suggests that other bases for decision were evident to all; is it sheer convenience that gives priority to this one?

Because non-neutral principles require judgments about conditions and circumstances, they are subject to bias when the disparities between competitors are small. Between Donald and George, however, the disparities in prognosis and social worth were very great; hence, bias would have been much less likely to arise.

To say that medicine might well pay greater attention to non-neutral distributive principles is not to deny that there will be disagreements over these principles, or occasions when relevant information is not available, or cases in which there are multiple disparities, some of which favor one competitor and some the other. But these are the hard cases. The case of Donald and George is *not* a hard case: both non-neutral principles could have been applied and would have favored Donald over George. Only a two-minute disparity in time of presentation favored George; a genuinely neutral principle would have permitted treatment of either one. In hard cases, retreat to neutral distributive principles cannot be avoided, but in this case the team retreated too soon. The society that resorts to easy strategies even before the choices become hard may fail to honor the fundamental moral commitments it makes.

49

The Doctor, the Patient, and the DRG

Jeffrey Wasserman

Lakeview Hospital has been reimbursed on the basis of "diagnosis related groups," or DRGs, since May 1980. The hospital's medical director, Jared Lapin, M.D., acts as a liaison between the hospital's managers and the medical staff. In addition, Dr. Lapin and Ellen O'Connor, director of finance, periodically review the performance of individual physicians from a financial viewpoint.

At a recent meeting, Dr. Lapin and Ms. O'Connor analyzed a lengthy computer report that matched, for each physician, the revenue the hospital received with the costs incurred for treating patients in each of the DRGs in one month. While studying the fifteen DRGs under Major Diagnostic Category number 14 (Pregnancy, Childbirth, and the Puerperium), they noticed that Dr. Daniel Weiner admitted seventeen patients who were later determined to be in DRG 373 (vaginal delivery without complicating diagnosis) but only two in DRG 371 (cesarian section, without complication and/or co-morbidity). Yet for the other three obstetricians on staff, fifty-eight came under DRG 373 and nineteen under 371. Across all deliveries, the costs of treating Dr. Weiner's patients exceeded the revenue received from the DRG rates. But the total cost incurred in providing care to the other obstetricians' patients was considerably below revenue and hence the hospital was able to earn a "profit."

The computer report also revealed that the reimbursement rate the hospital received for routine deliveries fell just short of covering all the incurred expenses, whereas the rate paid for cesarian sections was substantially greater than the actual cost to the hospital. The reason for Dr. Weiner's comparatively poor overall "financial performance," Dr. Lapin and Ms. O'Connor concluded, was that he performed many fewer cesarians than did his colleagues.

Dr. Weiner explained that he did not agree with his colleagues that once a woman had a cesarian delivery, all subsequent deliveries must be cesarian; he felt that most of these women could have normal deliveries. He cited a number of recent studies that found no differences in outcomes (in terms of health risks to both mother and child) associated with the different delivery modes. Dr. Lapin countered that the tradition of performing repeat cesarians was strong and that more time and research were needed before large numbers of physicians changed their practices. He noted too that, if a complication were to arise, the attending physician would likely be faced with a malpractice suit.

Finally, he pointed out to Dr. Weiner that the hospital was losing money on almost every patient he treated. "Dan," he said, "it's in all our interests to look out for the financial health of the hospital. And since it is unclear which of the two approaches benefits the patient more, I urge you to reconsider the way you handle these cases."

Was it ethical for Dr. Lapin to approach Dr. Weiner if there was no indication he was delivering poor quality care? How should financial considerations, both those related to the hospital and society at large, be weighed against physician judgment? What if Dr. Weiner could convincingly demonstrate that his patients were actually at less risk than those of his colleagues?

COMMENTARY
J. Joel May

The ethical question raised in this case is: what considerations are appropriate in making medical decisions? Certainly the question of what is good for the patient in the opinion of a competent physician is, and will continue to be, an important ingredient in making such decisions. Thus, Dr. Weiner's belief that, given no difference in outcomes, it is desirable not to expose obstetric patients to the trauma of surgery is a justifiable part of the calculus. Also, when outcomes are similar, patient preferences with respect to alternative forms of treatment should be considered. Finally, what the regimen of care will cost the patient (but not what it will cost the insurance carrier) is frequently a part of such a decision.

But, this case asks, is the financial impact of the chosen mode of care on the *hospital* an admissible ingredient? Hospitals, by virtue of their social purpose and their tax status, are expected to provide "charitable care" (that is, care that is not financially profitable to the institution) to those in need. But if a hospital were to provide "too much" such care, it would fail financially. Potential future patients would suffer reduced access to care. The hospital's obligation to all present and potential patients must be weighed against its obligation to provide "charitable care" in a particular instance. In this case, the hospital is faced with either losing a little money on each patient delivered normally or making "substantial" money on each patient delivered by cesarian. The hospital does have an obligation to point out that fact to its physicians and to urge them to consider including it as a relevant dimension of their decision-making process. Thus, it was not only ethical but appropriate for Dr. Lapin to call Dr. Weiner's "poor financial performance" to his attention.

The ultimate decision of how to treat patients, on the other hand, should remain with the physician. Were Lakeview Hospital to order Dr. Weiner to deliver such patients by cesarian section in order to improve its profitability and thereby reduce the options available to him, it would be acting unethically. The question raised in the case (of how financial considerations should be weighed against the physician's judgment) is therefore moot.

Financial considerations should be a part of a physician's judgment. Financial issues important to the individual patient (such as out-of-pocket expenditures for the procedure) have always been a part of such judgments. Because new financial dimensions of the question are related to institutional, community, or societal concerns, rather than individual patient concerns, does not preclude them from consideration. Nor should they be treated as if they were juxtaposed to medical judgment. Instead they should be incorporated into the decision-making process.

The final question concerns a hypothetical situation in which Dr. Weiner was able to demonstrate that his patients, delivered normally, were actually at less risk than those delivered by cesarian section. Herein lies a real ethical dilemma. The amount of reduction in risk to the patients is associated with a cost to the hospital. But if the patients (or the physicians on their behalf) are willing to incur additional risk, the hospital makes a profit. From the hospital's perspective, the decision must revolve around the cost it is willing to bear in order to reduce the risk. Since outcomes of medical treatment are never certain, and since risk can never be totally eliminated, a common denominator must be chosen to measure the extent of risk that is "appropriate" given the cost, and that, in turn, must be weighed against the relationship between the financial impact on the hospital and its ability to serve future patients.

Probably in the situation presented in this case, the fact that only a small financial loss is associated with the reduced risk would (and should) lead the hospital to encourage the least risky approach, even in the face of a loss of income.

In the past, financial considerations have played a small part in shaping or constraining physicians' judgments, and this has contributed to the inflation in hospital costs. Absence of cost constraints has also led to the provision of unnecessary (too much) care for some, perhaps at the expense of limiting or denying care to others.

Factoring cost implications into the calculus of medical decision making is not only desirable but essential in deciding fairly and equitably who shall get how much of what kind of care. Dr. Lapin should continue to identify such circumstances and bring them to the attention of the physicians. Dr. Weiner and his colleagues have an obligation to include such considerations when making medical judgments.

COMMENTARY
Daniel H. Schwartz

Some fifty years ago my professor of ethics drew two circles on the blackboard — a large one representing the common good, and a smaller one the individual good. Arrows pointed from each circle to the other, indicating conflict. The problem in ethics, he said, was to put the small circle inside the large one, so that the individual and common good could both be achieved.

The hospital administrator has the responsibility of putting a number of smaller circles — patients and physicians, students and researchers in a tertiary hospital, the hospital and its community — inside the larger one of societal good.

Case studies like this are designed to present hard choices for the hospital administrator in fulfilling that responsibility. But perhaps the choice in this case is not so hard after all. There is no reason why a hospital cannot provide quality care to patients and survive under a well-constructed DRG or other prospective payment system. Assuming that the hospital is doing a good job, it should both survive financially and permit Dr. Weiner to continue his practice of preferring normal deliveries over repeat cesarians. Physicians should be aware of the fiscal impact of their activities. They should also, in my opinion, practice the best medicine as determined by the leaders of their profession.

Changes in practice are familiar problems in the evolution of medical care and the DRG system is set up to adjust to medical advances. It is my understanding that the old view on repeat cesarians has changed and in most leading institutions it is no longer the rule. An NIH Task Force reached this conclusion a couple of years ago. In our own hospital about 70 percent of previous cesarians are handled by normal vaginal delivery. The original DRG is based on historical data but will change.

On the other hand, changes in cases designed to produce a "profit" under the DRG system would result in identifying the change in the particular hospital and physician's case mix. The hospital would get into more trouble by insisting that Dr. Weiner alter his approach than it would by permitting him to continue to avoid repeat cesarians. The State Health Commissioner, during the DRG demonstration, tells me that if Dr. Weiner changed his practice, it could result in a penalty to the hospital.

All of us in hospital administration (and many other fields) know that you win some and you lose some. A creative administrator will find an ethical way to compensate for the financial loss in Dr. Weiner's case by a variety of actions that will help, not harm, patients: more precise coding of complications and comorbidities; getting doctors to do better documentation in medical charts (which will improve patient care); reducing unnecessary laboratory tests; and other measures that will be stimulated by the DRG system. One of the ways we expect to deal with this problem is discharging patients earlier to our Home Health Agency, providing appropriate therapy in the home at less than a tenth of the cost of hospital care.

Finally, speaking of ethics, it should be noted that Dr. Weiner would receive a bigger fee from Blue Shield for a cesarian yet he prefers to do normal deliveries in these situations. Furthermore, Dr. Lapin is right that Dr. Weiner exposes himself to a greater possibility of a malpractice suit, since our legal system lags behind medical advances. The plaintiff's attorney is certainly going to say: "Why didn't you do a cesarian?" Dr. Weiner's ethical courage should be commended.

COMMENTARY
Joy Hinson Penticuff

Dr. Lapin asserts that "it's in all our interests to look out for the financial health of the hospital." Yet in this case he put one interest, the financial health of the hospital, ahead of other, more important interests, the physical and psychological health of women. The DRGs will produce bad medical care—that is, some mothers will be subjected to needless cesarian sections—if "traditional" medical practice is maintained despite scientific evidence that innovations produce improved patient outcomes. Dr. Weiner can convincingly demonstrate that vaginal delivery is just as safe for selected mothers and infants as repeat cesarian section. In spring 1982, the American College of Obstetrics and Gynecology published guidelines that described medical indications for trial of labor and vaginal delivery after previous cesarian section. The ACOG studies concluded: "As many as 50 to 75% of a carefully selected group of patients may achieve vaginal delivery after previous cesarian section."

Furthermore, a cesarian section is not just a surgical procedure. It is a birth experience, and as such, carries much symbolic meaning. There may well be a psychological trauma associated with cesarian section because the mother may consider it as a failure. Most mothers feel a sense of disappointment when they are unable to deliver their infant normally, and they frequently feel that what should have been a natural process has taken on a sterile, technical quality. Indeed, many mothers seek out cesarian support groups to cope with their feelings of inadequacy and frustration.

Cesarian sections are painful and interfere with the mother's initial interactions with her newborn infant. Breastfeeding techniques must be modified, since the usual positioning of the infant against the mother's abdomen causes discomfort. To subject the mother to this needless stress for the purpose of preserving the "financial health" of the hospital is outrageous.

In attempting to persuade Dr. Weiner to perform more cesarian sections Dr. Lapin was clearly in the wrong. The real problem here is that the reimbursement for vaginal deliveries in this hospital is too low, and the inducement to perform cesarian sections is too great. It is Dr. Lapin's duty in his role as liaison between the hospital's managers and the medical staff, to correct the faulty calculation of the DRG reimbursement schedule. He is incorrect in taking coercive action toward Dr. Weiner, which would increase the already alarming intrusion of medical intervention into what is a highly significant family process: the birth of a new baby.

Ironically, DRGs are being forced on consumers just when consumers are demanding that health care professionals consider the whole person, not just an affected body part. DRGs do exactly what consumers fear most—they categorize patients according to diagnosis. A patient does not want to be viewed as "the gallbladder in room 312," but as a unique individual with a particular medical condition.

And individuals do respond to illness in distinctive ways. While two mothers may stay in the hospital for the same number of days following cesarian sections, one mother's psychological experience and her need for support following that cesarian birth may be vastly different from that of the mother in the next bed. She may need assistance from her physician and nurses which cannot be calculated by a DRG.

DRGs were designed to decrease the cost of medical care. In this case, the faulty DRG reimbursement (giving incentive for performance of cesarian section over vaginal delivery) will drive up the cost of medical care because third-party payers will be paying for surgical deliveries rather than the less expensive vaginal deliveries. If one carries this logic to its natural conclusion, hospital administrators will coerce physicians into encouraging their patients to enter the hospital for a variety of unnecessary procedures just to ensure its own "financial health."

This case also shows the pressing need for consumers to be involved in the formulation of DRG reimbursement schedules. The best interests of individuals seeking health care *must* be the priority. Health care professionals who put the institution's financial interest above the best interests of the patient have sold their ethics to the highest DRG.

50
The HMO Physician's Duty to Cut Costs

William Edwards was thirty-nine when a serious, potentially life-threatening ventricular heart arrhythmia (irregular contractions) was diagnosed during a routine physical examination. The cardiologist first prescribed quinidine, but it failed to control the arrhythmia.

Diisopyramide was successful, but Mr. Edwards complained of severe blurred vision and dry mouth. When the medication was reduced, the side effects disappeared but the arrhythmia returned. At this point the cardiologist decided to combine the diisopyramide with propranolol, a common beta-blocker known to be effective in certain arrhythmias. This controlled the problem, without side effects.

Mr. Edwards continued with this medication regimen for five years until moving to a new town, where he joined a Health Maintenance Organization (HMO). He immediately consulted Dr. Sam Forester, a cardiologist.

Dr. Forester agreed that medication was needed, but he was concerned about diisopyramide, since severe problems had been reported in some patients. Moreover, Mr. Edwards and his original physician had never tried the obvious approach of using propranolol alone.

Both Dr. Forester and Mr. Edwards concluded that there were also risks in shifting to the single drug. Although it was generally safer than diisopyramide and probably should have been tried originally, there was a small chance of a fatal heart attack. On balance both agreed that the status quo was slightly better for the patient.

Dr. Forester then noticed the financial ledger for Mr. Edwards's care, which included the cost of the medication paid for in full by the HMO. The yearly cost of the diisopyramide was $430; the propranolol cost $26. He realized that even a significant increase in propranolol dosage, something that would involve little risk, would still reduce the HMO's medication bill by about $400.

Should Dr. Forester consider a change in medication, taking into account cost-saving for the HMO, or should he work solely on the basis of the welfare of the patient? If he should take into account the costs to the HMO, should he try to persuade the patient to agree to the change or should he simply refuse to authorize any further prescriptions for the diisopyramide? Does Mr. Edwards have any moral obligation to take costs to the HMO into account in choosing a medication regimen?

COMMENTARY
Robert M. Veatch

The traditional professional ethics of physicians—reflected in the Hippocratic Oath, the Declaration of Geneva, and elsewhere—is that the physician should always strive to do what he or she thinks will benefit the patient.

In this case that traditional ethical commitment is challenged. In effect, the question is: Should the physician divert his attention from the single-minded pursuit of the patient's welfare where the institution's or other subscribers' interests would be served by slightly compromising the patient? Specifically, a very small, but real increment of benefit is purchased for a very substantial cost. Does the patient-benefit principle apply in such cases?

Two ethical options are available, neither of which is very attractive. First, we could amend the Hippocratic commitment so that physicians should, at least in certain circumstances, take into account the welfare of others. We might give the physician the mandate to try to maximize total benefits instead of simply benefit to the patient.

That strategy produces at least two serious problems, however. First, physicians (like any other special social group) have unique notions about the comparative value of resource expenditures. In deciding whether to use Medicaid funds to pay for drugs, for example, a physician should have to compare the value of providing the drugs with the value of some remote nonmedical uses of the money. Asking health professionals to take these social trade-offs into account could introduce serious biases.

Second, if physicians include benefits to others in their calculations, patients have to be told that their physicians have conflicting agendas. The Hippocratic Oath would have to be removed from the waiting room wall and replaced with a sign that says, "Warning all ye who enter here. The physician will at times abandon your interests in order to benefit others and save them money." It is not clear that rational patients or physicians in an HMO would prefer this new mandate.

The other alternative is to give the HMO physician—in fact all clinicians—a special role-related ethic that exempts them from the general ethical duty to promote fair and reasonable distribution of resources. They would then be free to single-mindedly pursue the welfare along with the rights of the patient.

Then, however, someone else must decide to eliminate marginally beneficial care. Surely, in planning the HMO or insurance coverage, no rational persons would want all such care included. Assuming marginal care was eliminated for others as well as themselves, they would opt for a lower premium so they could spend the money on something they valued more. Mr. Edwards would reasonably prefer not to have the diisopyramide and other marginal treatments covered, if he could spend the savings somewhere else.

The most acceptable arrangement, therefore, would actively involve members of the HMO plan in decisions about whether certain marginal medical services are covered. Members might, for example, exclude heart transplant coverage, as Medicare does. They might decide to cover routine physical exams only every five years for people between twenty and forty even though they might reasonably benefit marginally from more frequent exams. They might cover only ten days of hospitalization for myocardial infarction even though a few more days would be marginally beneficial. These decisions should be made by the patients (the subscribers), however. Clinicians should not be put in the position of ruling on how much to compromise their patients.

The drug case poses an interesting problem. To the extent that the decision can be handled as a policy matter, it should be—like the physical exam frequency.

Judgments like the one in the diisopyramide case, however, do not lend themselves to policy. No obvious solution is apparent. Administrators, especially in profit-making HMOs, are not in any better position to make such decisions than clinicians.

An ethics committee comprising a representative sample of patients might be given the authority to rule based on the facts presented by the HMO professionals. In doing so the group would be acting as agents for their fellow subscribers with a mandate to eliminate marginally beneficial care. Theoretically, they might be asked to eliminate all care where the cost exceeded the benefit. That, however, would create serious tensions among members and would be unfair to the sickest members, exactly the group that has the greatest claim of justice for care, even inefficient care. If this ethics committee of HMO members cannot make these judgments, we may be forced to the bizarre conclusion that no one is in an ethical position to decide to eliminate such care.

That brings us to the role of Mr. Edwards. Does he have any moral responsibility to consider that the best drug regimen for him is one that offers only marginally more benefit for a much greater cost? Surely, it is both moral and prudent for Mr. Edwards to take all of this into consideration in endorsing, promoting, or participating in collective arrangements by which members establish policies that eliminate marginally beneficial, expensive care.

Does he have any obligation, however, to suggest eliminating his diisopyramide—in order that others may benefit from the savings? I am not convinced he has a strict moral obligation to do so. Such a contribution to his fellow subscribers seems supererogatory.

I am thus forced to conclude that, although the expensive drug should be eliminated, neither Mr. Edwards nor Dr. Forester is the proper person to make that decision. Surely the administrators of the HMO are in no better position to do so. If that decision can be made ethically at all, it should be made by the HMO members as a whole—at the policy level if possible, and by a committee of the members if not.

COMMENTARY
Morris F. Collen

In almost every patient encounter, a health care practitioner must consider first the quality of care he or she is prescribing—that is, whether a particular clinical decision will achieve an accurate diagnosis and/or bring about the desired benefit; and second, the costs resulting from this decision to the patient and/or to the organization financing the care. Thus, a very common problem in the practice of medicine is balancing the quality with the costs of medical care.

The physician often provides professional services on a fee-for-service basis to a patient with a disease for which there are alternative acceptable methods of treatment. The physician always considers the relative effectiveness of each treatment mode and should also consider the comparative total costs associated with each treatment. The physician should attempt to assess whether the patient can afford the most expensive treatments, and should discuss with the patient the comparative costs and effectiveness of the alternative treatments available, ideally to arrive at a mutually agreeable decision. As the fee-for-service practitioner knows, if the costs for the prescribed treatment exceed the immediate financial resources of the patient, then payment of the physician's fee may be delayed. Thus the financial success of fee-for-service practitioners is intimately linked to the financial solvency of their private patients.

Similarly, if the patient has prepaid for medical care services in a Health Maintenance Organization, the HMO physician knows that the immediate cost consequences of his or her clinical decision will have a direct impact on the HMO's finances. Furthermore, if the overall HMO costs exceed those that had been budgeted by the HMO for the year, then in the following year the prepayment dues (premiums) as direct costs to the patient and to all other subscriber-members of the HMO, will proportionately need to increase to restore the HMO's positive economic balance. If the HMO excessively increases its annual premiums, it will no longer be competitive with other health insurance programs in the community, its membership will likely decrease, and it will need to compensate by reducing personnel or decreasing the comprehensiveness of its prepaid services. Thus the financial success of the HMO physician is intimately linked to the financial solvency of his or her HMO.

Only under arrangements where the patient has no obligation to pay for any medical treatment (as in the Veterans' Administration hospitals or a charity clinic) and where the physician's salary is independent of revenues generated from professional services can individual physicians consider the effectiveness of care without taking into account the treatment costs. However, increasing budgetary restraints and public support for cost containment are introducing economic questions even into these medical practice arrangements.

Thus, in any doctor-patient encounter, under any financing arrangement, the doctor has some financial incentive—in addition to a moral obligation—to consider both the quality and the costs of the care being prescribed and to attempt to arrive at a good balance that can be justified and defended to other physicians and the doctor should try to persuade the patient to agree to that treatment which is acceptably effective at the lowest cost. Rarely, in a case such as this one, is any treatment 100 percent effective in curing the disease, so rarely is the choice clear-cut or simple. The physician should not refuse to authorize a treatment that the physician and the patient agree is best. Finally, physicians should be prepared to defend their judgment before their peers in the community within which they practice; and before a jury in court if their decision varies from the comunity's standard of practice.

51

The Noncompliant Substance Abuser

J.R. is a combative, young white female who presents in the Emergency Room disoriented, with a fever, chills, and a cough productive of yellow sputum. She complains of chest pain and shortness of breath.

J.R. is well known to the medical staff. She has had three previous admissions with endocarditis and interrupted her clinical course on two of those admissions by leaving the hospital against medical advice. On her most recent previous admission, her mitral valve was replaced with a porcine prosthesis. She also tested HIV positive (but was and remains asymptomatic for AIDS).

J.R.'s social history includes occasional prostitution, IV substance abuse (cocaine), and needle-sharing. Although J.R. had been referred repeatedly to the substance abuse shelter, she refused counseling.

With a diagnosis of pneumonia, *Staphylococcus aureus* bacteremia, and a mitral valve vegetation and mild insufficiency, J.R. is placed on appropriate IV antibiotics and hospitalized.

On the third hospital day, J.R. is much improved. She is calmer, less combative, and seems resigned to the clinical course as outlined to her by her attending physician (four to six weeks of IV antibiotic therapy).

On hosptial day 10 J.R. has a low-grade fever but otherwise feels much improved. She begins to show signs of irritability. She quarrels with her medical resident and nurse about the necessity of remaining in the hospital.

On hospital day 11 J.R. objects to receiving medical direction from the medical resident and demands to see her "real doctor." The attending physician is called. J.R. tells him that she can't stand being confined to the ward. She says that she feels well enough for discharge. The attending points out that the growth on her prosethic heart valve, while reduced in size, remains. He explains that the bacteria growing in her blood is especially dangerous and that a more extended clinical course is medically indicated. He warns J.R. that she risks death if she cuts off her clinical course prematurely. J.R. trivializes his warnings, saying, "I'm under a death sentence anyhow." On day 12, J.R. walks out against medical advice.

Two days later, J.R. again presents to the Emergency Room with a fever, shortness of breath, and a rapid heart rate. A repeat echocardiogram shows worsened mitral valve incompetence and heavier regurgitation. Replacement of the prosthetic valve is recommended. J.R.'s attending physician points out that contraindications of J.R.'s poor surgical risk status and her record for recidivism. A consultation with the hospital ethics committee is sought. After a thorough review, the committee offers the opinion that it would not be unethical to replace J.R.'s damaged heart valve. Surgery is scheduled.

J.R. tolerates surgery better than expected. Her course of antibiotics is resumed. In hope of achieving better compliance, J.R. is fitted with a PRN adapter (an indwelling catheter permitting direct IV access) and given instructions for self-administering her antibiotics at home. On the fifteenth day after surgery, J.R. is discharged, scheduled for a follow-up clinical appointment in two days. J.R. misses her appointment.

Four weeks after discharge, J.R. presents yet again in the Emergency Room, with a fever and shortness of breath. Clinical signs indicate that her second valve has failed. (J.R. admits to using the PRN adapter for cocaine.) An echocardiagram shows heavy mitral regurgitation and a perivalvular abcess. She is growing *Pseudomonas aeruginosa* in her blood. J.R. demands another valve, saying it would violate her civil rights to be refused. Would it be wrong to refuse her?

COMMENTARY
Christine Cassel and John La Puma

Patients like J.R. frustrate doctors and nurses no end. These patients are pejoratively referred to as "dirtballs," especially by residents. Sometimes attending physicians tell their residents that the best they can hope for in caring for such a patient is to learn how to insert a subclavian line when her blood pressure drops.

J.R. was an "undesirable" or "hateful" patient for several reasons: (1) she had a serious illness that would require prolonged hospitalization and intensive use of services; (2) she is HIV positive, for which there is no highly effective treatment; (3) she evidenced continued self-destructive behavior; and (4) she was medically indigent and inadequately insured.

The decision to operate on J.R. has been made twice, on the basis of medical distinctions: mitral valve rupture is a life-threatening complication of endocarditis. A decision not to operate on J.R. would be made on the basis of someone's, presumably the attending physician's assessment of socioeconomic and cost-benefit considerations in her care.

Faced with arguments about limited resources, it is always important to clarify whose resources are being considered and to what degree there is a scarcity of those resources. Here, the valves themselves are plentiful. Porcine valves are easily available, and not in fixed supply, as are human blood or human organ donors. A valve shortage does not limit J.R.'s care.

What might limit it is the shortage of financial resources. First, the Medicaid payment for J.R.'s care comes from a limited public purse, now faced with increasing numbers of poor people needing medical care, combined with state resistance to raising taxes to pay for this care. Funds spent on J.R. are likely to diminish availability of care for other needy people.

Second, concern exists about the overall amount of society's money that goes to health care. This concern is an important reason not to waste healthcare resources, but the definition of *waste* is complex in a fragmented reimbursement system like ours. Since most health-care providers are not working within a defined capitated system and are not asked to make actual tradeoff decisions between two different services, or even two different patients, how can we argue that a lifesaving procedure is a waste unless we believe that this specific patient's life is worth less than the average patient's life?

A scarcity of institutional resources may mitigate against valve replacement. But hospital beds are not scarce: low daily censuses have already forced many hospitals to close.

Yet, physicians are trained (and paid) to make medical distinctions, not social ones. Medical indications are different from issues of cost containment. We wonder if a physician would consider refusing the request of an impaired substance-abuser colleague—a young anesthesiologist, for example—who needed another valve replacement. Is there something morally different about the young physician's request? Is it primarily the young physician's means and peer group—our own—that separates his case from J.R.'s? In one study of 100 impaired physicians treated in Georgia, all were compelled to complete an in-patient training program; most went into remission and many returned to work after treatment.

What J.R. needs is treatment for two diseases, not one: prosthetic valve endocarditis and drug dependence. Successful treatment of one depends on the other. A recent national study documented a woeful shortage of drug treatment programs, many of which have been proven effective.

We would tell J.R. and her treating physicians that she should have the valve replacement, if she promised to complete an in-patient substance abuse program, just like the young anesthesiologist. If J.R. leaves the hospital AMA again, or breaks her promise, efforts at saving her life with intensive medical and surgical treatment will have been unsuccessful. Palliative care, with a limited treatment plan (symptomatic treatment for the discomfort for dyspnea and fever) is what we can and should offer then. But until we're willing to offer real treatment for J.R.'s underlying disease of drug dependence—and a routine referral to the city shelter is barely a start—treatment of her valve disease cannot be considered futile.

COMMENTARY
Lance K. Stell

This case challenges our capacity to control prejudicial impulses regarding unpopular forms of self-abuse. Our much-publicized war on drugs has created a social climate which selectively stigmatizes illicit drug use, making it respectable—no, laudable—to be especially harsh with refactory IV substance abusers. Having said this, however, it does not follow that we must never refuse heart valve replacements to substance abusers for fear of indulging prejudice. At some point, any reasonable person must begin to doubt the wisdom of additional heart-valve replacements for a patient like J.R. But when? Does it come only at the point where the expectable patient benefit from an additional surgical intervention equals zero? Somewhere short of this? Does the patient's extraordinary record of noncompliant, self-destructive behavior make a difference?

If a tissue graft may be withheld from an otherwise eligible heart transplant candidate partly because of expected noncompliant postoperative behavior, may a valve replacement be withheld on similar grounds? Presumably, the shortage of suitable organs and a determination that they do as much good as possible explains in part why noncompliant postoperative behavior matters in transplant cases. Resource scarcity does not present itself so dramatically in patients with substance-abuse-related endocarditis but it remains an issue nonetheless. Costs average $14,000 for treating endocarditis medically. Uncomplicated surgical replacement of affected valves averages $24,800. Since few substance abusers with endocarditis have full insurance coverage, their treatment expenses tend to be cost-shifted to others. Some observers may think that this provides another argument for socially guided health-care rationing. For present purposes, I leave questions of rationing aside, noting only in passing that some hospitals seems to have adopted a two-valve limit for IV substance abusers.

I think it would not be wrong to refuse J.R.'s demand for another heart valve. In general, health-care professionals have no obligation to offer treatment options that have proven to be ineffective in a patient. An otherwise effective therapeutic effort can be rendered ineffective by noncompliant patient behavior. A pattern of noncompliant, self-abusive behavior can justify a belief that otherwise effective therapy will be rendered ineffective by it. When such evidence exists, it is not wrong to withhold otherwise effective therapy until there is good evidence that it will be successful. J.R.'s history of noncompliance and drug-abuse count as sufficient evidence to believe that her future behavior probably would destroy any prosthetic valve that might be placed. Therefore it would not be wrong to refuse J.R.'s demand for another valve until and unless a change in her behavior makes a reassessment appropriate.

One might object that J.R.'s underlying medical problem, chemical dependency, is a chronic disease which, like diabetes, can be managed, but not cured. Refusing to offer surgery for the foreseeable complications of substance abuse is no differenct from refusing amputation of a gangrenous limb to a noncompliant diabetic, so it would be wrong to refuse amputation of a gangreneous limb to a noncompliant diabetic, so it would be wrong to refuse heart valve replacement to J.R. To refuse her amounts to punishing her for suffering from a common complication of her chronic disease. This is medically inappropriate.

Although the thrust of the objection does not rest on the analogy with diabetes, it is worth pointing out that there is an important difference between the moral resources of diabetics and substance abusers. No insulin-dependent diabetic can cure her disease by an act of will, yet at least some substance abusers do, by appropriate acts of will and perhaps with help, discontinue substance abuse.

The relevant part of the objection seems to rest on the claim that even an impressive record of noncompliance cannot justify refusing a surgical intervention which will likely be undermined by just that sort of noncompliance.

This strikes me as a dubious claim. Smokers are not candidates for heart transplantation. This is not because smokers are stigmatized socially, but because their addiction creates an unacceptable additional risk of allograft failure. J.R.'s record of noncompliance is similar in this respect.

The suggestion that refusing to offer J.R. a third valve replacement is punitive requires clarification. It likely means that regardless of the stated, justificatory reason for refusal, the real reason is punitive and discriminatory. Substantiating this claim would require showing that the reasons offered for refusal in J.R.'s case are inherently weak and that dispite their applicability in similar cases they are invoked only here. It would then be reasonable to explain J.R.'s treatment as motivated by widely held prejudices against substance abusers.

Everything important hangs on showing that the justification is inherently weak. I think J.R.'s record makes it permissible to refuse to offer her a third valve on the grounds that there is no obligation to offer patients interventions that will be ineffective. The controversial part of the argument concerns whether noncompliant, self-destructive behavior can be a relevant causal factor in judging efficacy. If it can, how much evidence must one have before the principle justifies refusal? Some ethicists think that a patient's noncompliant, self-destructive behavior can never serve in an argument to justify refusing an intervention. I think this absolutist position is too strong.

52

In Organ Transplants, Americans First?

Luiza Magardician, a twenty-year-old Rumanian citizen, arrived in New York in June 1985 in the hope of obtaining a kidney transplant. According to Reverend Dumitru Viorel Sasu of the Rumanian Orthodox Church of St. Dumitru in Manhattan, before her arrival here "all available methods of treatment were tried unsuccessfully in her country." The director of the National Kidney Foundation of New York-New Jersey says Ms. Magardician's chance of finding a kidney donor are bleak since "there is a bad shortage of donors in the United States, and U.S. citizens would usually come first." In addition, Ms. Magardician has reportedly exhausted her funds and could not afford hospital costs even if a donor were found.

In 1984, more than 8,500 Americans were waiting for kidney transplants; only half were expected to receive one that year. Should the decision to offer Ms. Magardician a transplant be made strictly on the grounds of her medical needs or should her country of origin or financial situation influence the decision? Should such decisions be made by individual hospitals or at the state or national level? Given the shortage of usable kidneys, what place should compassion, medical need, and justice play in allocating organs?

COMMENTARY

Jeffrey M. Prottas

Despite substantial improvements in the effectiveness of organ procurement efforts, the waiting lists for all transplants grow continually. More people wait longer for a transplant; some of them die waiting. All must accept medical treatments that are inferior in their own view and that of their physicians. Because organs are both valuable and in short supply their allocation among patients is a matter of important public concern. But only when two identifiable patients are candidates for the same organ does the issue of the treatment of nonimmigrant aliens arise.

When only one suitable recipient exists for a given organ there is no allocation problem; if Ms. Magardician is that recipient, no one denies that she should receive it. Her right of access to an organ is called into question only when a U.S. resident is also a medically suitable candidate. The issue is not one of citizenship, but of residence—membership in the community of potential organ donors. Unfortunately, with over 8,500 U.S. residents on lists awaiting a kidney transplant and thousands more awaiting nonrenal transplants, direct competition for an organ is more the case than the exception. The harsh fact is that, often, someone must be denied. On what grounds should that decision be made? I believe that membership in the community that supplies the organs is a legitimate criterion.

Every cadaveric organ available for transplantation in the United States is obtained through the generosity of members of the American community. Only the death of a young healthy person can make a suitable organ available, and only the willingness of family members to put aside their own grief can result in the organ retrieval. Every organ transplant starts in tragedy and kindness.

Organ procurement also requires a large investment in organizational, human, and financial resources. Over 110 organizations are at work locating and obtaining transplantable solid organs. These organizations represent the efforts of perhaps 1,000 men and women and over $100 million of public money.

In short, the American community (all those who live here) has committed resources and, more important, has demonstrated the altruism necessary to make organ transplantation possible. Under these circumstances members of this national community have a right not to be denied an organ transplant because that organ is being sent overseas or offered to a person who has traveled here specifically to obtain it.

An alternative to this policy that can be defended on the highest ethical grounds is that every individual be treated the same and that all nonimmigrant aliens seeking a transplant be placed on the nation's waiting lists without discrimination. But no nation operating an organ procurement system has seen fit to institute this practice. There is a sense that humanitarianism does not extend so far as to require a nation to share, to its own detriment, a scarce and lifesaving resource.

But what of Ms. Magardician? Even if we admit that she must take that kidney from a resident, isn't her need greater? The resident can in all probability remain on dialysis. And, if dialysis is a second best treatment for him or her, it is preferable to dying. Can we not set aside a percentage of organs on compassionate grounds?

First, I am very suspicious of generosity at the expense of other people. I will not have to go to dialysis treatments three times a week as a result of a decision to set aside a percentage of organs for immigrant aliens. But other residents will, and I would not ask that kind of unselfishness from anyone. Second, Ms. Magardician's situation is the same as that of most nonresident aliens. Since only the very rich can afford to treat end-stage renal disease without government support, almost all foreigners who come here explicitly for a transplant have as much claim on our compassion as she does. We cannot transplant them all. If some are more deserving of life than others, the solution is not a quota system but a decision-making process. This process would have to operate in a public manner, with explicit criteria and on a national basis. It is inappropriate to set aside a number of organs and ask individual hospitals to use them as they see fit.

Sending organs overseas or transplanting them into nonimmigrants is not sharing America's bounty but diverting its scarcity. As long as a shortage of organs continues in the United States, some individuals in need must be denied a transplant. Members of the community that make transplantation possible have a right to expect that their medical needs will be addressed and that allocation decisions will not adversely affect them.

COMMENTARY
Olga Jonasson

In North America, Europe, Australia, South Africa, and Japan, well-established programs in organ transplantation provide state-of-the-art therapy for highly selected patients with end-stage kidney failure. Transplantation is, however, unavailable in developing countries and in most of the impoverished areas of the world.

American medicine has a strong tradition and long history of generously sharing its medical technology and therapies. Foreign patients come to our medical centers in large numbers to obtain complex surgical procedures or medical treatment. It seems inconsistent with all our previous practices to exclude access to cadaver organ transplantation for patients from foreign countries.

Yet the reasons for reserving cadaver organs for American residents are compelling. Grossly insufficient numbers of organs are available for Americans who need transplantation; maintaining a patient awaiting kidney transplantation on dialysis is expensive, and thousands of patients wait for months or years until a kidney becomes available. Patients awaiting heart or liver transplantation, where no maintenance therapy is available to keep them alive, frequently die before an organ can be found. It is also commonly assumed (though unproven) that the public expects that the organs donated upon the death of a family member will be transplanted into an American resident. Lastly, the costs of public education campaigns encouraging organ donation and much of the costs of acquiring the organ are supported by tax dollars.

It is also probably true that several countries could mount adequate organ transplantation programs if necessary; the outlet provided by the centers in America and Europe that accept their citizens for transplantation removes the local incentive to establish centers, change laws, and educate the public.

Luiza Magardician came here with the expectation that she would find help in this generous country. In my experience, most of the foreign nationals who have come here for transplantation are like Luiza; they are ordinary folk, with no particular wealth or status and certainly without political clout or influence. Others have come with wealth and influence, and considerable pressure has been applied by institutions in this country and by our government to see to it that they receive a transplant, and as promptly as possible. This, of course, is completely unacceptable. But even people who are rich or powerful can be very sick. Organs should be distributed to rich and poor alike, on the basis of medical need.

Dealing with these issues has not been easy for the transplantation community. To close the doors to all foreign patients seeking transplantation is uncompassionate; to have a completely open policy is unfair to American residents. The Transplantation Society, an international multidisciplinary society with a broad membership from medicine and science, and the American Society of Transplant Surgeons (ASTS) have recently adopted similar positions condemning the commercialization of transplantation, wherein organs could be bought and sold. The ASTS also adopted a position, supported by a large majority of the membership, that at most 5 percent of all kidney transplants done in any center be in foreign patients, and that those patients be selected on the basis of the same medical criteria as all others.

The National Task Force on Organ Transplantation also addressed this issue, and was divided in its recommendations; the majority recommended the establishment of a quota (10 percent rather than 5 percent), but several members of the Task Force as well as many others in the field feel strongly that no organ should be given to a foreign patient unless no American resident is available as a recipient. I cannot agree with this view. It is inhumane to treat nonresidents as second-class patients, even if they voluntarily accept that status in order to gain a slight chance for an organ. They remain in this country, away from home and family, and often spend every asset they possess in the vain hope of obtaining treatment. Moreover, I am convinced that the public wants organs to be fairly allocated to sick patients, whether the recipient is or is not an American.

These decisions rest squarely with the transplantation community. It is their responsibility, as trustees of these precious organs, to develop and implement policies to provide organs to patients with equity and fairness; these policies must be publicly stated and defended, and carefully monitored.

The fact that Ms. Magardician has exhausted her funds poses another problem. Kidney transplantation costs about $30,000, if all goes well. She has no right to expect free care from any transplant center. Her government should be asked to fund her care; failing this, she must appeal to the Rumanian community in New York or elsewhere for support. Again, in my experience Americans are generous when faced with real need.

Clearly, a major reason for the serious discrepancy between need and availability is the failure of hospital personnel to identify potential donors and to offer the family the opportunity to give the gift of the organs. Policies of routine inquiry, guaranteeing that the families will be given this chance, would be important steps in meeting the needs of all deserving recipients.

COMMENTARY
John I. Kleinig

Ms. Magardician's situation is complicated by two factors: (1) she does not appear to have been accepted for assessment or treatment prior to leaving for

New York; (2) she did not make adequate financial preparations (might she not have organized community or church support?). We get a whiff of moral extortion—though perhaps she shouldn't be singled out unfairly: a "nag factor," advantaging the importunate, seems to influence even routine decisions.

More important is whether she should be eligible for any consideration, given the shortage of kidney donors and the understandable tendency to feel that "U.S. citizens [better: residents] would usually come first." Should Ms. Magardician's medical needs determine her eligibility, to the extent of putting her ahead of a U.S. resident who might also benefit from the same donor kidney? How might we decide?

At a general level we could, I guess, ask donors (or those who agree to donation for others) to specify whether—given the scarcity of the resource—they would be willing for the kidney to be made available to a nonresident. But without some principled reason for allowing this discretion, donors could claim a more extensive discretion about recipients (regarding color, sex, and the like).

Should it then be left to individual hospitals or states to determine the scope of eligibility? The constraints on arbitrary and invidious discrimination might be stronger, but if nonresidents as such are to be excluded from access to scarce resources, some argument will be needed to deflect the charge of medical jingoism.

What reasons might we have for exclusivism? We might answer differently for private and public transplant units: allowing the former to take whomever they wish, perhaps influenced by ability to pay. This *could* result in a large foreign clientele. Publicly funded units, being taxpayer supported, could argue the reasonableness of a "citizens first" policy.

A problematic assumption underlies both approaches, insofar as they disqualify nonresidents on the basis of their lack of residency. The assumption is that medical facilities and technology are "owned" in some morally strong sense by those who operate or finance them, justifying them in an exclusivist policy.

But like many sophisticated human products, transplant technology is the child not of local or even national effort, but of internationally shared endeavor. That U.S. residents are now able to receive relatively successful treatment for kidney failure owes a good deal to the work, among others, of French and Dutch researchers. A "this is for us alone" policy in scientific research would (and, where it occurs, does) greatly inhibit human progress; there is no overriding reason for its introduction at the point of application.

Of course, there are some reasons for favoring one's own, even as one might agree to donate only because the recipient is a close relative. National bonds, cultural and economic, count for something. Residents have a reasonable expectation that their contributions to their social environment will be reflected in services—particularly of a lifesaving kind. An open-door policy (whether in immigration, education, or medicine) would be destructive to much that has been labored for and is counted dear.

But the alternative to an open door need not be a closed one. In a world of scarce resources, a quota system, safeguarding for resident use perhaps 90 percent of donated organs, would be consistent with the conservation of national resources and values. At the same time, providing some foreign access to transplant units would acknowledge the transnational character of beneficent technology.

As a consequence some U.S. residents will miss out on lifesaving treatment because nonresidents have been given the use of scarce organs. Thus, there is surely some argument for viewing the quota system as only an interim solution, and for developing less problematic alternatives: International kidney donations? The export of successful transplant technology?

Where does this leave Ms. Magardician? If fairness in allocation is the issue, her way of pressing her case does not create a helpful precedent. If a quota system were already in place, we could determine whether, under its terms, she would have qualified for admission. In the absence of a quota system, any decision would probably be clouded by political factors. Whatever is decided, her case will constitute a strong argument for developing general criteria for nonresident eligibility.

53

The Anencephalic Newborn as Organ Donor

Mrs. Z., a young, pregnant woman with no children underwent an ultrasound examination. Her baby girl was overdue and the ultrasound revealed that she was anencephalic. There appeared to be no brain tissue present except for portions of the brain stem. The parents were told of this tragic diagnosis and immediately decided to volunteer the baby as an organ donor. The obstetrician in charge of Mrs. Z.'s care decided to contact a large, tertiary care facility nearby in order to ascertain their interest in utilizing the child as a donor.

Two-thirds of children who suffer from anencephaly are stillborn. Many of the organ systems in such children are underdeveloped, but it is possible to utilize both the heart and kidneys for transplantation to other children. The obstetrician and the pediatrician agreed that it would soon be necessary to induce labor. However, if organ procurement was to be undertaken, it seemed reasonable to transfer her to the large tertiary care hospital and to induce labor there.

The rest of the medical staff was uncertain whether to proceed. If they accepted the mother's wish to have the baby be an organ donor, were they under an obligation to try to resuscitate the infant if it was stillborn? What steps should they take to try and support the child considering that babies born with this condition normally receive no aggressive treatment in the neonatal nursery? Perhaps most confusing was the question of when death should and could be pronounced.

Should Mrs. Z. be transferred to the large medical center? Should the physicians accept the wishes of Mr. and Mrs. Z. to have their child serve as an organ donor? If they do, what steps would be morally permissible to help increase the chances of allowing the child to serve as an organ donor?

COMMENTARY
Michael R. Harrison

Mrs. Z.'s case is problematic because there are ethical and legal obstacles to taking organs from a prenatally diagnosed anencephalic newborn. Her case is also promising because the use of fetal organs may be a biologically sound and cost-effective treatment for otherwise hopeless childhood diseases, and because use of organs from this category of newborns could alleviate or solve the growing shortage of vital organs appropriate for children.

Under present definitions and laws, organs cannot be taken from a person who does not meet the currently accepted "whole brain" definition of death, which requires "irreversible cessation of all functions of the entire brain, including the brain stem." The liveborn anencephalic does not meet this definition; it is not "brain-dead" even though the cranial vault is incomplete and most of the cerebral cortex is absent. Even with this devastating and completely hopeless anomaly, the residual lower brain stem can maintain vital functions, although precariously, for hours or days. However, if vital functions are allowed to deteriorate until cardiorespiratory arrest, vital organs are irreversibly damaged, making them useless for transplantation.

The "whole brain" definition of death was adopted to protect the comatose patient whose injured brain might conceivably recover function. Obviously, this precaution need not and should not apply to an anencephalic who never had and can never have the physical structure necessary for higher brain activity or cognitive function. Failure of the brain to develop is clearly different from injury to a functioning brain, and was not considered when the brain-death definition was formulated.

One possible approach is to consider the anencephalic "brain-absent." By creating a new category, which is limited exclusively to anencephalics, we may be able to avoid revising presently accepted "brain-death" criteria to include anencephalics. I believe "brain-absent" will come to have the same medical-legal implications as "brain-dead." That is, life support can be withdrawn and organs can be retrieved. Of course, this will have to be recognized by society and confirmed by the courts.

There are advantages to treating the anencephalic fetus and newborn as a person who by virtue of biologic deficiencies (the absence of a brain) is analogous to brain-dead. First, this category can be narrowly defined and cannot be expanded to include individuals with less severe anomalies or injuries. Any attempt to make it possible to use organs from anencephalics should not relax or compromise the protection of fetuses and newborns with other, less devastating anomalies.

Another advantage is that an anencephalic fetus is considered a person, albeit one who is dying, a process that will be completed at or shortly after birth. Like the comatose patient on artificial life support, the anencephalic fetus requires maternal life support for maintenance of vital functions; but birth is inevitable, and birth will be death. If we accept the anencephalic as a person who is "brain-absent," we can recognize his devastating anatomic and functional deficiency without demeaning his very existence. Then it is easy to stipulate that organs can be taken only if this can be accomplished in a way that would not conceivably cause suffering and would not detract from the dignity of dying or abridge the right to die.

Prolonging gestation to get more mature organs or prolonging extrauterine survival to maintain organ perfusion would be inappropriate. In this setting removal of organs must be carried out with compassion, sensitivity, and respect for the anencephalic donor and the family; this is best accomplished in the operating room as is presently done for the brain-dead heart-beating cadaver. Finally, this approach makes sense of the presently accepted practice of allowing termination of anencephalic pregnancy at any gestational age.

Another approach to organ procurement from anencephalics might be to consider the anencephalic a product of human conception incapable of achieving personhood. Although it might be argued that the anencephalic lacks the biologic structure (forebrain) giving the potential for characteristic human activity, there are several reasons to avoid this approach. First, it is difficult to reach a consensus about personhood and what constitutes humanness, especially when the issue of gestational age is involved. Second, denying personhood denigrates the pregnancy itself and may lead to a less respectful approach to the grieving family and to medical care of the fetus and newborn. Finally, this approach raises a specter of abuse in which other fetuses or newborns, possibly with less severe handicaps, might be denied personhood. This frightening potential would require the most stringent safeguards, and is probably best avoided altogether.

If the anencephalic fetus were to be considered "brain-absent" and thus equivalent to "brain-dead" for legal purposes, Mrs. Z. would be ethically justified in allowing organ procurement after delivery. She and her physician should be able to arrange the timing and place of delivery to facilitate transplantation. After all, Mrs. Z.'s pregnancy provides fetal organ preservation and transport that is far better biologically and far cheaper than anything yet devised by the most accomplished organ harvest team.

Of course, the decision to end the pregnancy must be independent of and prior to any decision about using the organs for transplantation. The aim of perinatal management in this case is to evacuate the uterus as safely as possible for the mother and to allow fetal demise without discomfort. The newborn should be cared for by physicians independent of the transplant team and the condition of anencephaly (and therefore brain absence) confirmed by an independent team including a neurologist, bioethicist, and neonatologist. Prenatal diagnosis allows the family to choose beforehand whether they wish to see and hold the newborn as part of their grieving, and if and how organs can be procured.

If organ procurement from prenatally diagnosed anencephalics can be accomplished with safety for mother and respect for the fetal donor, Mrs. Z. should be able to salvage from the inestimable tragedy of fetal anencephaly the consolation of offering the gift of life to a dying child.

COMMENTARY
Gilbert Meilaender

There is in principle no reason why parents should not—after the death of a child—donate the child's heart and kidneys to suitable recipients. But how much we would like to know that this case does not tell us—in particular, what the parents were told, and what they think they are doing.

Having heard the diagnosis, they "immediately" decided to donate the baby's organs. What does this mean? Do they perhaps imagine that they are simply aborting a fetus—even though the child is already overdue? Do they feel guilt that, however irrational, causes them to want to *use* the baby to wrest some good from terrible circumstances? Have they thought about whether they will want to hold their child at least briefly and say goodbye to the infant who occupied their thoughts (and, who knows, perhaps their prayers) for nine months?

Questions ... none answerable at the moment. We can only reflect on the case and the questions. I presume that Mrs. and Mr. Z. and the health care professionals involved all wish to respect the life of Baby Z. This baby cannot live for long even if born alive. She will never have the "higher" human capacities of consciousness and self-awareness. But if born with brain stem activity she will be a living human being, though one born dying.

We can know human beings, whatever their cognitive capacities, only in their bodies, and that is the way we will know this baby—one of the weakest members of our species. She rightfully claims our care. But, of course, potential organ recipients also need care. Can we meet their needs while also caring for this child and respecting her humanity? If we can, we will surely want to do so, but from the outset we should be aware that this may not be possible. Our obligation is not to achieve all the good we can, as if our responsibility were godlike. It is, rather, to effect what good we can within the limits morality places upon us. Not only what we can *accomplish* but what we *do* counts.

One question the case raises admits, I think, of a fairly straightforward answer. Is there any reason why Mrs. Z. should not be transferred to the larger medical center nearby? *If* there is no other ground for objecting to the proposed organ donation, this need not be an obstacle. Transfer is primarily a matter of logistics. Were it feasible, it would be equally permissible to move potential recipients to the hospital where the donor is located. In this case the other direction of movement is called for, and that in itself does not seem objectionable.

As a guide to the more troubling issues raised by the case, we may take our cue from the first report published (in 1975) by the National Commission for the Protection of Human Subjects of Biomedical and Behavioral Research. That report dealt with the subject that had led to the formation of the Commission: research on the fetus. A different topic from the one in our case, to be sure, but related in certain ways.

Among the issues discussed and reported on by the Commission, one of the thorniest concerned research on the aborted, nonviable fetus *ex utero*. On the one hand, the Commission held that such dying subjects could not be harmed in the sense of "injured for life." Since this altered the meaning of "harm" in subtle but very significant ways, the report suggested that the class of experiments carrying only "minimal risk of harm" might be larger for these nonviable fetuses than for other experimental subjects. On the other hand, the Commission held that the integrity of the dying subject was not to be violated. It concluded that "out of respect for the dying subjects, no nontherapeutic interventions are permissible which would alter the duration of life of the nonviable fetus *ex utero*."

That particular recommendation did not receive the support of the Secretary of HEW [Health, Education and Welfare, the former title of the Department of Health and Human Services], but it was a sound moral instinct. A similar principle can guide us through the case at hand. We should care for Baby Z. as we would normally care for an anencephalic child who is born dying. The anticipated organ donation should not lead us to prolong her life or subject her to medical interventions—unless we would do so in any case, apart from the desire to transplant her organs. That is what it would mean to respect her as a dying subject and not just to use her life as a means to someone else's good. But—subject to the instruction of those with more medical knowledge—I suspect that acceptance of this principle will create difficulties for the planned organ donation.

How would we ordinarily care for this baby at her birth? The case suggests a standard, and it seems to me the right one: she would receive "no aggressive treatment in the neonatal nursery." She is born dying, and proper care for her does not entail useless attempts to sustain her life. Ordinarily, then, we would not and should not provide respiratory assistance to her, assistance that could only prolong her dying. Ordinarily we would not and should not resuscitate such an infant if she were stillborn. And ordinarily, I suspect, we would rely on the normal clinical signs to determine death.

But if the heart and kidneys of this child are to be available for transplantation, we might want to resuscitate her even if she were stillborn. If her organs are to be suitable for donation, we might want to provide (while she still lives) exactly the sort of assistance we normally eschew—respiratory assistance, with death determined not by ordinary clinical signs but by absence of brain activity. In other words, the anticipated organ donation tempts us to treat in ways we otherwise would not—which is, I fear, a temptation to use this child simply as a means to another (admittedly desirable) end.

If the transplantation can be carried out without significantly altering the way we would otherwise treat this baby, I see no reason to disapprove and much reason to approve it. But if transplantation requires significant change in the normal care of Baby Z., we ought to have serious moral reservations. To intervene in this baby's living and dying in ways we normally reject (because we think it an indignity to a dying subject) would be to do here what we normally think it wrong to do—and to do so for reasons entirely unrelated to the care of Baby Z. What we *accomplish* thereby would be good; what we *do* would not.

54

Can the Fetus Be an Organ Farm?

Mr. R., a twenty-eight-year-old engineer, has been on dialysis for three years, and is growing desperate because of the restrictions it places on his life. He can not work regularly because of the amount of time he has to spend in a dialysis center, and he feels weak and is suffering from many of the debilitating side effects of the treatment.

Mr. R. has already investigated the possibility of obtaining a transplant. However, he had been adopted as an infant and does not know his natural family. In addition, tests show that he has a rare tissue type that makes it highly unlikely that a suitable cadaver kidney can be found.

Mr. R.'s physical and mental state continue to deteriorate and his wife suggests a solution to the transplant surgeon. She will, she says, become pregnant, and after five or six months, have an abortion. The kidneys from the fetus could then be transplanted in her husband.

The surgeon knows that technically such a transplant could be performed, and that the graft would probably not be rejected. He also knows that Mr. R. has threatened to commit suicide if he has to remain on dialysis for an indefinite period.

Should he agree to transplant the kidneys of a deliberately conceived and aborted fetus?

COMMENTARY
Mary Anne Warren

I would argue that if the relevant factors were only those described, then the surgeon ought to agree to the woman's plan to provide her husband with the kidneys of a fetus conceived for that purpose, and aborted at five or six months. I say "if" because I want to consider the morality of the action apart from any of the legal, professional, or personal complications that might arise if such a plan were actually carried out in today's world.

Even more than the typical abortion case, this case forces us to focus on the moral status of the (five- or six-month-old) fetus, that is, on whether or not it should be considered a human being with a full-fledged right to life. For none of the more plausible arguments intended to show that abortion is morally permissible even if the fetus has the same right to life as an adult human being apply in this case; it is not a matter of self-defense on the woman's part, nor an exercise of her right to retain control of her body by refusing to submit to an unwanted pregnancy. Unless, therefore, one supposes that mere biological parenthood confers the right to kill one's offspring, at any age, one must conclude that if a fetus of this age is a human being with full moral rights, then the woman's proposal is tantamount to murder. On the other hand, if a fetus does not have a significant right to life, then the plan raises no serious moral problem, and provided that the operation has a good chance of saving her husband's life without seriously endangering hers, it should certainly be performed.

It is clear that if we are to make a reasoned judgment about the moral status of fetuses, and of nonhuman animals, alien life forms, intelligent machines, and other problematic entities, we must develop a criterion for the possession of moral rights that is species-neutral. That is, it will not do to make "genetic humanity" (mere genetic affiliation to the human species) either a necessary or a sufficient condition for the possession of full moral rights. To make it necessary is to beg the question against all nonhuman entities, even those which may prove to have intellects and sensibilities comparable or superior to our own; while to make it sufficient is to beg the question against abortion, particularly in a case like this one.

My candidate for a species-neutral criterion for the possession of full moral rights is what I call *personhood*. A person, to speak very roughly, is an entity that has the (actual, not merely potential) capacity for consciousness, complex and sophisticated perception, rationality, self-awareness, and self-motivated behavior. Such entities have rights by virtue of the fact that they have definite, preconceptualized preferences with respect to their own present and future states; they have desires, hopes, plans, and fears. Above all, they normally desire to go on living, or at least not to be killed in a way not of their own choosing. This is why killing people against their will is intrinsically bad, and in most cases morally wrong.

But fetuses, one might say, as yet have no will; they do not desire life, or anything else, any more than trees or amoebas do. Neither the mere *potential* to become a person, nor preconscious organic existence, not even a degree of sentience unaccompanied by the other aspects of personhood, can generate a right to life comparable to that of a person. Hence I think that there can be no serious moral objection to killing a fetus, an entity far below the threshold of personhood, in order to save the life of an adult human being.

I realize, of course, that most people will resist such a conclusion. Fetuses, especially those as old as five or six months, elicit our sympathy, and tempt us to endow them with moral rights, not only because they are potential people, but because they look disconcertingly like people; their physical features are recognizably human. But this sympathy is misplaced, unless there is a good deal more conscious activity in the fetal "mind" than we have any reason to suspect. While a fetus of five or six months may, perhaps, possess some flickering of sensation, or some capacity to feel pain, this is equally true and probably even more true of creatures like fish or insects, which few would doubt the propriety of killing in order to save human lives. In such cases, a proper respect for the right to life requires that it not be respected where it does not exist.

COMMENTARY
Daniel C. Maguire

One of the most neglected ways to resolve an apparently irresolvable ethical dilemma is to ask: are there viable alternatives to that which is proposed? In this case, there is one alternative that seems to transform the dilemma of Mr. and Mrs. R., making the intentional abortion for a transplantable kidney morally out of order. The alternative is: allow the baby to be born, and then see whether its tissue type is a suitable match. Since the mother's genes enter into the baby's genetic endowment, it is possible that the kidney will be incompatible with the father's rare type.

If the match is good and if the baby has two kidneys, one could be removed and given to the father. The greater maturity of the organ would likely enhance the prospects for successful transplant. Allowing the baby to be born changes the *what* of the case significantly, making the transplant proposal medically and morally more promising. The mother's plan to conceive a baby who might or might not have the right tissue type and to terminate the life of the fetus in any event is not the same case as bearing a baby who might, among other things, be a suitable donor for its father.

There are many reasons for having a baby, and, of course, the baby makes its own sweet case for living when it arrives. But, having a baby as a potential donor does not appear either evil or frivolous. And, medically, a born baby seems to have more realistic credentials as a donor. Even if the baby were not the right tissue type, its birth might possibly give Mr. R. more zest for life helping him to bear his terrible affliction.

But suppose Mr. and Mrs. R. insist that they do not want to have a baby, they only want to have a kidney. In reply I would point out the difficulty of having one without the other. More technically, I would say that they do indeed want a baby, but as a means not as an end. This is not self-evidently immoral.

In addition to these points against the abortion, I confess an extreme uneasiness in contemplating the very idea of the uterus as an organ farm or the fetus as an organ bank. Maybe my uneasiness is simply a shrinking before the unaccustomed, a horror of the new, or weakness of the masculine mind in the face of a tragic but moral option. Maybe the death of the fetus makes sense in a world where laying down one's life for a friend is the supreme moral achievement. The death of the fetus might be more easily entertained since it is preconscious, and not in the same human situation as a fully personalized adult.

On the other hand, my uneasiness may be the yield of moral intelligence. Ethics begins in awe and moves on to articulation, argument, and debate. Even in the midst of debate, the mind of the moralist should be attentive to the awe that is its foundation. In this case, my uneasiness, plus the facts and alternatives, conspire to make me very certain in offering a negative moral judgment on the proposed abortion.

One question remains: what right have we to presume the permission of the baby in donating its kidney to its father? Shouldn't the autonomy and privacy of the baby be protected until it grows to adulthood and can consent to such a dramatic donation?

A baby is not born outside the pale of human solidarity. It is a horrid individualism that sees the baby born into a "state of nature" with no debts or beneficent relationships to the social body until it "consents" to participate in the social contract. A baby is not an alien untouchable or a mere candidate for human communal existence. "Person" is a relative term and even baby-persons are intrinsically related to other persons.

Relationship to the other and the capacity for sharing are present before we are aware of them, since they relate to our elementary humanity and not just to our subsequent maturity and volition. Part of the awesome grandeur of parental care is the right and duty to interpret sensitively what a baby's humanity entails. And it may entail the surrender of a paired organ when that surrender is "a gift of life." The inability to permit this has its roots in an isolationist-individualist anthropology that ostracizes the baby from genuine humanness under guise of protecting its nonadult status.

Notice that the issue here cannot be discussed merely at the level of consent—whether personal or proxy. It involves the foundation upon which one's entire ethics is based.

COMMENTARY
Carol Levine

The conception and birth of a wanted child have always been among humanity's most powerful affirmations of life and its intrinsic value. When a pregnancy is unwanted, and abortion is contemplated, it is usually because of some serious reason—contraceptive failure, rape or incest, severe medical problems in the mother, probable genetic defects in the offspring, or economic deprivation. In these cases the rights and interests of the already existing person must be weighed against those of the fetus. Abortion in such cases need not be condemned; neither, of course, should it be celebrated.

The scheme proposed in this case study, however—planned conception followed by planned abortion for the sole purpose of producing a body organ—is a perversion of both acts. Creating life in order to destroy it mocks both religious and humanistic concepts of the value of an individual. Manipulating the procreative process in this way transforms it from a natural and positive act to a callous and calculating one that transcends the permissible limits of human interference.

And one need not be opposed to abortion in all cases to be opposed to it in this one. The fetus is not an adult or even an infant; neither is it a chicken or a carrot. As what I would consider a potential person, it has at the very least the right to be treated with respect and dignity, and not as a source of spare parts for another's body. In carrying out this scheme, Mrs. R. would not only be using her unborn child solely as a means and not as an end, but she would also be permitting herself to be used in the same unethical way.

But would this violation of the moral imperatives of valuing life and treating persons as ends and not means be acceptable because of another, more compelling principle—saving the life of another human being? There may be situations in which it is the highest form of altruism to sacrifice one's life to save another's, but that is not at issue here. It is harder to imagine situations in which one person may be allowed to sacrifice the life of another, even potential, person, to save a third, but even that is not at issue.

Consider the facts. Mr. R. is not dying—he is only threatening to kill himself. Two medically accepted therapies are available for his kidney disease. He has tried dialysis, and finds it too restricting. Now he wants a transplant, and no near relatives or suitable cadaver organs are available. But even if the aborted fetus's kidney were available, success is by no means guaranteed. With present medical knowledge, such a transplantation is technically feasible, but it is not certain that the kidney tissue will match or that if it does, the graft will take over his failed kidney function. Rejection rates for kidneys from related donors are much lower than for cadaver organs; even so, a third fail within five years.

Transplantation itself involves a not inconsiderable risk of death. Even the successfully transplanted patient faces the frequently serious medical and psychological effects of continuous immunosuppressive drug therapy. It is quite likely that the best Mr. R. could hope for is a few years' respite from dialysis, and then what? Another conception? Another abortion? Another transplant?

Mr. R. finds dialysis intolerable, but thousands of other patients like him have learned to accept it. For some it is even the treatment of choice: it is more predictable, safer, and less damaging to the body over the long run than repeated transplants.

But Mr. R. does not feel his life on dialysis is worth living, even though he has a supportive wife to share his difficulties. In a desperate attempt to give her husband the reason to live that she alone apparently cannot provide, Mrs. R. is willing to use her body to produce the kidney he wants. Can her offer be considered entirely voluntary, or must it inevitably be suffused with the guilt and bitterness she must feel knowing that her husband values her not as a marriage partner, or as the mother of his child, but as an organ incubator? Threats of suicide can be very persuasive, but they are at the same time coercive.

I believe that the transplant surgeon should refuse to participate in the abortion scheme. Instead, he should try to help Mr. R. to understand and adjust to the practical alternatives. Some psychiatric counseling seems in order for Mr. R. as well as marriage counseling for the couple. Adding the burden of a morally unacceptable act to a serious medical problem and a troubled marital relationship would only deepen their despair.

55

A Prisoner in Need of a Bone Marrow Transplant

J.B., who is serving a prison term for third-degree murder, is being considered for an early pardon and release so that he can undergo a bone marrow transplant. He is suffering from chronic myelogenous leukemia (CML). Without the transplant, doctors say he will probably die within five years. With a transplant, J.B. has a 50 to 60 percent chance of long-term remission.

Ordinarily, inmates who need medical care are hospitalized and then returned to prison. But officials would prefer to release J.B. before his transplant, because they say they cannot afford the $100,000 to $200,000 estimated costs of surgery. If J.B. is released, he will probably qualify for public aid, since bone marrow transplants for CML are no longer considered experimental in his state.

Should J.B. be granted an early release on the grounds of his medical condition? If an early release is not feasible, does the prison system have an obligation to pay for his care? In or out of prison, is it fair for him to receive a publicly funded transplant when others who need a transplant might have to pay for it out of their own pockets?

COMMENTARY
Robert L. Cohen

Does the fact that a prisoner has chronic myelogenous leukemia disease (CML) meet the criteria for medical parole? Assuming that J.B. was incarcerated for a crime that he actually committed, that he received due process in his trial and sentencing, and that he has more than five years left to serve, the decision to grant medical parole should be based on prognosis and current degree of debilitation.

Prognosis is a relative issue because a very long anticipated survival would moot the question of medical parole. The five years survival prognosticated in this case seems to me long rather than short in the context of medical parole, and would argue against early release. If J.B.'s physical condition were marked by a severe degree of debilitation, and it seemed to the relevant officials that he was physically unable to pose any threat to the community, this would argue for medical parole. Continued incarceration would no longer serve the "correctional goals" of deterrence and punishment effectively (a severely debilitating terminal illness being punishment enough). However, from the record we are given, J.B. does not appear to be in a state of terminal debilitation. An early release therefore would not be appropriate.

Indeed, the chance of prisoners to receive medical parole is determined by other factors as well. Prisoners' social status, their access to influential legal and political supporters, and the perceived "seriousness" of the crime for which they have been incarcerated are the most critical issues. It may be that the aging of the prison population, as well as an increase in the number of terminally ill prisoners secondary to cancer and AIDS will result in expanded availability of medical parole. If such were to occur, driven by the economic pressures upon state departments of correction caring for terminally ill people, it would be a good thing.

Based on the principle that all individuals deserve equal access to medical care, which prison officials in this case seem to support, the question of who should pay for J.B.'s transplant is a real one. In practical terms, the state is obligated for the cost of care, since an incarcerated individual has no effective way of paying for his or her own medical services. The fact that J.B. would be eligible for Medicaid as a medically disabled person if released from prison, whereas he is not as a state prisoner, is a cost sharing problem, not an ethical one. These questions could be raised only in a system in which medical services are not universally available and where payment precedes the provision of necessary care. It is to our country's dishonor that universal access to care that is free at the point of delivery has not been codified as law.

The final question raised is the fairness of J.B.'s receiving a bone marrow transplant while incarcerated. Such a transplant would be publicly funded, and might place him at an advantage to others equally in need of a bone marrow transplant but who might have to pay for it "out of their own pockets." The normal course of events is in the opposite direction: availability of scarce and expensive medical technologies is often determined by market forces. Those with the greatest economic resources have the greatest access to these expensive and scarce procedures. In any case, the availability of bone marrow transplantation as a treatment for CML represents the fruit of publicly funded research and should be available to all, regardless of their ability to pay. I do not think it will be unfair for J.B. to receive a bone marrow transplant if that were clinically indicated.

COMMENTARY
Jeffrey Paul

Presuming punishment for a crime necessarily involves forfeiture, temporarily or permanently, of some of the criminal's rights (personal liberty, for example), which rights ought to be circumscribed by the state and to what extent? To determine what degree of circumscription is appropriate for a certain category of criminal, we must first assess the moral seriousness of the crime and analyze the social purposes that are to be served by assigning punishment. Such purposes have traditionally included retribution, incapacitation, reform, and deterrence.

Given the deliberate character of third-degree murder, a suitably severe punishment may deter some prospective criminals from committing it. Any punishment that deters others from unjustifiably taking an innocent life and does not *inappropriately* transgress the rights of the criminal should be incorporated into his sentence.

What counts as an appropriate transgression of those rights? Where deterrence, reform, incapacitation, and retribution are collectively employed to determine the requisite punishment, the retributive component must set the morally appropriate boundaries for such transgressions.

Thus, to ask what rights the perpetrator of third-degree murder surrenders is to ask what retribution is morally appropriate for a certain type of criminal. Because the crime involves violation of the victim's right to life, it can be argued that the criminal surrenders the right to life, or at least the right to life at liberty, by committing it. But because the crime here is murder in the *third degree*, the moral culpability of J.B. is less than that of someone who commits murder in the first or second degree. J.B. thus has surrendered neither his right to life nor the whole of his right to liberty. The punishment assigned to him therefore should not involve taking his life or permanently abrogating his liberty (in the form of life imprisonment, for example). However, given that his crime involved violation of another's right to life, neither is the state obligated to do everything in its power to sustain his life while he is incarcerated.

Against this it might be claimed that J.B. has only been denied a life at liberty temporarily, that his punishment assumes his eventual release, and, thus, that provisions must be made to maintain his existence until that time. Yet this does not address the goals of retribution, deterrence, and reform.

Arguably, imprisonment for third degree murder requires the state to take only technologically and economically *ordinary* measures to assure the criminal a life at liberty after he serves his term. One of the rights the third degree murderer surrenders by his crime is that of access to extraordinary care for disease that, untreated, would be fatal.

This argument for retribution is further supported by one that appeals to the deterrence value of denying such criminals access to extraordinary life-saving treatment. If prospective murderers know that, should they contract a potentially fatal disease during their prison terms, they may die because they may be denied extraordinary treatment, some murders may be prevented. Moreover, those who contract such illnesses during their terms but survive their sentences to seek treatment when released may learn something from such a harrowing experience. Denying extraordinary care might, that is, also reform such criminals.

Clearly a punishment that includes both a temporary denial of liberty and access to technologically or economically extraordinary lifesaving measures precludes a criminal's entitlement to a publicly funded transplant of the kind contemplated in this case. Having partially surrendered his rights, the criminal may justifiably be denied access to public funds for treatment. If the goals of deterrence and reform are also served, this increases the moral desirability of denying access.

Thus J.B. should not be granted an early release on the grounds of his medical condition, nor should the prison system pay for his care. The severity of his crime militates against either, and should preclude his eligibility for any publicly funded treatment.

HEALTH CARE POLICY

56

Drinking on the Job

Boyd Anderson was a company man. He started working at Tone Master Radio in 1945, just as it was beginning to expand. Over the next twenty-five years the company became a huge conglomerate. Anderson worked his way to the top, becoming vice-president of the western division in 1970.

Shortly thereafter the company brought in an aggressive young president to revive lagging sales. He lasted only a year, but in that time he replaced Anderson and transferred him back to the company's main office, where he was given only limited responsibilities, a small office, and a part-time secretary.

Anderson had become accustomed to meeting clients at lunch and having a few drinks. When he had to face the humiliation of being useless to the company, he began to drink more heavily. He lobbied for new positions within the company but failed. Month after month the mail brought only rejection letters from other firms. His drinking became more and more uncontrollable.

Offered a minor overseas post with the firm, he refused it, in part because his family was not able to go with him, but largely because he was afraid his drinking would become known. By this time his self-confidence was gone. The company had been his life, and it was clear that his career was over.

In 1973 at the age of fifty-eight he was told to accept special early retirement. Within a month he was found in an alcoholic convulsive coma. He went through several episodes of drying out and drinking again. Nothing worked.

At this point he sued the company for $1.1 million for retroactive medical disability, claiming his job had made him an alcoholic. He claimed not only the disability pay, but payment of his medical and psychiatric expenses and back pay. He argued during a hearing, "My God, you give your life to the company, then you discover that they think you're washed up. The mental strain is just too much. Drinking was part of my business life. The company should bear the responsibility."

What kind of responsibility, if any, should the company bear for Anderson's drinking problem? If it is not found legally liable for his expense, does it still bear a moral responsibility?

COMMENTARY

Herbert Fingarette

Insofar as Anderson's problems were caused by his excessive drinking, he is morally responsible for them. He should also be legally liable for their costs unless he is specifically insured.

Until he was demoted, Anderson voluntarily accepted his company position, including (presumably without protest) the custom of luncheon drinks. Over a period of many years he drank at lunch without drinking to excess.

What changed things? The company president reassigned him to a less important position. Understandably, he was unhappy. He then began drinking excessively. Plainly, it was the demotion and resulting unhappiness that were decisive in triggering his excessive drinking, not the long-established custom of drinking at lunch.

Can Anderson reasonably justify his claims against the company? He can claim that his alcohol abuse was job-related. But the risks and damages at issue here are not specific to a particular job. They are risks associated with working for hire generally—one risks being demoted or fired, either of which is likely to make one unhappy. So Anderson's drinking is not "job-related" in any specific way that would entail company responsibility or financial liability. After all, an employer cannot be held responsible for keeping an employee happy or for the untoward consequences of the imprudent actions of an unhappy employee.

Anderson could try to base his claim on the fact that he is an "alcoholic," that "alcoholism" is a "disease" that he acquired while on the job, that his self-damaging behavior is a "symptom," and that therefore he is not responsible for his behavior or its consequences.

But even if Anderson has a "disease" and so is not responsible, meaning in this context "at fault," this does not imply that the *company* should be held responsible or liable. Anderson's vulnerability to disappointment and the resulting "disease" are his bad luck, if they are not his fault. Why should the company automatically have to pay?

Moreover, the assumption that Anderson is not responsible, because diseased, is unsound. We often hold a person responsible for imprudent conduct that brings about a disease; additionally, we may hold a person responsible for failing to take steps to prevent the disease from doing damage to oneself or others, or for taking steps to limit or cure the disease. The word "disease" is not an incantation that gives blanket relief from all responsibility for the damages it does.

However, one might assume that "alcoholism" is a very special disease in that it destroys one's "will power" and renders one incapable of acting responsibly. But this is contrary to the assumption shared by medically oriented treatment programs, as well as by such major alcohol-abuse programs as AA. Such programs rely on the alcoholic's initiative in seeking and entering treatment, or they use inducements to elicit voluntary entrance and then rely on the alcoholic's self-discipline which requires a large amount of "will power."

Finally, is it true that "alcoholism" is a "disease"? Consider the following facts: there is no scientifically accepted basic understanding of the origins, causes, or nature of "alcoholism"; nor is there a scientifically demonstrated method of "cure"; nor is there even any generally satisfactory analysis of what is meant by "alcoholism." The slogan "alcoholism is a disease" represents not a scientific discovery or a generally accepted scientific hypothesis; it represents the *faith* of many health professionals that a "solution" to the problems of alcohol abuse will someday be found by medical science.

But not every social problem is rooted in physical disease. At present, the evidence to be found in the enormous literature on alcohol and drug abuse reasonably allows one to suppose that there is not a single causal process, but a complex set of problems having biological, psychological, social, and cultural dimensions.

More to the present point, no one can satisfactorily explain in specific and scientific terms why Anderson started to drink excessively, why he kept it up, or what would get him to stop. He is to be pitied. It is a misguided pity, however, that assures him that he is a helpless victim, with no responsibility for his drinking problems. It is morally corrupting, and legally unsound, to assure him that it is the company's fault. It is simple deception to give him to understand that these assurances are grounded in a modern scientific understanding of alcohol abuse.

COMMENTARY
Luther A. Cloud

Alcoholism is a disease, and has been accepted as such by the American Medical Association and by virtually every major medical and scientific body in the world. Criteria for the diagnosis of the disease of alcoholism were published in 1972 by the National Council on Alcoholism and are in use by the medical profession.

Boyd Anderson's claim, however, is being made on a faulty premise. Since alcoholism is a physiological disease entity, it would be manifestly impossible for the company to have "given" Anderson that disease, just as it would have been impossible for them to have given him a cancer or have caused him to have a weak heart.

Anderson's job *did not require* him to drink. He was required to take out clients and entertain them. His drinking was a matter of his own choice. About one out of ten individuals who drink appears to have a biochemical or physiological "predisposition" to alcoholism. Obviously, Anderson was one of these individuals.

He contracted alcoholism, not as a result of his drinking per se, but because of a physiological difference which, coupled with his drinking, gave him the disease of alcoholism. The company can hardly be blamed for this situation.

Anderson might have had a valid claim if he had based it on the manner in which the company handled the situation that resulted from his alcoholism. Instead of telling him "to accept early retirement," the company would have been better advised to offer him a firm but fair choice between accepting treatment for his disease (alcoholism *is* treatable), or accepting the alternative early retirement.

Treatment for the disease of alcoholism should have been covered by the group health insurance policy just as it would cover treatment for any other disease.

Many firms have programs which offer alcoholic employees a choice of accepting the disciplinary consequences of the poor job performance caused by their alcoholism. These companies consistently report long-term, stable recovery rates from 70 percent to 85 percent and occasionally even higher. Any company that does not have such a program leaves itself open to suits like Anderson's, which can be extremely costly to the company, even if it wins in the end.

COMMENTARY
Sally Guttmacher

The issue of legal liabilities is the least interesting raised by this case. It seems unlikely that many courts would recognize Anderson's claim. Anderson, it can be argued, accepted the rules, and willingly took risks for the possibility of substantial rewards. Yet he claims that in the course of his work he became damaged by as well as dependent on the company. In effect, Anderson declares illegitimate the rules he had previously accepted and seeks compensation through the only means possible—the legal system.

His case is weak. Unlike occupational disease such as black lung where the line of causality is clear, self-destructive behavior (suicide, drug addiction, chronic excessive eating, drinking, or smoking) is generated by a combination of factors—some work-related and some not. In addition, most would argue that chronic excessive drinking is to some extent voluntary. Perceiving the alcoholic simply as a victim of his "disease" denies the notion of his autonomy, an approach that may actually impede rehabilitation.

The more subtle and engaging questions emerge from viewing self-destructive behavior as a response to, or even sometimes a rebellion against, the inhumane and pathological conditions of our lives. How does self-destructive behavior become a commonly selected option for dealing with stress or failure? And who bears the moral responsibility for this situation? How are such disorders related to work in our society, and how might work be restructured to decrease the risk of such outcomes? Finally, why are there so few real options outside the work situation through which an individual can develop self-esteem and taste success?

Even though it may be difficult to argue that an individual corporation should be held *legally* responsible for a pattern of behavioral response that is clearly a product of broadly based social habits, these habits are not mere accidents. They are covertly encouraged, for example, by being presented as a legitimate way for adults to deal with stress. (One needs merely to note in one evening of commercial television viewing the proportion of scenes involving social interaction in which alcohol and cigarettes are common props.) Through a myriad of such linkages—each perhaps weak in itself, but powerful in the aggregate—the corporation acquires responsibility in its broader role as part of the ruling segment of the society that establishes "the rules of the game" and even creates and encourages life styles for its own benefit.

Therefore, a given corporation cannot be permitted to retreat conveniently behind the claim that it, too, is the victim of the iron laws of the market. This may be a legal defense, since laws are codifications of the rules of the game, but it fails as a moral defense given the rudimentary facts that modern corporations exist chiefly to make profits. To the extent that these profits are at the expense of the well-being of workers or of consumers, corporations can be charged with behaving immorally.

Certainly, within the current rules many will argue that the corporation acted fairly, even humanely, in its dealings with Anderson. While there is some merit in this view, the motivation behind the corporation's action is another question. With relatively high levels of unemployment many workers carry the status of expendable, easily replaceable commodities. That Anderson was offered other options by the company is not simply testament to corporate compassion, but rather an indication that he belongs to a special class of workers who, because a substantial investment goes into their training, are perceived as (human) capital. Thus, as with fine-tooled machinery, some trouble is taken to see that they continue to function in some productive capacity. At the very least, the company will make an effort to see that those with problems, such as Anderson, are handled in ways that do not demoralize the others.

Because Anderson must bring the case to court and bear the burden of proof, the issue becomes depoliticized. Accepting this way of proceeding, moreover, ratifies the view that problems such as alcoholism simply represent the unintended, unforeseen, and unwanted consequences of an essentially well-functioning system. This is a curious response to a problem that now affects 10 percent of our work force, a statistic that may be interpreted as an indicator of a serious malfunction in our way of life.

With these rates in mind, we must ask who bears the risks in our society, and, if these risks are too great, who has the power to restructure the system and decrease the risk? By presenting the problem as a question of individual corporate responsibility, we lose sight of its broader implications. And by permitting corporations in general to shift the price and responsibility for the human wastage that is a by-product of our whole economic system onto public institutions, we ignore the need for a basic reorganization in the structure of work.

57

Health Risks and Equal Opportunity

Robert E. Stevenson

Mark Dalton, a thirty-two-year-old technician, was hired six months ago by a large chemical company. He has proven to be highly skilled and works at a rate exceeding his co-workers. Recently, after he took a sick leave, the employee health department nurse was surprised to learn that he is suffering from chronic renal disease. His entrance medical questionnaire did not mention any problem.

Since his job requires exposure to chemical solvent vapors at levels permissible by OSHA regulations, the company physician counseled him that continuing exposure to the vapors could exacerbate the disease.

Company management found a job for which he would qualify at the same rate of pay; but two current employees, one of whom is female, who are eligible for promotion are interested in the job. Both have better training and longer service with the company than Dalton.

Management has grounds for dismissing Dalton on the basis of false representations about his health. If he is given the available job to protect his health, it is likely that the woman employee who is better qualified will file a complaint charging discrimination with the Equal Employment Opportunity Commission.

Should Dalton be fired? Given the safer job? When three workers have a valid claim to a job, one based on health, one on seniority, and the third on equal opportunity, which should prevail?

COMMENTARY
Deborah G. Johnson

This case raises a set of questions about the relationship between employers and employees. Just what rights and obligations each party has with respect to the other is a matter that is only vaguely understood and only partially defined by law. Nevertheless, assumptions proliferate on both sides. Employers assume, for example, that employees should have a certain amount of loyalty to their employers; and employees assume that they should have the right to an appeal if they are treated unfairly in evaluation and promotion.

In this case, if Dalton knew of his condition and failed to report it on his application form, then he falsely represented himself and the company's commitment to him is voided. In a sense, the application form becomes part of the tacit contract between employer and employee. The company agrees to employ the individual, to provide certain benefits in exchange for work of a certain type and quality, but the employer agrees to do this on the assumption that information given by the applicant is true. The company would not have hired Dalton if they had known of his condition; thus, it does not have a duty to continue to employ him. But, this does not mean that they must or should fire him. Since he misrepresented himself, it is morally permissible to fire him, but continuing to employ him does not violate a moral norm.

Companies that hire individuals to work in environments that are unsafe or pose a threat to health have a duty to inform those workers of the risks involved. Failure to inform workers whose health is at risk or will be at risk is a violation of employees' bodily integrity. Violating employees' rights to control what is done to their bodies is roughly the same as placing people at risk in an experiment without their consent. However, companies should not make decisions for their workers. To do this would be to deny the autonomy of individual workers and to disregard their ability to judge what is in their best interests. Each worker should decide for himself or herself whether or not to take the risks involved. Workers can do this only if they are given information about the risks, and therefore companies have an obligation to so inform workers.

In this case, since levels conform to OSHA standards, the company has fulfilled its obligation by counseling Dalton that continuous exposure to the vapors would be dangerous to his health. If Dalton is a mature, sane individual and wants to continue working, the company may continue to employ him. Of course, if Dalton chooses to take the risks and his condition worsens . subsequently, the company should not be considered liable for compensation. Dalton would have accepted the responsibility for his condition by accepting the job knowing the risks.

If Dalton prefers another job in the organization, the company may provide such a job but, as already indicated, they are not obligated to do so. It might be good for Dalton and might be good for the company but morality does not demand that these goods be brought about. The company would have an obligation to find an alternative position for someone who developed a renal problem while working for the company, and this obligation would be even stronger if the condition was caused by the work environment, but this is not the case with Dalton. In this instance, if people already employed by the company are qualified for an available job, then the company has a stronger obligation to promote these employees according to rules that are operative in the company.

This analysis suggests that companies have obligations to their employees but that these obligations are voided if workers misrepresent themselves. It suggests that the company has no obligation to act paternalistically, that is, to protect employees from themselves (which is what the company would be doing if it refused to let Dalton work at a job of his choice, even when he knew the risks involved). Rather, the obligation is to provide information to employees so that they can make autonomous decisions. But circumstances might arise when the claims of individual employees would compete.

While Dalton's claim to the job does not compete with the claims of the other workers, the rights of a worker with seniority may well conflict with those of a woman. I do not think we can decide in advance how companies should resolve all such cases. The merits of each claim must be weighed in the light of given circumstances. Who has the stronger claim will depend on such matters as the type of job available, the merit of the employees, the company's past record on discrimination, and the firm's stated policy on seniority. This does not mean that companies should disregard a claim to equal opportunity. On the contrary, a commitment to equal opportunity means an obligation to consider the strength of an applicant's claim on the basis of relevant criteria.

COMMENTARY
Knut Ringen

English and American common law traditionally have held that the employer is responsible for the conduct of work, including the provision of a safe and healthy workplace. This common law principle underlies the Occupational Safety and Health Act of 1970.

However, absolutely safe and healthy workplaces do not exist today, and they will not exist in the future. Given the reality of residual risks, particularly associated with chronic diseases, safety and health in the workplace must be a responsibility shared by employer and worker.

How can this responsibility be shared fairly? Employers through their associations continue to insist that they should have absolute control of the workplace, including the right to restrict information about hazardous substances. For this reason, many workers, who are forced to be responsible to some extent for their own health, are not informed about the hazards that they are exposed to in the workplace.

However, we can assume that Dalton was knowledgeable about the risks. This case therefore raises the following issues of responsibility:

- Did the worker act irresponsibly in not revealing the chronic renal condition at the time of employment, and should he therefore be fired?
- Should the worker be moved to another job for health reasons?
- If moved, should he be given precedence over other candidates for the available alternative job?

Legally, a worker is required to give truthful answers to preemployment medical questions. In reality, however, the worker should be allowed some leeway, just as the employer is given leeway in providing a safe and healthy workplace. Most workers know that they will not be employed if they provide information about having a chronic disease, because the employer does not want to risk being held liable if the worker gets sick. Thus, even where there is no association between type of work and the worker's chronic disease, the mere presence of the disease (or even a personal disease risk factor) may preclude employment. We must expect that some workers who understand this situation will not be totally candid in answering their preemployment medical questionnaire. However, we would expect the technician to be more responsible for assessing the risk and potential hazard than a less informed worker.

Justification for firing the technician on these grounds thus may or may not exist. We cannot know for sure if the worker knew of his renal condition at the time of employment. We also cannot be sure that he knew the condition could be exacerbated because of his work. The company physician seems to acknowledge that the contribution of workplace exposure to the disease progression is potential, but not certain. Given this caveat, justification could exist for the worker not to admit his chronic disease. It would be unreasonable to expect him to jeopardize a specialized career by revealing medical conditions that he might judge unrelated to his work.

Medical removal protection is central to the current debate on occupational health regulations. This principle was legally promulgated for the first time in OSHA's initial occupational safety and health standard for asbestos exposure and it is an essential element of the recent standard to protect workers from exposure to lead (43 *Federal Register* 52952, 1978). Under the lead standard, a worker may be removed from his or her regular employment on the basis of an examining physician's medical opinion or when the measured level of lead in the worker's blood is high enough to indicate a "material impairment to health or functional capacity." When removed under this provision, the worker will receive compensation in the form of maintained earnings, seniority, and other benefits.

Although the lead standard requires only temporary removal of the workers and may not necessarily apply to permanent displacement, it clearly signals a new direction for the protection of worker rights. It represents a means of last resort to protect individual workers where the established permitted level of exposure to risks is inadequate. OSHA standards, including the lead standard, allow some exposure because it is not feasible to achieve a zero level and they may be fairly adequate for most workers. However, individuals who are especially susceptible to a given toxic effect will suffer disease even when exposure falls within accepted limits. It is these individuals that the medical removal provision will protect.

A few employers voluntarily offer job security and medical removal. In a few union contracts (notably the Steelworkers) medical removal is part of the benefit program. However, most workers know that they will lose their jobs and suffer other adverse employment effects because of an abnormal medical finding. The workers realize that once fired for medical reasons they will have a very hard time obtaining similar types of work and may even be investigated by companies that monitor workers' compensation claim files (see *Business Insurance*, June 9, 1980, p. 27). And workers have long known intuitively what was documented recently by the Department of Labor Interim Report to Congress on Occupational Diseases. According to that report, only 1 to 5 percent of job-related diseases are covered under current workers' compensation programs.

The ethical employer should also recognize the limitations of existing OSHA standards and the inequity of firing for medical reasons the worker who is denied general health protection under existing standards because of unique susceptibility. In other words, the same latitude that is allowed the firm in operating at levels of exposure that will fail to protect everyone should apply to the workers who cannot tolerate those exposures. In this case, the employer acted correctly in voluntarily providing medical removal protection.

Finally, the case raises the issue of preferential treatment. If the lead standard is cited as the precedent, preferential treatment would probably favor the worker with the medical condition. The worker is not at fault for the medical condition, and to deny alternative employment would be to place the burden on him. Also, various medical problems today qualify for affirmative action under federal law, and medical removal could fall into this category.

58

Who Pays for AZT?

In October 1987 the U.S. Congress appropriated $30 million to subsidize the purchases of AZT by individuals who do not have insurance coverage for the drug or who are not eligible for Medicaid. Congress provided the funding on an emergency basis for one year only, with the expectation that the states would act to continue the subsidization program under local auspices. Congress has since extended the federal program twice (with an additional $20 million appropriation), to give the states additional time to devise programs of their own. State legislatures are beginning to consider local funding of such programs.

Congress approved the AZT subsidy program because of the efficacy of the drug and its prohibitive cost. AZT is the only drug approved for use in the United States that has been shown to be effective in ameliorating the effects of AIDS. Although there are no complete studies on the effects of AZT, interim improvements in the health of many patients with symptomatic HIV infection have been significant. AZT both prolongs and improves the quality of the lives of persons with AIDS. AZT reduces the number of opportunistic infections and the rate of relication of the HIV virus in the patient's system. It also increases the number of healthy helper cells. As a result of taking AZT, some patients either remain healthy enough to contine to work or regain their health sufficiently enough to return to work.

Despite its helpful properties, AZT is highly toxic. Some patients cannot tolerate the drug at all; others can tolerate it only for a short while (less than one year). In addition, if taken off the drug, patients who had been helped by AZT experience a rapid decline in their health.

Moreover, AZT is not curative. Thus, despite AZT's availability, AIDS remains a fatal disease.

Although it is the only AIDS drug approved for use, AZT is prohibitively expensive. The purchase price of AZT is approximately $650 per month, or $7,900 per year at full dosage. Although Medicaid eligibility standards differ from state to state, each has categorical (e.g., blind, aged, permanently and totally disabled) and financial (i.e., income and assets) tests that applicants must meet. The federal AZT program has no categorical requirements, and it leaves financial standards up to each individual state. In each state, it is easier to qualify for the AZT program than it is to qualify for Medicaid.

Many persons with AIDS work in service industries where their income keeps them at or just above poverty level. But many patients taking AZT are not eligible for Medicaid: even if they meet Medicaid's financial status requirements (even one month's bill for AZT can devastate a patient's resources), AZT keeps them healthy enough not to be "permanently and totally disabled," and they generally do not meet other Medicaid categories (blind, aged, AFDC recipient).

A proposal to fund the subsidization of AZT purchase is now up for debate before one state legislature. How should it decide?

COMMENTARY
Robin Levin Penslar

The prohibitive cost of AZT clearly calls for some kind of government assistance. Arguments in support of state aid can be based on four principles: equitability, humanitarianism, financial savings, and precedent.

The principle of equity unquestionably demands a government-supported AZT purchase program. AZT is an FDA-approved drug that is available to persons with the financial means to purchase it, with medical insurance or who are on Medicaid; it is also the only FDA-approved drug currently available to help persons with AIDS. The only legal therapy for AIDS is therefore available to the wealthy and the disabled, but not to persons in financial need. In fact, the purchase of AZT may be what makes the program's participants financially needy. It would be fundamentally unjust to deny access to AZT to persons who cannot afford to purchase the drug, but do not qualify for Medicaid.

An argument based on humanitarian principles is equally compelling. One immediate justification for continuing the AZT program is a moral imperative to help sufferers of this devastating disease in all ways possible. To respond that AZT does not cure but merely prolongs life or alleviates suffering, and that we should therefore not interfere with the inevitable, would be callous and unbefitting civilized society.

Second, all persons deserve to live in dignity, one element of which is the opportunity to continue to carry our a productive life for as long as possible. Quite apart from any cost savings realized by keeping persons out of the welfare system, humanitarian considerations weigh heavily in favor of doing what we can to allow everyone to participate as fully as possible in society. For many AIDS patients, AZT presents the only means that enables them to participate in society.

Fiscal considerations on two levels support government assistance for persons who are medically and financially needy, but do not qualify for Medicaid. On the first level, use of AZT prolongs patients ability to continue work and thus reduces their need for reliance on Medicaid and other government programs such as food stamps, diability, AFDC, and subsidized housing. Such persons remain productive members of the economy and society in general, producing goods and services and paying taxes.

On the second level, the use of AZT may reduce the cost of delivering care to the AIDS patients because they appear to suffer fewer opportunistic infections and thus require less hospital care. It has been estimated that the use of AZT reduces the direct costs of treating AIDS by $11,000 per patient year, and reduces the costs of treating AIDS-related Complex by $25,000 per patient year.* The combined savings amounts to $386 million on the national level for the first year's use of AZT. Thus, once patients who have been taking AZT do become eligible for Medicaid, it may well be that Medicaid will pay out even less claims. Even for those patients who do not go on Medicaid, fewer medical resources are directed toward the care of AIDS sufferers and can be used for other needs, at least in the short run. Thus, the direct outlay of funds for the AZT program may well be offset by cost savings in other state- and federally funded programs. The uncertainties of the financial implications of a state-level AZT program are not so great as to justify a refusal to continue assisting those in need.

Finally, the role of precedent in devising new medical programs is worth noting. By providing emergency funding, the federal government made clear that an important element of fighting AIDS is assisting persons in purchasing AZT. Furthermore, programs already exist in many states to help patients with such diseases as hemophilia, sickle cell anemia, and renal disease who are in need but are not eligible for Medicaid. Some states have also provided special assistance for the purchase of extraordinary expensive prescription drugs in at least one other setting: organ transplants. Medicaid in those states will pay for the costs associated with a transplant including the continued purchase of immunosuppressive drug therapy. It is unquestionably an appropriate response, well within the scheme of government medical assistance programs,

---

*Source: Paul A. Snyder, Burroughs Wellcome Co. Attachments to letter dated October 21, 1988.

to make AZT available to persons who are medically needy but do not qualify for Medicaid.

A nagging background question remains: With most other illnesses, patients must use up their own financial resources and be permanently disabled before they can obtain government assistance; why should AIDS be any different? It is possible, however, to distinguish AIDS from other diseases. First of all, AIDS is an illness unlike any other illness: At present no other communicable diseases hold such a destructive potential for our entire populace. It is true that AZT does not cure AIDS, but the longer patients survive, the greater the possiblity that other, curative, drugs or treatments will be developed.

Another criticism of giving AZT programs priority is that in many states a whole array of health care programs is also in desperate need of support. Nonetheless, the severe and devastating nature of AIDS, together with the relatively low cost of and potential savings generated by the program should give AZT funding the highest priority in state public health expenditures.

A related issue is whether, within the framework of caring for persons with AIDS, an AZT program is the best way to spend scarce health care funds. Are there other programs on which funds would be better spent, such as making twenty-four-hour home nursing care or hospice facilities available? States are attempting to develop comprehensive schemes to ensure adequate delivery of care to persons with AIDS; the resources they have to work with are not unlimited. Until policy makers can see where the AZT program fits in a comprehensive plan, funding should continue.

COMMENTARY
Richard D. Lamm

We are rapidly sailing into a new and morally painful world of American medicine. The central characteristics of this new world is that we have invented more medicine than we can afford to pay for. Even if we could successfully remove all the inefficiencies from American medical system, we are still confronted by a new painful reality: Infinite medical needs have run into finite resources.

This should not really suprise us. One of the universal historical truths is that resources are limited relative to wants. But it still comes as a painful realization. Americans are really good at avoiding reality. We pretend that we don't ration medicine, yet thirty-seven million Americans are not covered by health insurance and the Robert Wood Johnson Foundation has found in a recent year that a million American families had one or more members who were denied access to health care.

It is said that "maturity is a recognition of one's limitations." I suggest that maturity in American society involves recognizing our limitations and moving realistically to set priorities in all aspects of American life, particularly health care.

What yardsticks should we use when we prioritize medicine? Thoughtful people who have wrestled with this question suggest there are generally two standards: (1) improving the length of people's lives, and (2) improving the qualtity of people's lives. Setting medical priorities is a multilateral equation. These decisions will not only be morally painful, but immensely difficult as we compare one beneficial procedure with another beneficial procedure. The agony of choice can be seen in the recent decisions by Oregon and Virginia not to pay for soft tissue transplants but, instead, to spend the money on prenatal care and basic health care for the medically indigent. While politically thoughtful people recognize that it is better to cover basic health care for the many rather than high technology medicine for the few. As George Annas has warned us, "we have been doing more and more to fewer and fewer people at higher and higher costs for less and less benefit." Yet as difficult as the transplant/basic health care tradeoff is, it is easier than most that lie in our future.

To prioritize American health care spending we have to ask basic questions: "How do we buy the *most* health care for the *most* people?" "In a world of limited resorces, what procedures are the most cost effective?"

Providing AZT to AIDS sufferers is very unlikely to meet these tests. In a nation that doesn't cover the basic health care for all its citizens, doesn't vaccinate all of its children, doesn't provide prenatal care to all of its women, it is very unlikely that public policy can justify paying approximately $8,000 a year a person for a drug that does not cure but only alleviates symptoms. This is not a moral judgment, but instead a judgement of health policy. We wish abstractly that we could do everything for everybody, but if we can't and if we must set priorities, there are many, many medical procedures that we now deny people that will have a higher priority than AZT. AZT does improve the quality of people's lives but the disease is terminal. Until we cover basic health care for pregnant women and indigent children, it is unlikely to make many people's priority list.

As in most states there is a strong movement in Colorado to get state government to pay for AZT. Much of the political discourse is out of the 1960s, as those who object to AZT as a medical priority are painted as "uncaring" or "conservative." So many of our memories and political institutions were built in the 1960s when America doubled its wealth every thirty years and we thought we could do everything. The reality of the times in which we live is that we can't do everything. Being in government today is like sleeping with a blanket that is too short. We simply cannot cover everything. We must make choices, however painful.

Excluding AZT from a list of priorities is not a matter of not caring, but of understanding that the "opportunity costs" of those dollars are much higher elsewhere in the system. When we let go of the illusion that we can pay for everything and start to set priorities, too many other health procedures will have higher claims on our limited dollars. The debate over AZT thus becomes a harbinger of many similar decisions that we are going to have to make in the future. Those people who argue that limited dollars can be put to a higher use than AZT should not yield one inch of moral ground. We care just as much as the advocates of AZT; we are just demanding that limited dollars be expended in a way that will bring the highest amount of well-being to the maximum number of our citizens.

59

When Is Home Care Medically Necessary?

E.N., a seventy-five-year-old retired widow and member of the Optima HMO, lives alone in a subsidized apartment complex for the elderly. For the past six years she has had mild congestive heart failure and atrial fibrillation, well controlled by medication and a salt-restricted diet. However, for approximately three years she has shown a gradually progressive loss of short-term memory and orientation that has impaired her ability to understand and carry out the treatment program.

In April and May 1990, a home care nurse made four visits to Ms. N. to assess her capacities. Ms. N. categorically rejected the idea of nursing home placement. The nurse set up a system to help Ms. N. take her medications on schedule and arranged for a neighbor to shop for her and visit each day. On this regimen Ms. N. seemed to be doing well.

No nursing visits occurred in June or July. On 1 August, Ms. N.'s neighbor reported that Ms. N. was having difficulty breathing and was complaining of pain. Ms. N. was admitted to the hospital for three days for treatment of congestive heart failure. While it appeared that she had been taking her medication, the doctors believed that she may have been taking it irregularly and that she had apparently gone off the salt-restricted diet. The episode of hospitalization might have been prevented if the home visits had been continued.

After Ms. N.'s discharge on 3 August, the nurse made weekly home visits to check on her status and to review whether the regimen was being followed. By 6 September she seemed stable and well, so she was not seen again until 25 September, when her physician found her in congestive failure again with shortness of breath and edema. Once again he instituted a series of home visits. With slight adjustment of the medications and five home visits to ensure cooperation with the regimen the congestive heart failure cleared. By mid-October, Ms. N. was again relatively well.

Like many insurers, Optima covers "medically necessary" services. Specifically, home care services are covered if they meet the following criteria:

- the service is an essential part of active treatment;
- there is a defined medical goal that the Member is expected to gain;
- the Member is homebound for medical reasons;
- the service is not "for custodial care."

Now that Ms. N. was stable again, the nurse and doctor wondered if continued services would be authorized. Checking on whether the regimen was being followed appeared to be very useful for Ms. N.'s well-being, but would Optima judge the home care to be medically necessary under the terms of the insurance?

COMMENTARY
Lachlan Forrow

Should Ms. N. receive ongoing visits from a home health care nurse? Unquestionably.

These home care visits are undeniably "medically necessary." Ms. N. has a serious, potentially life-threatening *medical* condition. In effect, Optima has set up and conducted a "natural experiment": in less than six months, a single, specific change in her clinical regimen (the discontinuation of home care visits) has *twice* been followed by a serious worsening of Ms. N.'s medical condition, once requiring hospitalization. Optima has thus proven the medical necessity of home care and should have no doubts about its continuation. The only thing to be learned from another cycle of discontinued home care is the *extent* of harm—perhaps mortal—that will ensue.

The evidence that this specific aspect of her care is *medically necessary*, i.e., that it is part of a direct causal chain that ensures her medical well-being, is thus considerably stronger than the evidence for the vast majority of the services (ranging from routine examinations for the common cold through ultrasound examinations during pregnancy and bypass surgery for coronary disease) that Optima (or any other insurer) provides to any of its members. In the language of Optima's subscriber agreement, ongoing home care is clearly "an essential part of active treatment" aimed at "a defined medical goal" (avoidance of life-threatening congestive heart failure) for an Optima member who "is homebound for medical reasons."

Optima may claim that home care, though *necessary* to Ms. N.'s survival, is not *medically* necessary because the personnel needed to provide most of that care (checking on compliance, etc.) need not have special *medical* background or expertise: a neighbor could do as well. In fact, however, in other institutional contexts, insurers do not place decisive weight on this distinction between "medical" and "nonmedical" personnel. For example, insurers routinely cover the costs of nonmedical hospital personnel who transport patients, bathe them, or prepare and deliver their meals. When tasks are clearly essential to the effective functioning of a health care institution, they are naturally viewed in that context as part of the "medically necessary" services that comprise a patient's care.

What is "medically necessary" is context-dependent in yet another way. Optima may insist that society is committed to providing the services Ms. N. needs through agencies other than those that provide health care. In fact those services are not available in Ms. N.'s case. Insurers committed to providing "medically necessary" services must be responsible for delivering them in the real world facing Ms. N., not in the some hypothetical arrangement in which different agencies fulfill their commitments to do what's necessary. When Optima knows that such cooperation is not forthcoming, it cannot leave medically necessary services unprovided.

It is true that Optima was forthright about its view of the social division of responsibility when it explicitly excluded custodial care from its benefits package. Nevertheless, in Ms. N.'s case, where there are no other custodians and the home care is clearly medically necessary, Optima, like any insurer promising medically necessary care, cannot hide behind narrowly construed contract language. Doing so puts clinicians in an impossible situation.

Clinicians, whether they work for HMOs like Optima or on a fee-for-service basis for indemnity insurers, cannot allow the insurers to evade the obligation to provide medically necessary services. They must resist policies that violate the fundamental norms of the provider-patient relationship. At least on this point, Hippocrates had it right: "Into whatever houses I may enter, I will come for the benefit of the sick, remaining clear of all voluntary injustice..." The objection here is not specific to managed care in an HMO. Any insurer who covers "medically necessary" services must provide the home care on which Ms. N.'s survival may depend.

COMMENTARY
Norman Daniels and James E. Sabin

The home care is not only beneficial to Ms. N., but providing it may reduce overall costs to Optima as well as support clinicians' morale. Nevertheless, the care does not come under the benefits promised in the Optima HMO contract, which explicitly preclude "custodial care." A concerned family member or neighbor would be able to check on Ms. N. to make sure she fills the prescriptions and takes the medications. Within the terms of the insurance the home care cannot be described as "medically necessary."

The caretakers' wish to provide the home care is praiseworthy, but it would be wrong for them to obtain the care by gaming the system and quite unwise for Optima to make an exception to the benefit contract to provide the noncovered custodial care. Optima's decision regarding Ms. N. must be generalizable within the HMO and consistent with similar coverage decisions elsewhere in its program. Sticking by a reasonable, consistent policy is not merely bureaucratic contractualism but a prerequisite for treating all patients in the plan equitably, and a necessary bulwark against the corrosive deception and case-by-case gaming so pervasive in health care today. Optima—and wider society—should ask its clinicians to do the best possible for their patients within a reasonable and fair set of guidelines and coverage policies, not to engage in deception to bring about what they believe to be the right course of action in a particular case.

Despite its straightforward biotechnical appearance, the concept of "medical necessity" is packed with nonbiotechnical assumptions and implications that bear on Ms. N.'s case. Clinicians typically use "medical necessity" to convey that a proposed intervention provides a necessary link in a causal chain that will lead to the desired outcome. In this sense, penicillin is "medically necessary" for treating streptococcal pharyngitis and appendectomy for appendicitis, and by analogy, home care for Ms. N.

But as actually used in making insurance determinations, "medical necessity" also carries powerful, unstated assumptions about the proper division of labor in society. In the case of Ms. N. the key assumptions involve how responsibility is allocated among clinicians, patient, and family, on the one hand; and between the health care system and other institutions in society, on the other. Unfortunately, Ms. N. has no family. The best alternative would be a commitment by Ms. N.'s neighbors to look after her. Because this commitment is supererogatory, Optima can encourage it but cannot expect it. If neighborly supervision is not forthcoming, our individualistic social values require that Ms. N. must pay for the home care herself if she can.

When family, supererogatory neighborliness, and personal means are not present, responsibility for providing the custodial home care Ms. N. needs falls to the social sector—the state and local community. American society has established agencies to meet its obligation for provision of this kind of service. In the current climate of tax rollbacks and "read my lips" morality, however, these agencies are often poorly funded and hard-put to carry out their mandate. As a result, they may try to pass the buck of their responsibility elsewhere—e.g., to the health care sector.

Organizations like Optima should resist "medicalizing" the custodial services Ms. N. needs, just as they should not medicalize the provision of food and shelter. Because people think their entitlements to "medical" services are even stronger than their entitlements to social welfare services, providing medical coverage for "custodial" home care (or food or shelter) can unwittingly undermine the attitudes of mutual support among friends and family that form a necessary communal background to society. Overmedicalizing supportive services can be corrupting even for the recipient, whose independence would be weakened if she no longer saw it as necessary for her to try to elicit help from a neighbor or pay for the services if she could. Neither private insurance nor public programs could survive if "moral hazard" weakened individual, familial, and neighborly sources of support.

Just as overmedicalizing delivery of services can create "moral hazard" and undermine support at the level of individual, family, and neighborhood, it can do the same at the level of social organizations. If Optima picks up the slack created by underfunded social agencies, its members pay a hidden tax for services the state is committed to providing but is refusing to pay for. From the perspective of clinicians focusing only on Ms. N.'s cardiac well-being, beneficence is the applicable value and it may be seen as requiring the home care. But from a wider social perspective, failing to confront our collective refusal to meet our obligations to the Ms. N.s of society can be seen as moral cowardice. Putting a Band-Aid on a festering wound is not good medical or social care.

In view of this analysis, Ms. N.'s nurse and doctor should first seek the needed custodial home care from the appropriate social agency. If services are not forthcoming, Optima should undertake prompt advocacy via such means as high-level organizational contacts with state government, joining with other advocacy groups, and going to the media to expose the inadequate funding of community-based social services. If all else fails, it may seem that Optima is uniquely situated as a Good Samaritan to provide them. It may even seem to be abandonment if Optima refuses, although the actual abandonment flows from leadership in the political sector. But if Optima can be counted on to act like the Good Samaritan, we will find more and more cases of society refusing to meet its obligations to other Ms. N.s. Because "custodial care" is not "medically necessary" treatment covered by medical insurers in our current system, Optima's caretaking responsibility in this case is to advocate for social responsibility.

60

Palliation in the Age of Chronic Disease

Sixty-one-year-old A.T. has recently been confined to a wheelchair by progressive osteoarthritis in his right hip, which causes him considerabe pain. Formerly an active individual—an avid walker and weekend sailor—A.T. is equally distressed by his lack of mobility and loss of independence. A hip replacement, for which his insurance company would pay, would relieve his pain, increase his mobility, and significantly improve the quality of his life. He has thus decided to proceed with elective surgery.

A.T. considered himself in excellent health except for the degenerative joint disease, which has recently decreased his stamina. He was therefore surprised to learn that a preoperative blood count suggested that he had chronic lymphocytic leukemia (CLL) and associated moderate anemia. A thorough workup confirmed the diagnosis of State III CLL, which is associated with a life expencetancy of approximately twelve to fourty-two months. A.T.'s physicians can correct his anemia with periodic blood transfusions and believe that his CLL poses no significant acute contraindication to the proposed surgery.

Would hip replacement be considered inappropriate therapy for A.T.? What are the limits of palliation in the age of chronic disease?

COMMENTARY
Joseph J. Fins

At first glance this case is just a little too easy. Despite his shortened life expectancy, it's hard to imagine anyone would wilfully deprive A.T. of a hip replacement that would reduce his pain and improve the quality of his life.

But lurking just beneath the surface of this easy entitlement is a question about how far we should go in pursuit of palliation.

A seventeenth-century usage of *palliation* is "to cloak or disguise." Surgery does exactly that in A.T.'s case: hip replacement will allow this otherwise terminally ill patient a surgical veneer so that he may pursue his previous life for a short time. For a year or perhaps two he will again be independent and without chronic pain, yet chronic and progressive illness will inevitably bring death. In light of this, is surgery a deceptive cloak—or one that provides warmth and new life?

The traditional view, which made this case seem so simple, is that A.T.'s surgery is cut from cloth of the life-giving sort. As physicians we have always wanted to cheat death and turn back the clock one moment at a time. It would be counter to our historical nature to see A.T.'s surgery as anything but life-promoting. One can imagine a gleeful physician watch his rehabilitated patient walk without pain or hear once more of A.T.'s weekend sailing exploits.

At the heart of such a physician-patient celebration is the briefly suppressed knowledge that this is their *last* victory before the final battle with leukemia. Given the surgery's success, both can willingly suspend disbelief and momentarily embrace the idea of a "cure." This sort of deception can continue as long as A.T. remains relatively asymptomatic from his leukemia. It persists because both physician and patient have a stake in their final victory together.

Under the cloaks of such benevolent collusion a physician may fail to recognize that even technically successful surgery may not win the penultimate battle for a patient's life. If circumstances dictate that the pain relief and independence sought through surgery will be rapidly overtaken by a progressive leukemia, then despite its feasibility surgery might be injurious. The injury comes not from a failed hip replacement but rather from a failure to meet a patient's inflated preoperative expectations.

Confronted with the facts of this case it would be all too easy to see the surgery as therapeutic and fail to appreciate that it may ultimately be palliative in nature. When healing or making whole are even remotely or briefly within reach surgery seems appropriate. But when it is generously offered in the context of irremediable illness, the largess of the offer is misleading and evasive.

The distinction that should guide our understanding of A.T.'s case then is whether surgery can achieve therapeutic or palliative goals. Given a three-year life expectancy, the surgery is clearly therapeutic. At six months we are less sure. Because palliation is a kind of masquerade, it is inherently deceptive; we have trouble judging it.

Palliation was once synonymous with end-stage cancer care in which efforts were circumscribed and limited to morphine, radiation, or hospice care. Time frames were short and goals were limited. But in our age of chronic illness, therapies once reserved for "curative" treatments can now be used in the service of palliation. We must not mislable palliative services because they happen to employ advanced technology—an intervention should be defined as therapeutic or palliative based on the clinician's intent, not the sophistication of the technology employed.

Blurring the distinction between curing and caring raises important concerns in an era when palliation is no longer inexpensive and outcome instruments are perceived to be important. If a formerly "curative" therapy is used palliatively, outcome measures may categorize it as a failed therapy unless we recognize that it was never intended to cure. A cost-benefit analysis of A.T.'s successful hip replacement might find it exorbitantly expensive if he were to live for (only) a year. But, if the intent were recognized as being palliative, the surgery's success could be measured on more apropriate grounds that take into consideration the patient's independence and pain relief.

Proper palliative care serves the goals of medicine. At a time when we are ever more concerned with providing access to basic care to all, it is important that palliative measures receive their due. Moreover, patients whose chronic diseases are the product of tertiary care are entitled to palliative efforts that might temper their conditions. The same individuals who came to expect acute care from their physicians have every right to expect commensurate care for their resultant chronic conditions.

The possibilities for confusion about palliation are limitless unless physicians recognize that they will care for more patients like A.T. with technologies they once reserved for making people well. By clearly distinguishing therapy and palliation, we can ensure that patients receive the care they require, even when cure is no longer possible.

COMMENTARY
Daniel Callahan

There is something maddening about cases of this kind. Why do I say that? There is, in principle, no way of giving a sensible answer to the dilemma posed by A.T.'s case. It is not that we lack sufficient details about the clinical situation; they seem clear enough in this case. What we lack is any sense of economic context in which the case is set.

If A.T. is not given his hip replacement, what would the money saved be used for? Or put another way, if A.T. is given what he needs, what will be taken from the needs of someone else to pay for it? Or, as an economist might put it, what are the "opportunity costs" of spending money on Mr. A.T.'s hip replacement? Might we not spend it better on, say Mrs. A.T.'s need for reconstructive surgery after a masectomy for her breast cancer, or for their grandson L.T.'s need for a well-trained mathematics teacher in his third grade class?

Yet increasingly, in the name of cost containment and the effecent use of scarce resources, cases like this are being discussed. My instinct is to say we should refuse to discuss them altogether, or even to take them seriously, unless that can be done within a meaningful economic context and rational health care system. As the case is given us—knowing nothing about the context—the argument could reasonably go many ways. What are the standards of comparison to be?

I could argue, for instance, that A.T. should be denied the hip replacement because that money could surely be spent on someone even more in need of relief from pain and suffering than he is. Or I could argue, as the British seem to do, that even if high-technology medicine should in general be restricted to nonelderly patients, hip replacement displays a good cost-benefit ratio simply because the costs of caring for a bedridden or otherwise immobile patient will likely be even higher. Still again, I could argue (consistent with my general views) that caring and palliation should always have the highest priority and that, on those grounds alone, the hip replacement is justifiable (while an expensive experimental treatment to save his life from the leukemia would be less so).

Yet I believe each of those arguments becomes meaningless without understanding the economic context in which the problem arises. I assume that this patient is an American. If so, then as Norman Daniels long ago enlightened us, there is no good reason for A.T. or his physician to give up any expensive treatment in our open-ended, crazy health care system. There is rarely any assurance the money saved will be put to better use.

In the end, just these kinds of cases show how necessary it is that we move to a closed universal health care plan, and that as part of it we put in place a priority system of the kind being advanced in Oregon. Unless we have come to some collective decisions on relative priorities in the health care system as a whole (or at least within coherent sub-parts), we will have no basis whatever for sensibly deciding cases like that of A.T. I think it would be perfectly appropriate to take age into account in a priority system—but utterly inappropriate to do so in an ad hoc way with economically contextless decisions.

Unless we know how the money might otherwise be spent, we know nothing of value about such cases. We should refuse to talk about them and just urge A.T.'s physician to get the hip replacment for his patient however he can, no holds barred. The present system in fact rewards those physicians and patients who act as if only the needs of this patient here and now count. Their behavior is rewarded both because our present system legitimates, in the name of health, the most unbridled self-interest, and also because, if self-interest is not pursued, any sacrifice made may result in no alternative good whatever. Of course that is about as silly and unfair a way to run a health care system as can be imagined. It just happens to be the way we do things in this country.

Selected Bibliography

Part Six: Allocation and Health Care Policy

Aaron, Henry J., and Schwartz, William B. *The Painful Prescription: Rationing Hospital Care.* Washington, DC: Brookings Institution, 1984.
Annas, George J. "Fetal Protection and Employment Discrimination—The *Johnson Controls* Case," *New England Journal of Medicine* 325 (5 September 1991): 740–43.
Bayer, Ronald, Caplan, Arthur L., and Daniels, Norman, eds. *In Search of Equity: Health Needs and the Health Care System.* New York: Plenum Press, 1983.

Callahan, Daniel. *Setting Limits: Medical Goals in an Aging Society.* New York: Simon and Schuster, 1987.

Callahan, Daniel. *What Kind of Life: The Limits of Medical Progress.* New York: Simon and Schuster, 1990.

Childress, James F. "Who Shall Live When Not All Can Live," *Soundings* 53 (Winter 1970): 339–55.

Churchill, Larry R. *Rationing Health Care in America: Perceptions and Principles of Justice.* South Bend, In.: University of Notre Dame Press, 1987.

Daniels, Norman. *Just Health Care.* New York: Cambridge University Press, 1985.

Draper, Elaine. *Risky Business: Genetic Testing and Exclusionary Practices in the Hazardous Workplace.* New York: Cambridge University Press, 1991.

Evans, Roger W. "Health Care Technology and the Inevitability of Resource Allocation and Rationing Decisions," *Journal of the American Medical Association* Pt. I 249 (15) (15 April 1983): 2047–53; Pt. II 249 (16) (22/29 April 1983): 2208–19.

Fried, Charles. "Equality and Rights in Medical Care," *Hastings Center Report* 6, no. 1 (1976): 29–34.

Fuchs, Victor R. *The Health Economy.* Cambridge: Harvard University Press, 1986.

Menzel, Paul T. *Strong Medicine: The Ethical Rationing of Health Care.* New York: Oxford University Press, 1990.

New York State Task Force on Life and the Law, *When Others Must Choose: Deciding for Patients without Capacity.* New York: NYS Task Force, 1992.

Outka, Gene. "Social Justice and Equal Access to Health Care," *Journal of Religious Ethics* (Spring 1974): 11–32.

President's Commission for the Study of Ethical Problems in Medicine and Biomedical and Behavioral Research. *Securing Access to Health Care,* vols. I-III. Washington, D.C.: U.S. Government Printing Office, 1983.

Task Force on Organ Transplantation. *Organ Transplantation: Issues and Recommendations.* Washington, D.C.: U.S. Department of Health and Human Services, Public Health Service, Health Resources and Services Administration, April, 1986.

Winslow, Gerald R. *Triage and Justice.* Berkeley: University of California Press, 1982.

Glossary

Advance Directive An advance directive is a declaration by a person that stipulates the forms of medical treatment to be provided by caregivers and/or designates someone to act as a proxy should the person at some future date lose decision-making capacity. In written form, an advance directive is often referred to as a "living will."

Autonomy Derived from Greek words meaning "self-rule." In bioethics, autonomy typically refers to the patient's right of self-determination concerning medical care. Autonomy may be used in various senses including freedom of action, effective deliberation, and authenticity. It supports such moral and legal principles as respect for persons and informed consent.

Beneficence The principle of beneficence involves duties to prevent harm, remove harm, and promote the good of another person. In bioethics, beneficence refers to the obligation of health care professionals to seek the well-being or benefit of the patient.

Best Interests A decision-making standard used in the absence of an advance directive or when a substituted judgment is not possible, best interests involves more objective, societally shared criteria about what reasonable persons would probably choose in a particular situation.

Casuistry Derived from *casus*, "case" or "occasion," casuistry is a method of analyzing ethical issues by comparing the particular case in hand with paradigm cases whose moral status is agreed upon. In focusing on individual dilemmas rather than global ethical theories or principles, the casuist seeks to interpret moral obligation in ways that take adequate account of the particular case's unique moral, social, political, and personal characteristics.

Competence Competence refers to a patient's capacity to make decisions about the provision of medical care for him or herself. It is an element of informed consent, and involves comprehending information, choosing in accordance with one's values, and communicating a decision. The decisions of competent patients are usually respected, while a determination of incompetence may warrant paternalistic and coercive measures, such as involuntary commitment.

Conscience Moral agents often appeal to conscience in making ethical judgements about particular cases. The content of conscience is informed by basic moral

293

values. In medical ethics, health care professionals may refuse to perform certain procedures, for example, abortions, sterilizations, or withdrawal of life-sustaining treatment, based on fidelity to conscience, a phenomenon known as "conscientious objection."

Deontology   Derived from the Greek *deon* or "duty," deontological moral theories (along with utilitarianism) form a philosophical basis for contemporary bioethics. A deontological position holds that the moral worth of an act is not limited to assessing the character of the agent of the consequences or the performance of the act, but that there are intrinsic features of acts that are at least as relevant and may even be decisive for moral deliberation. The principles of autonomy, respect for persons, and distributive justice are typically grounded in a deontological theory.

DNR Orders   Do-Not-Resuscitate orders are directions not to initiate cardiopulmonary resuscitation (CPR) in the event of cardiac or respiratory arrest. DNR orders raise ethical questions about when life-sustaining treatment should be withheld and who should make that decision.

Ethics   Ethics is systematic reflection on the norms, principles, or values that do or should guide human conduct or action, and as such can be distinguished from morality, which is the practice or conduct itself. Bioethics is a form of *applied normative* ethics that involves the application of general ethical principles and rules to specific moral problems that arise in medical practice, the provision of health care, and scientific research.

Euthanasia   Etymologically, euthanasia means easy or gentle death. Contemporary usage is often ambiguous, and modifiers are used to make the intended sense clearer. "Active" euthanasia refers to the direct killing of a patient, and is typically contrasted with "passive" euthanasia, which involves the withdrawal of medical technologies in order to allow the underlying disease process to take its natural course. "Voluntary" euthanasia (either active or passive) means that the action is undertaken at the behest of the patient, and should be distinguished from "nonvoluntary" euthanasia where the patient has not made or is not capable of making such a request, and "involuntary" euthanasia, where the action is performed against the patient's wishes.

Extraordinary/Ordinary Means of Treatment   Historically, extraordinary and ordinary means of treatment have been distinguished according to whether (a) a proposed medical intervention has a reasonable chance of succeeding, and (b) the benefits of the intervention outweigh the burdens. The distinction is based on a moral or professional obligation to provide ordinary treatments, but no obligation to provide extraordinary treatment. The extraordinary/ordinary distinction has been criticized recently for focusing attention on treatments for diseases rather than patient interests, leading to decisions about the provision of treatment based on what is routine or customary in medical practice. The terminology optional/obligatory has been proposed as a preferable, patient-centered, standard for such judgments.

Informed Consent   Except in emergency situations, physicians are morally and legally required to obtain the patient's informed consent to invasive medical procedures. The elements of informed consent include professional disclosure and patient comprehension of information, and patient voluntariness and competence to consent.

Justice   As a general moral concept, justice requires that persons be given what they are due. Theories of justice have specified different criteria upon which such a determination can be made, for example, societal benefits might be distributed to persons based on equality, need, effort, merit, or contribution to society. In bioethics, distributive justice is especially important in decisions about the fair allocation of health care resources.

Nonmaleficence   The principle of nonmaleficence prohibits the infliction of harm, injury, or death upon others, and supports more specific moral rules such as the prohibition of killing. Nonmaleficence is related to the maxim *primum non nocere* ("above all, or first, do no harm"), which is widely used to describe the duties of health care professionals. The duty not to harm others is typically considered more stringent than the duty to benefit others and it also imposes moral limits on autonomy.

Paternalism   Paternalism assumes a parent (father)-child relationship in which an authority figure acts to benefit the subordinate party even against his or her desires or choices. Medical paternalism normally involves the refusal of a health care professional to accept the wishes, judgments, or acts of a patient on the grounds that the health care professional knows best. Paternalism is widely viewed as morally suspect because of its assumptions of moral inequality in the professional-patient relationship and because it violates patient autonomy. However, paternalism is usually considered warranted if the patient's capacity for autonomous choice and competent decision making is restricted or impaired.

Personhood   Philosophers and theologians frequently propose criteria—for example, sentience, consciousness, or purposive action—that specify when a living entity is or becomes a person. The concept of personhood is critical in many bioethical debates. Divergent views of personhood are assumed in arguments over the moral status of the human fetus and animals, and over the determination of death.

Professional Ethics   Ethical standards are important in defining the boundaries of a profession such as medicine or nursing. Most professions have developed codes of ethics that identify the responsibilities of the professional in special relations with patients or clients. These standards are viewed as obligatory upon members of the profession, and may not be applicable to nonmembers or to relationships outside the professional setting.

Proxy Consent   When a patient has been determined to be incompetent and incapable of giving informed consent to the provision of medical teatment, a proxy may be appointed to make decisions for the patient. The proxy, frequently a family member or relative, may be appointed by the court or designated by the patient through an advance directive.

Quality of Life   Quality of life is often contrasted with quantity or sanctity of life and indicates that there are moral limits to the use of life-prolonging medical interventions. It is portrayed as a patient-centered moral criterion, emphasizing the worth of the patient's own life to him or herself.

Respect for Persons   The moral principle respect for persons is based on the maxim that a person should never be treated simply as a means, but always as an end. At a minimum, it requires providing reasons or moral justification for actions that infringe upon the liberty and life plans of others. Respect for persons supports moral rules, such as privacy, confidentiality, and truthtelling.

Rights   Rights are justified claims upon others for action or forebearance. "Negative" rights are rights to noninterference by others, such as the "right to life," to undergo an abortion based on the right of privacy, or to refuse medical intervention. "Positive" rights are claims on others for assistance, such as federal or state funding for access to abortion, or the right to health care.

Risk-Benefit Analysis   Risk-benefit analysis weighs the probability and magnitude of potential harm against the probability and amount of potential benefit. Various measures of harm and risk are used. This form of analysis is widely used to set standards of safety and health for the workplace and to assess medical technologies.

Sanctity of Life   The principle of sanctity of life assumes that the moral and religious value of life transcends judgments about its quality. In bioethics, the sanctity of life principle is associated with conservative, life-prolonging positions in debates over such matters as abortion, infanticide, suicide, and euthanasia.

Slippery Slope Argument   A "slippery slope" or "wedge" argument raises questions about the precedents that may be set and the consequences that may follow if a particular practice is accepted. In its *sociological* version, the slippery slope argument suggests that if X is accepted, then Y will follow as a matter of due course. The legal acceptance of active, voluntary euthanasia, for example, is often predicted to erode society's respect for the value of life so that moral barriers against nonvoluntary or involuntary euthanasia would be undermined. In its *logical* version, the slippery slope argument suggests that the acceptance of X already contains an implicit justification of Y, even if in practice Y never occurs. For example, arguments that support the use of infants with anencephaly as organ donors might seem also to validate harvesting organs from patients in a persistent vegetative state.

Substituted Judgment   In a case of substituted judgment, a proxy decision maker makes a decision about medical treatment for an incompetent patient based upon his or her understanding of what the patient would have decided if competent. The "substituted judgment standard" has been important in influential legal decisions and is typically contrasted with the "best interests standard."

Supererogation   Supererogatory acts are those considered "above and beyond the call of duty." Such acts, like a rescue that imposes substantial risk to the rescuer, are not considered morally obligatory and failure to perform them would not be regarded as morally wrong. The moral agents who do perform them are often praised for their heroism. Judgments about supererogatory action are often role dependent: because of commitments to standards of professional ethics, the ethical expectations of lifeguards or physicians to save life are often higher than those imposed upon normal citizens.

Triage   Drawn from a French term for "sorting," triage is important in emergency medicine and in procedures for determining which patients should receive scarce medical resources. Patients may be classified according to whether they will probably (1) survive without immediate medical treatment, (2) die even with immediate treatment, or (3) survive only with immediate treatment.

Utilitarianism   Utilitarianism is a philosophical theory that assesses the moral worth of acts according to their extrinsic features, particularly their outcomes and consequences. In a utilitarian position, the morally justifiable act is that which produces the greatest amount of value over disvalue. Utilitarianism supports a range of ethical principles, including nonmaleficence and beneficence, and methods of moral assessment, such as risk-benefit analysis.

9. Vol. 15, No. 6, December 1985, pp. 13-15
10. Vol. 20, No. 5, September-October 1990, pp. 42-44
11. Vol. 17, No. 1, February 1987, pp. 22-23
12. Vol. 15, No. 1, February 1985, pp. 17-19
13. Vol. 14, No. 4, August 1984, pp. 26-27
14. Vol. 20, no. 3, May-June 1990, pp. 31-35
15. Vol. 15, No. 5, October 1985, pp. 29-31
16. Vol. 16, No. 1, February 1986, pp. 24-25.
17. Vol. 20, No. 1, January-February 1990, pp. 33-34
18. Vol. 21, No. 3, May-June 1991, pp. 21-23
19. Vol. 15, No. 2, April 1985, pp. 22-23
20. Vol. 10, No. 2, April 1980, pp. 25-27
21. Vol. 18, No. 1, February-March 1988, pp. 21-22
22. Vol. 12, No. 5 October 1982, pp. 27-29
23. Vol. 17, No. 4, August-September 1987, pp. 18-19
24. Vol. 8, No. 1, February 1978, pp. 13-14
25. Vol. 9, No. 4, August 1979, pp. 12-13
26. Vol. 5, No. 3, June 1975, pp. 9-10, 47
27. Vol. 10, No. 5, October 1980, pp. 21-22
28. Vol. 14, No. 1, February 1984, pp. 24-26
29. Vol. 22, No. 3, May-June 1992, pp. 26-27
30. Vol. 17, No. 3, International Supplement, June 1987
31. Vol. 17, No. 6, December 1987, pp. 33-35
32. Vol. 12, No. 4, August 1982, pp. 26-28
33. Vol. 14, No. 3, June 1984, pp. 22-24
34. Vol. 18, No. 2, April-May 1988, pp. 24-26
35. Vol. 11, No. 6, December 1981, pp. 21-23
36. Vol. 11, No. 4, August 1981, pp. 20-21
37. Vol. 16, No. 4, August 1986, pp. 31-33
38. Vol. 19, No. 4, July-August 1989, pp. 16-18
39. Vol. 19, No. 1, January-February 1989, pp. 26-28
40. Vol. 21, No. 1, January-February 1991, pp. 32-34
41. Vol. 5, No. 1, February 1975, pp. 49-51
42. Vol. 12, No. 3, June 1982, pp. 18-19
43. Vol. 19, No. 2, March-April 1989, pp. 32-24
44. Vol. 6, No. 2, April 1976, pp. 13-15
45. Vol. 20, No. 4, July-August 1990, pp. 30-32
46. Vol. 9, No. 3, June 1979, pp. 19-20, 26
47. Vol. 7, No. 6, December 1977, pp. 21-22
48. Vol. 12, No. 2, April 1982, pp. 24-25
49. Vol. 13, No. 5, October 1983, pp. 23-25
50. Vol. 15, No. 4, August 1985, pp. 13-15
51. Vol. 21, No. 2, March-April 1991, pp. 30-32
52. Vol. 16, No. 4, October 1986, pp. 23-25
53. Vol. 16, No. 2, April 1986, pp. 21-23
54. Vol. 8, No. 5, October 1978, pp. 23-25
55. Vol. 17, No. 5, October-November 1987, pp. 26-27
56. Vol. 8, No. 6, December 1978, pp. 16-18
57. Vol. 10, No. 6, December 1980, pp. 25-26
58. Vol. 19, No. 5, September-October 1989, pp. 30-32
59. Vol. 21, No. 4, July-August 1991, pp. 36-38
60. Vol. 22, No. 1, January-February 1992, pp. 41-42